Contents

Preface to the First Edition

The aim of this handbook is to provide junior medical staff and nurses who work in neonatal intensive care nurseries with details of how to manage very ill and premature babies. We feel that there is need for a pocket-sized handbook that could readily be referred to in emergency situations. This book, however, should not replace but rather supplement the readily-available experience of consultants.

The line diagrams illustrating practical procedures were drawn by Mr Brendan Ellis of the Department of Medical Illustration, Royal Victoria Hospital, Belfast. We are also grateful to our mentors in Belfast, Cardiff, Toronto, Cleveland and San Francisco for their teaching and inspiration. Our thanks are also due to the numerous longsuffering junior doctors and senior nurses who have helped to put our plans into action and who have never failed to point out difficulties.

Lastly our thanks are due to Mrs Lynda Thompson for typing and retyping the manuscript.

June 1981

Henry L. Halliday
Garth McClure
Mark Reid

Preface to the Third Edition

Another 4 years have elapsed between editions of this handbook, and in this time considerable developments have occurred necessitating changes in our text. On the medical politics front the Report of the Royal College of Physicians on 'Medical Care of the Newborn in England and Wales' has helped to highlight deficiencies in services for the newborn and set down guidelines for improvements.

Medical advances include the greater evaluation and usage of surfactant replacement therapy for babies with respiratory distress syndrome, and the improvements in non-invasive imaging techniques discussed in detail in the second edition. AIDS has been a new and unwelcome problem and we have devoted a section to its effects on perinatal care. Because of advances in paediatric subspecialities we have asked our colleagues to review some chapters and our thanks are due to Dr Angela Bell for improving Chapter 16 (Neurological Problems); Dr Brian Craig (Chapter 17, Cardiovascular Problems); Dr Maurice Savage (Chapter 19, Genitourinary Problems); and Dr Dennis Carson (Chapter 20, Metabolic and Endocrine Problems).

Equally as important is a nursing input for a handbook such as this and we have encouraged Sisters Sheila Lamont and Phil Farrell to write short notes on nursing aspects of management at the end of most chapters. We hope that this innovation will increase the appeal of the handbook, whose aim remains to assist junior medical staff and nurses who care for ill and preterm babies.

We remain indebted to Lynda Thompson and Florence Herbert for their secretarial help and to Brendan Ellis for his line drawings.

March 1989

Henry L. Halliday
Garth McClure
Mark Reid

Introduction

Perinatal mortality rate in the UK has declined during the past two decades from over 30 per 1000 births to under 10 per 1000 births in 1988. A significant contribution to this reduction has been made by the development of neonatal intensive care.

This book is intended to be a guide to neonatal intensive care for junior medical staff and nurses. We have defined neonatal intensive care as the need for assisted ventilation, blood gas monitoring, intravenous feeding and close observation of severely ill newborn infants. This manual will not deal with routine neonatal care or special care of the newborn, except where it relates to intensive care. We think it imperative that junior paediatric staff coming to work in neonatal intensive care should have both a background in general paediatrics and a knowledge of neonatal and perinatal physiology. We suggest that a useful introduction to newborn medicine is *The Newborn Child* by Vulliamy and Johnston (1987). There are also many larger texts of neonatal medicine which should be used for reference (e.g Klaus and Fanaroff, 1986; Avery, 1987; Fanaroff and Martin, 1986; Avery and Taeusch, 1984; Roberton, 1986). For an introduction to obstetrics related to the newborn we recommend *Perinatal Medicine* (McClure *et al.*, 1988).

We intend that this manual be carried in the coat pocket so that it may be readily referred to in emergencies. The manual, however, will not replace sound clinical experience gathered over many years. We believe that a useful maxim to follow is that *if you are in any doubt about what to do next, ask someone senior.* Neonatal intensive care is an area of medicine where emergency management, rapid diagnosis and minute-to-minute monitoring of patients are necessary. It is often essential that doctors with experience at either senior registrar or consultant level help with these critical decisions. To seek help from a senior colleague is not an admission of defeat, but rather part of the learning process that should lead the junior paediatrician to become proficient in dealing with problems of the high-risk newborn. This learning process takes months and indeed years so that consultants expect to be questioned until your confidence and competence has increased.

Neonatology should not begin with the birth of the infant, but earlier during pregnancy, so the manual begins by discussing prenatal diagnosis and high-risk pregnancy. Neonatal paediatricians must work in close harmony with obstetricians to provide the best possible perinatal care. All high-risk pregnancies and labours are indications for attendance at the delivery of a paediatrician skilled in neonatal resuscitation. Resuscitation is perhaps the cornerstone of neonatal care and the prevention or early and effective treatment of asphyxia will often reduce the need for further intensive care in the neonatal period. We have written a chapter on common procedures in the newborn which is illustrated with many line drawings. We hope that this will be helpful to the paediatrician newly arrived in the neonatal nursery, but experience of procedures is best gained by observing senior colleagues.

The book provides a number of protocols for management of many disorders of the newborn, some common, like respiratory distress syndrome and transient tachypnoea of the newborn, and some uncommon, like pulmonary haemorrhage and persistent fetal circulation. Infections with the group B haemolytic streptococci and *Listeria monocytogenes* are becoming increasingly common and carry a high mortality. We have also devoted a chapter to the very low birth weight infant as we feel that present mortality and morbidity in this group of infants is unacceptably high. These babies develop an almost unique set of problems and we believe that there is a need to discuss them in a separate chapter. Since the first edition we have added chapters on prenatal diagnosis, the normal newborn, metabolic and endocrine problems, congenital malformations and recent developments in investigation. Since our second edition in 1985, surfactant replacement for respiratory distress syndrome has been shown to not only save lives but reduce the incidence of major complications. The introduction of this treatment promises to become the largest single advance in neonatal care for decades.

We hope that this book will also be useful to intensive care nurses and other persons involved in the care of the newborn. The management protocols that we describe are based upon our present knowledge and experience. However, we reserve the right to alter this advice in the light of new experience and research. We are aware that there is always more than one way to manage any particular situation and so we have left room at the end of the book for the reader to make his own notes. We would also appreciate any advice or comment from readers. We suggest that you fill in the telephone numbers of the following persons and departments in the space below for easy reference:

Consultant paediatricians	______________
Senior registrar	______________
Special care baby unit (SCBU)/intensive care unit (ICU)	______________
Labour ward	______________
X-ray department	______________
Biochemistry laboratory	______________
Bacteriology laboratory	______________
Haematology laboratory/blood bank	______________
Physiotherapy department	______________
Pharmacy	______________
Porters	______________

GLOSSARY

Neonate — A newborn baby from birth to age 28 days. The first 28 days of life is the neonatal period and a death occurring in this time is referred to as a *neonatal death*

Infant — A baby during the first 12 months of life

Perinatal death — Death of a fetus after 28 weeks of pregnancy (stillbirth) or the death of a newborn in the first 7 days after birth

Term — An infant is at term if born after 37 weeks gestation and before 42 weeks gestation (259–294 days)

Preterm infant — One born before 37 completed weeks of pregnancy (< 259 days)

Post-term infant — One born after 42 weeks gestation (> 294 days)

Low birth weight (LBW) infant — One whose birth weight is 2500 g or less

Very low birth weight infant (VLBW) — One whose birth weight is 1500 g or less

Extremely low birth weight infant (ELBW) — One whose birth weight is 1000 g or less

Small for gestational age (SGA) — An infant is small for gestational age if birth weight is below the 10th percentile for gestation. In order to determine if the infant is small for gestational age, birth weight should be plotted on an appropriate growth chart (see p. 45). Also called small-for-dates

Appropriate for gestational age (AGA) — An appropriate for gestational age infant is

	one whose birth weight lies between the 10th and 90th percentiles for gestation
Large for gestational age (LGA)	A large for gestational age infant is one whose birth weight is greater than the 90th percentile for gestation
Intensive care	The provision of life-support systems such as assisted ventilation or continuous positive airways pressure, monitoring of heart rate and respiration, monitoring of blood gases and intravenous feeding for ill newborn infants
Special care	The provision of care to infants who are at special risk and who require special observation but do not need life-support systems. Twenty-four hour laboratory and radiology services should be available

REFERENCES AND FURTHER READING

Avery, G. B. (1987). *Neonatology: Pathophysiology and Management of the Newborn*, 3rd edn. Philadelphia: Lippincott.

Avery, M. E. and Taeusch, H. W. (1984). *Schaffer's Diseases of the Newborn*, 5th edn. Philadelphia: W. B. Saunders.

British Paediatrics (1985). Categories of babies requiring neonatal care. *Arch. Dis. Child* **60**: 599.

Fanaroff, A. A. and Martin, R. J. (1986). *Behrman's Neonatal-Perinatal Medicine: Diseases of the Fetus and Infant*, 4th edn. St Loius: C. V. Mosby.

Klaus, M. H. and Fanaroff, A. A. (1986). *Care of the High-risk Neonate*, 3rd edn. Philadelphia: W. B. Saunders.
McClure, G., Halliday, H. L. and Thompson, W. (1988). *Perinatal Medicine*. London: Baillière Tindall.
Roberton, N. R. C. (1986). *Textbook of Neonatology*. Edinburgh: Churchill Livingstone.
Vulliamy, D. G. and Johnston, F. B. (1987). *The Newborn Child*, 6th edn. Edinburgh: Churchill Livingstone.

1. Prenatal Diagnosis

Recent developments have allowed many disorders of the newborn to be diagnosed prenatally. Pre-pregnancy counselling and risk estimation should be a routine part of the care of all prospective parents. During the pre-pregnancy visit a couple can be given advice about conception, diet and health risks, such as smoking, drug taking and alcohol ingestion.

Where a couple have previously had an abnormal baby, prenatal diagnosis may be used to determine normality of the fetus and reassure the parents. If an abnormal fetus is detected then pregnancy may be terminated or if the defect is amenable to surgery this can be planned in advance. Many of the tests used for prenatal diagnosis are invasive and increase the risk of subsequent spontaneous abortion. This means that only those mothers at high risk should be tested. The methods available for prenatal testing are shown in Table 1. Amniotic fluid taken at amniocentesis may be used for chromosome analysis (takes 2–3 weeks), diagnosis of neural tube defects (raised alpha-fetoprotein) and detection of some inborn errors of metabolism. Amniocentesis can be performed before 16 weeks by an

Table 1. Tests for prenatal diagnosis.

1. Serum alpha-fetoprotein
2. Amniocentesis:
   - alpha-fetoprotein
   - chromosome analysis
   - inborn errors of metabolism
   - rhesus
   - contrast media
3. Ultrasound: structural defects
4. Fetoscopy:
   - structural defects
   - fetal blood sampling
   - fetal tissue sampling
5. Chorion villus biopsy

experienced operator using ultrasound to locate the placenta. There is a risk of 0.5% spontaneous abortion following amniocentesis. Table 2 shows some conditions that can be detected prenatally. The commonest chromosomal abnormalities are the trisomies, Down's syndrome, Edwards syndrome and Patau's syndrome (see Table 119). Indications for chromosome analysis are maternal age 37 years and above (see Table 120), previous child with chromosome disorder, parent carrying a balanced chromosome abnormality and for fetal sexing to identify males at high risk of genetic disease, e.g. Duchenne muscular dystrophy or haemophilia. This latter is performed when the mother is a carrier.

Fetal tissue may also be obtained by chorion villus biopsy in the first trimester but the complication rate is higher than that of amniocentesis. Use of amniocentesis at 11–12 weeks may mean that chorion villus biopsy is less often used.

Raised maternal serum alpha-protein may be used to screen for neural tube defect. However, false positive results occur in multiple pregnancy, threatened abortion, intrauterine death, fetal omphalocele, Turner's syndrome, congenital nephrosis, duodenal atresia, cystic hygroma and, most importantly, if the dates are wrong. Raised serum levels should always be repeated. Ultrasound scanning may show the defect. If there is doubt then amniocentesis should be carried out when an elevated alpha-fetoprotein level will indicate neural tube defect unless other defects are present or the liquor is blood stained.

Ultrasound may be used to diagnose certain structural defects, e.g. short-limbed dwarfism, major cardiac anomalies, intrathoracic cysts or tumours, hydronephrosis, renal agenesis, hydrocephalus, hydranencephaly, holoprosencephaly and omphalocele. For postnatal management of abnormal antenatal renal ultrasound scan see chapter 19.

Over 50 inborn errors of metabolism may be detected prenatally (see Table 2). These may be diagnosed after culture of cells obtained from chorion villus biopsy, amniotic fluid or fetal blood obtained at fetoscopy. Fetal blood sampling is usually performed at about 18 weeks and is useful in the diagnosis of metabolic disorders and haemoglobinopathies. Chorion villus biopsy in the first trimester may also be used for fetal chromosome analysis and for identification of certain haemoglobinopathies using DNA recombinant techniques.

Table 2. Conditions that can be detected prenatally.

1. *Chromosome abnormalities*:
   - Down's syndrome
   - Edwards' syndrome
   - Patau's syndrome

2. *Neural tube defects*:
   - Anencephaly
   - Spina bifida
   - Iniencephaly
   - Encephalocele
   - Hydrocephalus
   - Holoprosencephaly
   - Microcephaly
   - Hydranencephaly

3. *Anatomical abnormalities*:
   - Skeleton and limbs
   - Heart
   - Bladder and kidneys
   - Brain
   - Duodenal atresia
   - Omphalocele/gastroschisis
   - Tumours: neck, thorax, abdomen
   - Diaphragmatic hernia

4. *Inborn errors of metabolism*:

Lipid storage diseases	*Mucopolysaccharidoses*	*Amino acid disorders*
Tay–Sachs' disease	Hurler's syndrome	Homocystinuria
Gaucher's disease	Hunter's syndrome	Cystinosis
Niemann–Pick disease	Sanfilippo's syndrome	Maple syrup urine disease
Fabry's disease	Morquio's disease	Methylmalonic acidosis
Generalized gangliosidosis	Mannosidosis	Arginosuccinic aciduria
Farber's disease	Mucolipidosis	Citrullinaemia
Wolman's disease		Non-ketotic hyperglycinaemia
		Tyrosinaemia
		Propionic acidaemia

5. *Others*:
   - Lesch–Nyhan syndrome
   - Xeroderma pigmentosum
   - Galactosaemia
   - Glycogen storage disease Type II, IV
   - Congenital nephrosis
   - Thalassaemia/sickle cell disease
   - Acid phosphatase deficiency
   - Adenosine deaminase deficiency
   - α_1-Antitrypsin deficiency
   - Congenital adrenal hyperplasia
   - Menkes' disease
   - Osteogenesis imperfecta
   - Haemophilia A and B
   - von Willebrand's disease
   - Severe combined immunodeficiency

REFERENCES AND FURTHER READING

Dornan, J. C. and Reid, M. Mc. C. (1988). *Genetic Problems and Congenital Malformations in Perinatal Medicine* (eds, McClure, G., Halliday, H. L. and Thompson, W.). London: Baillière Tindall.

Ferguson-Smith, M. A. (1983). Early prenatal diagnosis. *Br. Med. Bull.* **39**: 301.

Kelnar, C. J. H. and Harvey, D. (1987). *The Sick Newborn Baby*, 2nd edn. London: Baillière Tindall.

Parness, I. A., Yeager, S. B., Sanders, S. P. *et al.* (1988). Echocardiographic diagnosis of fetal heart defects in mid-trimester. *Arch. Dis. Child* **63**: 1137.

Thomas, D. F. M. and Gordon, A. C. (1989). Management of prenatally diagnosed uropathies. *Arch. Dis. Child* **64**: 58.

2. Examination of the Normal Newborn

All newborn should be examined at least twice before discharge from hospital. The first examination is carried out soon after birth to assess adaptation to normal extrauterine life, and to exclude major malformations requiring urgent surgical correction (p. 302). At this initial examination, the baby should also be measured, with a note of birth weight in grams, and crown–heel length and occipitofrontal circumference (OFC) in centimetres. These measurements should be plotted on appropriate percentile charts (see Appendix VIII). Assessment by Apgar score is discussed in Chapter 4 and assessment of gestational age in Chapter 6.

The second or discharge examination should be carried out on the fourth or fifth day after birth and should include the following:

Skin

Look for pallor, jaundice, cyanosis and abnormal skin lesions.

Heart and lungs

Record heart rate and respiration rate. Normal heart rate should be between 110 and 160 beats/min and respiration rate less than 50 breaths/min. Listen for murmurs, accentuated second pulmonary heart sound or crepitations. Check for presence of femoral pulses and note the presence of hepatomegaly.

Head and face

Remeasure occipitofrontal circumference, check size and tension of anterior fontanelle. If OFC is greater than 90th percentile or below 10th percentile then hydrocephalus or microcephalus is possible. Examine the eyes for conjunctivitis, cataracts, aniridia and coloboma. Look at the ears for accessory auricles, malformation or low set position. Check the mouth for the presence of cleft palate.

Abdomen
Palpate for hepatosplenomegaly, abdominal distension, renal masses or imperforate anus. Check the umbilical stump for signs of infection, single umbilical artery or small omphalocele.

External genitalia
In the female, look for enlargement of the clitoris or increased pigmentation. In the male look for hypospadias, undescended testes and hydrocele.

Limbs
Check for dislocation of the hips using Ortolani–Barlow manoeuvre. With the baby lying on his back, adduct and flex the hips. The examiner's hands should be placed with the thumbs inside the thighs opposite the lesser trochanters and the tips of the middle fingers over the greater trochanter. A gentle attempt is made to push each femoral head backwards and forwards into or out of the acetabulum. This will test for stability of the hips. The flexed hips should now be abducted and dislocation can be diagnosed if there is a definite movement of the femoral head into the acetabulum, often referred to as a 'clunk'. If abduction is limited the hip should not be passed as normal and further investigation with ultrasound is indicated. If in doubt refer to consultant paediatrician or orthopaedic surgeon.

Also look for deformities of the feet such as talipes equinovarus or metatarsus adductus. Look also for extra digits.

Back
Look for clues to spina bifida occulta such as swelling, dimple, hairy patches. Look for dermal sinus.

CNS
Influenced by sleep state. Try and observe in a quiet, awake state. Abnormal postures include neck retraction, frog-like posture, hyperextension or hyperflexion of limbs, and asymmetry. Check muscle tone for increase or decrease and asymmetry. Check tendon reflexes for absence, exaggeration or

asymmetry. Look for abnormal involuntary movements, e.g. jitteriness, seizures or asymmetry. Listen for a high-pitched or weak cry. Check primitive reflexes (Moro or startle, sucking, rooting and tonic neck). Assess visual fixation and reaction to sound.

NURSING POINTS

1. General inspection and examination in labour ward
2. Check for patency of anus, each nostril and pass stomach tube
3. Check cord for security of ligatures
4. Check eyes for discharge
5. Measure temperature, heart rate, respiration rate, weight, length and occipitofrontal circumference
6. Note whether baby has stooled and voided urine
7. Check that identity bands are on and legible
8. Check that vitamin K has been given (orally for all babies and intramuscularly for risk group, i.e. preterm, small for gestational age, breast fed)

REFERENCES AND FURTHER READING

DHSS Guidelines (1986). *Screening for the Detection of Congenital Dislocation of the Hip*. London: DHSS.

Halliday, H. L., McClure, G., Reid, M. Mc. C. and Thompson, W. (1988). Normal pregnancy. In: *Perinatal Medicine* (eds McClure, G., Halliday, H. L. and Thompson, W.). London: Baillière Tindall.

O'Doherty, N. (1985). *Atlas of the Newborn*, 2nd edn. Lancaster: M. T. P. Press.

Roberton, N. R. C. (1988). *A Manual of Normal Neonatal Care*. London: Edward Arnold.

Thomas, R. and Harvey, D. (1984). *Colour Aids: Neonatology*. Edinburgh: Churchill Livingstone.

Vulliamy, D. G. and Johnston, P. B. (1987). *The Newborn Child*, 6th edn. Edinburgh: Churchill Livingstone.

3. High-risk Pregnancy

A high-risk pregnancy is one that is complicated by reason of maternal illness, obstetric disorder or drug therapy, and from which one may anticipate an ill or immature infant. High-risk pregnancies should be identified as early as possible in the antenatal period and in labour the fetus should be monitored to detect fetal distress. It is essential that a neonatal paediatrician skilled at resuscitation be present at the delivery of an infant from a high-risk pregnancy and labour.

Some of the the causes of high-risk pregnancy are listed in Table 3. Appropriate management of these conditions requires good communication between nursery and labour ward staffs. Nursery house staff should always be aware of any potential problems in the antenatal and labour wards with regular meetings to discuss these in advance so that adequate preparations may be made to receive the infant.

Table 4 lists some maternal illnesses that can seriously affect the newborn.

DIABETES MELLITUS

Good maternal control reduces risk of neonatal macrosomia and hypoglycaemia. Maternal postprandial blood glucose <7 nmol/l or fasting <5 mmol/l is the aim. Long-term diabetic control may be assessed by maternal haemoglobin (Hb) A_1 levels (<7%). Good pre-pregnancy control lowers congential malformation rates. With Hb A_1 at booking over 10%, about 24% of babies will have major malformations compared to only 3% if the Hb A_1 is less than 8%. Poor control causes hyperglycaemia in mother and fetus with fetal hyperinsulinaemia and subsequent neonatal hypoglycaemia.

Asymptomatic hypoglycaemia is common (50%). Doubt exists as to whether asymptomatic hypoglycaemia is harmful.

Hypoglycaemia occurs early (Fig. 1) so check glucose strip test at birth and at 30 min and begin treatment early (see

Table 3. Causes of a high-risk pregnancy.

Maternal conditions:
1. Age: elderly primigravida (>35 years) or <17 years
2. Hypertension and pre-eclampsia
3. Diabetes mellitus
4. Rhesus isoimmunization
5. Drug therapy: steroids, β-adrenergic drugs, excessive narcotics, magnesium sulphate
6. Maternal infection: rubella, herpes simplex, syphilis or chorioamnionitis (fever and chills)
7. Previous birth of a child with a hereditary disease, respiratory disorder or neonatal death
8. Maternal illness (see Table 4)

Labour and delivery conditions:
1. Antepartum haemorrhage
2. Prolonged rupture of membranes (>24 hours) (see p. 24)
3. Forceps or vacuum delivery
4. Abnormal presentation (breech, brow, face or transverse)
5. Caesarean section
6. Prolapsed cord
7. Maternal hypotension (especially epidural or bleeding)
8. Fetal distress:
   abnormal fetal heart rate
   scalp pH < 7.25
   meconium staining

Fetal conditions:
1. Multiple births
2. Premature delivery (<37 weeks) or post-term (>42 weeks)
3. Growth retardation
4. Immature lecithin/sphingomyelin ratio (L/S < 2:1)
5. Polyhydramnios (oesophageal atresia, etc.)
6. Oligohydramnios (Potter's syndrome of renal agenesis)

Table 4. Maternal illnesses complicating pregnancy.

1. Diabetes mellitus
2. Thyrotoxicosis
3. Idiopathic thrombocytopenic purpura
4. Disseminated lupus erythematosus
5. Myasthenia gravis, myotonic dystrophy
6. Drug therapy and alcohol addiction
7. Other endocrine disorders: Cushing's, Addison's, Simmonds', hyperparathyroidism, adrenal hyperplasia
8. Cyanotic heart disease
9. Malignant disease
10. Epilepsy
11. Renal failure
12. Psychiatric illness
13. Open tuberculosis
14. Others: ulcerative colitis, sickle cell anaemia

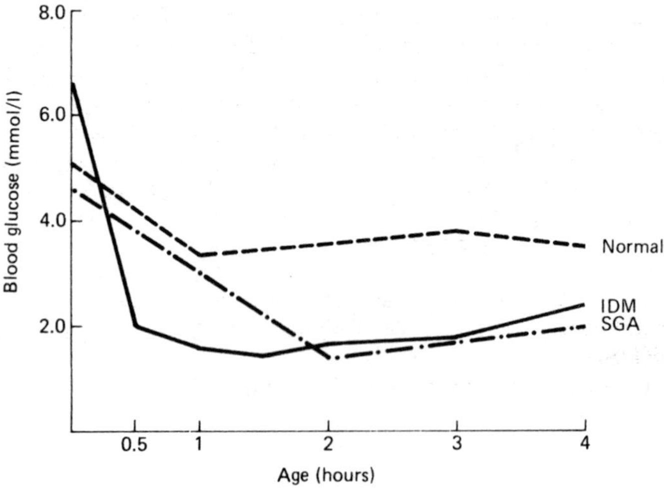

Fig. 1. Changes in blood sugar after birth in three groups of infants: normal, infants of diabetic mothers (IDM) and small for gestational age (SGA) infants.

Table 5. Indications for admission of the infant of the diabetic mother to the SCBU.

1. Preterm baby – gestational age <36 weeks
2. Macrosomic baby – >95th centile weight for gestational age
3. Obvious congenital abnormality e.g. cardiac, central nervous system or skeletal
4. Respiratory distress persisting >1 hour
5. Cyanosis in room air
6. Hypoglycaemia persisting after first feed (<1.5 mmol/l – see below)
7. Babies with severe asphyxia or traumatic delivery (Apgar score <5 at 5 min)
8. Subsequent problems developing on post-natal ward e.g. hypoglycaemia, hypocalcaemia, severe jaundice

pp. 57, 172). Most infants of diabetic mothers (IDMs) can be admitted to postnatal wards with their mothers. Table 5 lists indications for admitting IDM to special care nursery. Babies on the postnatal wards should be fed early and often beginning within the first hour and 3 hourly thereafter until blood glucose levels are stable (see Fig. 1). Blood glucose should be checked by stix methods every half an hour for 2 hours and then 3 hourly for 24–48 hours. Levels below 1.5 mmol/l constitute hypoglycaemia and necessitate an immediate feed and recheck within an hour. If blood glucose falls below 1.1 mmol/l a blood sample should be sent to the laboratory and the paediatrician informed. Persistent levels below 1.1 mmol/l or the development of symptoms warrant intravenous fluids (p. 173).

Other problems of IDM:

1. Birth complications: asphyxia, shoulder dystocia
2. Increased incidence of respiratory distress syndrome (RDS)
3. Congenital malformations (congenital heart disease and sacral agenesis)
4. Transient tachypnoea of the newborn
5. Increased jaundice and hypocalcaemia
6. Polycythaemia
7. Hypertrophic cardiomyopathy
8. Others: renal vein thrombosis, small left colon

THYROTOXICOSIS

Sometimes caused by long-acting thyroid stimulator (LATS), an IgG antibody that crosses the placenta and may cause temporary neonatal thyrotoxicosis.

Tachycardia, weight loss, hyperthermia, congestive heart failure, goitre, exophthalmos, seizures and diarrhoea occur. Onset of symptoms may be delayed because of the effects of maternal antithyroid drugs on the fetus.

Close observation, cord blood for LATS, T_4 and TSH estimations required.

May need:

Digoxin and diuretics (see p. 237)
Potassium iodide, 10%, 8 mg/kg/day, 8 hourly
Carbimazole 0.5–1 mg/kg/day, 8 hourly
β-Blocker, e.g. propranolol 2 mg/kg/day, 8 hourly

LATS half-life about 6 weeks and therapy not usually needed beyond this. No long-term effects on infant but developmental follow up needed.

IDIOPATHIC THROMBOCYTOPENIC PURPURA

This is caused by transfer of a maternal anti-platelet antibody and three-quarters of babies will be affected by thrombocytopenia with 6% neonatal mortality. Severity of thrombocytopenia in newborn is usually proportional to that of the mother at time of delivery, but mothers previously treated by splenectomy may have normal platelet counts and give birth to affected infants.

Petechiae and bruising common; bleeding may occur from umbilicus, nose, gastrointestinal and genitourinary tracts, injection sites or into the brain. Risk of haemorrhage greatest within 3 days of birth or when platelet count is below 20 000/mm^3.

Steroids are used if the platelet count is below 20 000/mm^3 but efficacy remains unproven. Steroids may protect against severe haemorrhage even though platelet count does not increase. Platelet transfusions have a short-lived benefit if severe bleeding occurs. Recently, infusion of immunoglobulins has been shown to increase platelet count, perhaps by acting as a blocking antibody.

Neonatal illness self-limiting is usually recovered by 6 weeks; discharge from hospital if platelet count is above 50 000/mm^3.

For other causes of neonatal thrombocytopenia see p. 287.

DISSEMINATED LUPUS ERYTHEMATOSUS (DLE)

Increased risk of abortion, stillbirth and preterm delivery, especially if renal involvement is present.

The baby rarely develops DLE but may have LE cells transiently.

The baby may also show complications of maternal drug therapy or thrombocytopenia, anaemia, leucopenia and skin rashes, especially of the face. Endocardial fibroelastosis and heart block can occur.

MYASTHENIA GRAVIS

One-quarter of babies may be affected with temporary myasthenia, presumably mediated by antibodies that cross placenta. May present with respiratory difficulty, feeding problems and hypotonia. Onset may be delayed.

Symptoms are relieved by test dose of edrophonium (Tensilon) 1 mg intramuscularly. Maintenance with prostigmine 1–5 mg orally with feeds (see p. 302).

MYOTONIC DYSTROPHY

This is an autosomal dominant disorder and babies of affected mothers can be severely affected; stillbirth, preterm labour, severe birth asphyxia and respiratory failure are quite common presentations. Affected babies may have hypotonia and a myopathic facies but do not show myotonia. Long-term outcome is variable with some babies improving and others having developmental delay or remaining ventilator dependent. Often the diagnosis in the mother is made only after the neonatal illness.

DRUG AND ALCOHOL ADDICTION

Drug addiction is common in some cities of the British Isles, e.g. London, Edinburgh, Liverpool and Dublin.

Heroin addiction is associated with repeated maternal infections (including septicaemia, hepatitis and AIDS), fatal overdoses, poor attendances at antenatal clinics and poor nutrition. Pre-eclampsia is a common complication. About half of all heroin addicts will deliver preterm and the infant is usually small for gestational age; may be meconium staining.

Heroin stimulates production of surfactant so incidence of RDS is less than expected at each gestational age.

Neonatal withdrawal symptoms usually appear within 24–48 hours after birth, though late symptoms can occur. Early signs: tremors, high-pitched cry, regurgitation of feeds, irritability, sneezing, increased tone, loose stools, sweating and tachypnoea. Later signs: vomiting, diarrhoea, dehydration, circulatory collapse and seizures. Infants born to alcoholic mothers may also develop similar withdrawal symptoms and may need sedation.

Treatment depends on symptoms:

Seizures:

Chloral hydrate (sedation) 50 mg/kg/day
Phenobarbitone (anticonvulsant) 5–8 mg/kg/day

Irritability:

Paregoric (opiate replacement → slow withdrawal) 0.3 ml/kg/day (2 drops/kg/dose, 4 hourly)
Chlorpromazine (can precipitate seizures) 1.5–3 mg/kg/day
Swaddling may be helpful

Serology for syphilis, serum hepatitis and AIDS (after consent) should be performed.

Drugs in breast milk may also affect the baby (see Table 6 and p. 160).

Fetal alcohol syndrome (FAS) is characterized by growth retardation, hirsutism, microcephaly, eye abnormalities, elongated upper lip, absent philtrum, developmental delay, lowered intelligence and postnatal growth retardation. Congenital heart lesions and renal anomalies have also been found. The amount of alcohol required to cause these findings is

Table 6. Drugs affecting the fetus.

Drug	*Effect on the fetus and newborn*
Alcohol	Fetal alcohol syndrome Withdrawal: seizures, hyperactivity
Aminoglycosides	Ototoxic, nephrotoxic
'Aminopterin'	Abortion, skeletal abnormalities
Amphetamines	Generalized arteritis, developmental delay
Androgens	Virilization ? Congenital anomalies
Aspirin	Platelet dysfunction, risk of kernicterus, prostaglandin inhibition
Azathioprine	Reduced immunocompetence
Barbiturates	Multiple abnormalities Withdrawal, haemorrhage
Cannabis	Chromosome breakage, skeletal anomalies
Cigarettes	Stillbirth, reduced birth weight and head growth, ? hyperactivity, ? heart defects (PDA)
Chlorpropamide	Fetal death, prolonged hypoglycaemia
Corticosteroids	? Teratogenic
Cytotoxic drugs	Multiple abnormalities
Danazol	Virilization
Dicoumarol	Fetal death, haemorrhage, abnormal facies, retardation
Diazepam	Hypotonia, hypothermia, apnoea Withdrawal: irritability, ? cleft lip and palate
Diazoxide	Hyperglycaemia, ? diabetes, genital anomalies, hypertrichosis
Diethylstilboestrol	Vaginal carcinoma and adenosis
Glutethimide	SGA, irritability, hyperthermia, diarrhoea
Hydralazine	? Cleft palate
Indomethacin	Prolonged labour, premature ductus closure, pulmonary hypertension
Iodine	Goitre, altered thyroid function
Isoniazid	Pyridoxine deficiency
Isotretinoin (Roaccutane)	Abortion, multiple anomalies

Table 6. Drugs affecting the fetus (continued).

Drug	*Effect on the fetus and newborn*
Lithium	Respiratory distress, lethargy, congenital heart disease, goitre
Lysergic acid diethylamide (LSD)	Probably teratogenic
Magnesium sulphate	Respiratory depression, hypotonia, seizures
Narcotics (morphine, methadone, heroin, codeine, pentazocine)	Apnoea, hypothermia, withdrawal
Nitrofurantoin	Haemolysis
Oestrogens	Later vaginal adenosis and adenocarcinoma, uterine abnormalities in females; hypospadias, possible subfertility in males
Oxytocin	Increased bilirubin, hyponatraemia
Paradione	Fetal death and multiple abnormalities
Paraldehyde	Apnoea, cerebral and respiratory depression
Phenobarbitone	? Teratogenic, haemorrhagic disease
Phenothiazines	Apnoea, hypotonia or hyperactivity, withdrawal, extrapyramidal signs, ? chromosome breakage
Phenytoin	Cleft lip and palate, congenital heart disease, skeletal anomalies, haemorrhage, ? retardation
Primidone	Teratogenic
Progestogens	Virilization
Propranolol	Prolonged labour, bradycardia, hypoglycaemia, respiratory depression
Pyrimethamine	Do not combine with sulpha drugs or dapsone
Quinidine	Fetal death, thrombocytopenia, retinal haemorrhage
Quinine	CNS and skeletal anomalies, thrombocytopenia, deafness, small optic nerve
Radioiodine	Hypothyroidism
Reserpine	Nasal stuffiness, bradycardia, hypothermia
Retinoids	*see* isotretinoin
Ritodrine	Fetal tachycardia, hyperglycaemia
Salicylates	Fetal death, haemorrhage, prolonged labour, premature ductus closure, pulmonary hypertension

Table 6. Drugs affecting the fetus (continued).

Drug	*Effect on the fetus and newborn*
Scopolamine	Apnoea at birth especially in preterm
Steroids	SGA, adrenal and immunosuppression, surfactant induction, DNA reduction
Streptomycin	Deafness
Sulphonamides	Kernicterus, thrombocytopenia
Tetracyclines	Multiple anomalies, bone and teeth
Thalidomide	Phocomelia, heart defects, gut defects
Thiazides	Thrombocytopenia, hypokalaemia, haemolysis
Tridione	As for Paradione
Tolbutamide	Thrombocytopenia, prolonged hypoglycaemia
Vaccines	Avoid live viral and attenuated bacterial vaccines, i.e. BCG, measles, mumps, Sabin polio, rubella, smallpox, yellow fever
Valproate	? Multiple anomalies, ? neural tube defects
Vitamin K (water soluble)	Jaundice
Vitamin B_6 (pyridoxine)	Withdrawal seizures
Vitamin D (in excess)	Hypercalcaemia, may cause syndrome of elfin facies, aortic stenosis, retardation
Warfarin	Haemorrhage, nasal hypoplasia, stippled epiphyses, CNS defects, microcephaly

After Hill (1979)

usually over 1 litre of spirits per week but the syndrome has been reported with lower intakes.

Incidence of FAS in the USA and Northern Ireland is about 1:750 births. Forty per cent of heavy drinking women give birth to FAS babies. Some risk occurs at two drinks per day but substantial risk at five or more drinks per day.

AIDS

Pregnancy may increase the risk of AIDS developing in HIV-positive women and termination of pregnancy has been advocated. Approximately two-thirds of HIV-positive mothers give birth to seropositive babies and about 25% of these babies will retain antibodies past 15 months to develop clinical AIDS. Fetal infection can also occur causing an embryopathy (growth retardation, microcephaly, box-like head, hypertelorism, short, flat nose, long palpebral fissures and patulous lips) although this has recently been doubted. Women at risk should be screened after consent, and the following are considered to be high-risk groups: intravenous drug abusers, prostitutes, women from central Africa, partners of bisexual or haemophiliac men.

Medical and nursing personnel should avoid self-innoculation with blood or infected secretions. Precautions as for hepatitis B should be employed (p. 196) and breast feeding discouraged in developed countries.

MANAGEMENT OF PROLONGED RUPTURE OF MEMBRANES >24 HOURS

1. Maternal swabs: cervix, rectum. Avoid maternal antibiotics unless pyrexia, rising white cell count, foul discharge or tender uterus. If mother colonized with group B streptococci give chemoprophylaxis with ampicillin or penicillin during labour
2. Admit baby to special care nursery if:
    (a) Low birth weight
    (b) Asphyxiated
    (c) Early respiratory distress
3. Well LBW baby:
    (a) Superficial cultures of skin, umbilicus, rectum, external ear
    (b) Culture and Gram stain gastric aspirate
    (c) Blood culture
    (d) White cell count and platelets

   Consider antibiotic cover with penicillin or penicillin plus aminoglycoside
4. Ill infant: as for LBW baby plus chest radiograph, lumbar puncture and bladder tap for culture and cell counts. Start antibiotics (Appendix V)

REFERENCES AND FURTHER READING

British National Formulary (1989). *Prescribing in Pregnancy.* London: British Medical Association and the Pharmaceutical Society of Great Britain.

Dornan, J. C., Halliday, H. L. and McClure, G. (1988). High-risk Pregnancy. *In: Perinatal Medicine* (eds, McClure, G., Halliday, H. L. and Thompson, W.). London: Baillière Tindall.

Halliday, H. L. and Traub, A. I. (1988). Metabolic and endocrine disorders. In: *Perinatal Medicine* (eds, McClure, G., Halliday, H. L. and Thompson, W.). London: Baillière Tindall.

Halliday, H. L., Reid, M. Mc. C and McClure, G. (1982). Results of heavy drinking in pregnancy. *Br. J. Obstet. Gynaecol.* **89**: 892.

Hill, R. M. (1979). *Perinatal Pharmacology.* Evansville, Indiana: Mead Johnson.

Lang, M. A. (1985). The nursing management of neonates born of diabetic mothers. *Pract. Diabetes* **2**: 16.

Lissauer, T. (1989). Impact of AIDS on neonatal care. *Arch. Dis. Child* **64**: 4.

Rylance, G. and Houtman, P. (1988). Drugs and the neonate. *Hospital Update*, June, p. 1726.

4. Asphyxia and Resuscitation

Effective resuscitation is extremely important because of consequences of asphyxia (Table 7).

RESUSCITATION SHOULD BE PERFORMED BY THE MOST EXPERIENCED PERSON AVAILABLE

The goals of resuscitation are:

1. Clearing the airway
2. Expansion and ventilation of the lungs
3. Ensuring adequate cardiac output
4. Minimizing oxygen consumption by preventing heat loss

The ability of newborn to withstand asphyxia depends on:

1. Systemic arterial pressure
2. Cardiac glycogen stores

In asphyxia, shunting of blood occurs through:

1. Foramen ovale
2. Ductus venosus

Table 7. Sequelae of asphyxia.

1.	Cerebral hypoxia, oedema and necrosis
2.	Seizures (from raised intracranial pressure or cerebral necrosis)
3.	Increased incidence of intraventricular haemorrhage in preterm
4.	Renal failure: tubular necrosis
5.	Shock lung and/or respiratory distress syndrome, pulmonary haemorrhage
6.	Heart failure, 'anoxic cardiomyopathy'
7.	Disseminated intravascular coagulopathy
8.	Pulmonary hypertension/persistent fetal circulation
9.	Bowel perforation and necrotizing enterocolitis
10.	Adrenal haemorrhage
11.	Metabolic disturbances: hypocalcaemia, hyponatraemia (inappropriate ADH), hypoglycaemia or hyperglycaemia, disordered temperature control, metabolic acidosis

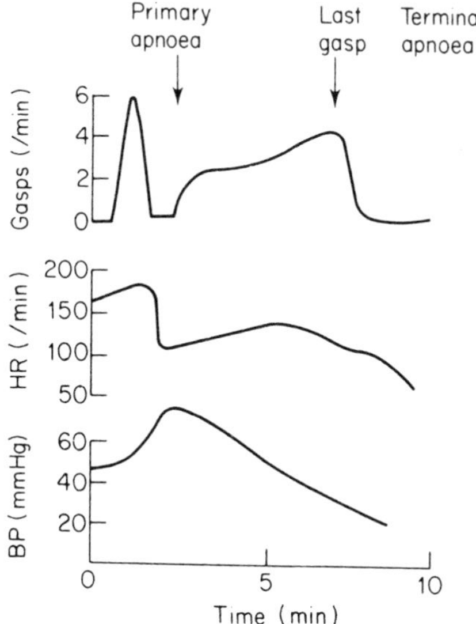

Fig. 2. Changes in respiration, heart rate and blood pressure during asphyxia. If resuscitation is delayed after the last gasp, irreversible brain damage will occur. From Dawes (1968) with kind permission of Year Book Medical Publishers.

These mechanisms maintain circulation to brain, heart and adrenals.

Figure 2 demonstrates changes in respiration, heart rate and blood pressure following acute asphyxia. Primary apnoea occurs soon after the onset of asphyxia. During the phase of primary apnoea, circulation is not greatly compromised so that heart rate remains above 100/min and blood pressure is maintained. The newborn will respond to simple measures of resuscitation. Primary apnoea is followed by repeated single gasps which increase in rate after 4–5 min before the last gasp occurs. After the last gasp, secondary or terminal apnoea occurs and the infant is pale and shocked with heart rate less than 100 /min and poor tone. This whole sequence of asphyxia probably extends over 10–12 min, after which time irreversible brain damage is likely to result. The duration of asphyxia may be estimated retrospectively as approximately half the time taken from the onset of respiration to the

Table 8. Assessment at birth and resuscitation.

1. Anticipate problems, get to labour ward early and review maternal history
2. Check resuscitation equipment and drugs. This includes radiant warmer, oxygen supply with bag and mask of appropriate size, suction apparatus with sterile suction catheter, laryngoscope with neonatal blade and endotracheal tubes of sizes 2.5, 3.0 and 3.5 mm
3. At birth start the stop-clock
4. On receiving the baby, gently aspirate mouth and pharynx, then the nose, while listening to the heart rate with stethoscope
5. *Keep warm under radiant heater and dry with warm towel*
6. By 1 min ensure completion of an initial assessment to give a 1 min Apgar score. Heart rate and tone are most important
7. Oxygen by face mask. If necessary ventilation with bag and mask → ventilation by endotracheal tube → ventilation with cardiac massage
8. Drugs, bicarbonate 2 mmol/kg intravenously diluted 4:1 with 5 or 10% dextrose, naloxone 10–20 μg/kg intravenously, glucose 3 ml/kg of 10% solution may be used if indicated
9. Consider other problems:
   - pneumothorax
   - diaphragmatic hernia
   - choanal atresia (p. 153)
   - oesophageal atresia
   - Pierre Robin syndrome (p. 153)

attainment of regular spontaneous breathing. The equipment needed for resuscitation is shown in Appendix XIV. Table 8 shows a suggested sequence of assessment and resuscitation of the newborn. Do the simple things first and progress from Step 1 to Step 8. The sequence can be simply remembered as ABCD:

A Airway
B Breathing
C Circulation
D Drugs

It is important to keep the baby warm by preventing heat loss from evaporation and radiation as cooling causes increased metabolic rate and oxygen consumption. Careful drying of the baby and use of a radiant warmer are vital in preterm and severely asphyxiated babies.

The Apgar scoring system of newborn assessment at birth

Table 9. Apgar scoring system.

Signs	0	1	2
Heart rate	0	<100	>100
Colour	Blue or pale	Blue at peripheries	Pink
Respiration	0	Weak, gasping	Strong and regular
Responses to suction	0	Slight	Cries
Tone	0	Fair	Active

was developed over 35 years ago and is now universally applied (Table 9). Asphyxia is only one of many causes of low Apgar scores and the following factors need to be taken into account: maternal sedation and analgesia, cerebral malformations, neuromuscular diseases, prematurity, congenital heart disease, congenital infection and respiratory obstruction (see below). A mnemonic for the Apgar score is:

A Appearance, i.e. colour
P Pulse, i.e. heart rate
G Grimace, i.e. response to suction
A Activity, i.e. tone
R Respiration, i.e. respiration

The Apgar score (AS) should be assessed at 1 and 5 min after birth:

1 min, AS >7 no further resuscitation
1 min, AS 5–6 bag and mask ventilation
1 min, AS <4 intubation (Table 10)

Table 10. Indications for endotracheal intubation.

1. Terminal apnoea at birth
2. Apgar score 4 or less at 1 min
3. Delayed apnoea
4. Thick meconium staining
5. Extreme immaturity

Sometimes an infant will appear well at birth with a high 1 min Apgar score but later become apnoeic. Delayed apnoea or progressive worsening of the Apgar score may be due to:

1. Excessive maternal analgesia during labour
2. Respiratory obstruction: mucus and blood, choanal atresia, Pierre Robin syndrome
3. Intrauterine infection (pneumonia)
4. Excessive suctioning of the pharynx leading to reflex bradycardia

Intubation and aspiration of meconium from below the cords of an infant born through thick meconium-stained amniotic fluid decreases the risk of severe meconium aspiration syndrome. Do not wash out the lungs as this liquefies the meconium allowing it to pass distally. If the baby is vigorous at birth, attempts at intubation may be more harmful than the small risk of severe meconium aspiration.

Extremely immature infants fare better if their respiration is assisted early in postnatal life and before severe RDS presents. We usually intubate all babies of less than 1200 g at birth for their initial resuscitation.

Techniques of intubation and cardiac massage are described in Chapter 5, pp. 76, 107.

INDICATIONS FOR CARDIAC MASSAGE

1. Absent heart beat at birth unless maceration or extreme immaturity (weight less than 500 g) or gross congenital anomaly
2. Heart rate under 50/min at 1 min } unless increasing
3. Heart rate under 80/min after adequate ventilation } unless increasing

CORRECTION OF ACIDOSIS

Use of alkali in resuscitation remains controversial. Sodium bicarbonate should not be given unless ventilation is adequately established as respiratory depression may occur with rising $P\text{CO}_2$.

Alkali should not be given if there is hypovolaemic shock until this has first been corrected by plasma expansion.

Administration of bicarbonate has been associated with

intraventricular haemorrhage in the very immature infant.

Bicarbonate should be diluted, 8.4% sodium bicarbonate is diluted 4:1 with 5% dextrose to give a solution containing 0.25 mmol/ml of bicarbonate. Use 2 mmol/kg as a stat. dose and repeat once more if necessary so that a total daily dose of 8 mmol/kg is not exceeded in the preterm infant.

The adverse effects of acidosis in the newborn are:

1. Decreased myocardial contractility when pH below 7.1
2. Increased pulmonary vascular resistance with right-to-left shunting
3. Decreased cellular metabolism affecting especially the brain

Indications for alkali therapy in resuscitation are:

1. pH <7.1 if this can be measured
2. Apgar score <3 at 1 min
3. Apgar score <5 at 5 min } unless rapid improvement

In the labour ward, bicarbonate should be given intravenously either directly into the umbilical vein or into a peripheral vein.

ASSESSMENT OF CARDIAC OUTPUT

Should be carried out after establishment of adequate ventilation.

An infant with hypovolaemia has:

1. Pale and limp appearance
2. Tachycardia (not always present)
3. Poor capillary filling
4. Low blood pressure (Fig. 3)
5. Low packed cell volume if haemodilution has occurred

May be consequence of fetal haemorrhage due to:

1. Vasa praevia (do Apt test on APH in labour)*
2. Breech
3. Twin-to-twin transfusion

---

*Apt test: dissolve two to three drops of bloody specimen in 5 ml of water in a test tube, add 1 ml of 1% sodium hydroxide. If adult blood, colour will turn from pink to yellow-brown in 1 to 2 min; if fetal haemoglobin, colour will remain pink, i.e. fetal haemoglobin resists alkali denaturation.

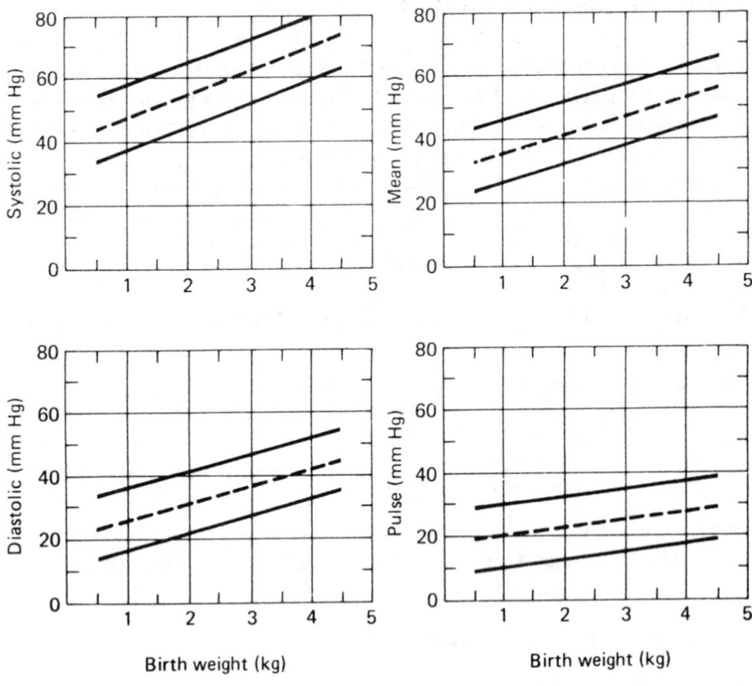

Fig. 3. Blood pressure by birth weight with 95% confidence limits. From Versmold *et al.* (1981) with kind permission of the authors and the editor of *Pediatrics*.

4. Caesarean section
5. Fetomaternal transfusion (do Kleihauer test on mother)

Treatment of hypovolaemic shock involves volume expansion 10–30 ml/kg with fresh blood or from placenta; 5% salt-poor albumin or plasma.

Correction of metabolic acidosis with bicarbonate before plasma expansion may lead to severe shock or collapse. Hypotension after birth may be caused by:

1. Blood loss
2. Septicaemia
3. Acidosis
4. RDS
5. Fluid loss, e.g. necrotizing enterocolitis (NEC), gastroenteritis

PERINATAL CARDIAC ARREST

Management is far from simple. The difficulty lies in the estimation of how long the circulation has ceased and whether the resulting hypoxaemic and ischaemic damage to vital organs, especially the brain, is reversible.

Intubate and ventilate while performing cardiac massage unless gross congenital abnormality or maceration are present.

If spontaneous heart beat is not regained within 3 min then 0.3 ml/kg of 1.10 000 adrenaline should be given by endotracheal tube. This avoids intracardiac injection.

Infants who respond to this therapy within 10 min showing regular, spontaneous heart beat and developing spontaneous respirations before 30 min usually have a good prognosis.

If the infant shows no response, CALL A SENIOR COLLEAGUE since half of infants failing to regain regular, spontaneous respirations within 30 min after the return of spontaneous heart beat will die within 1 week and the remainder will survive with gross handicaps, although there are occasional exceptions.

Further management of the baby following severe asphyxia is described on pp. 34, 221.

OTHER DRUG THERAPY

Naloxone is an opiate antagonist which effectively reverses respiratory depression due to pethidine and other similar analgesics. This drug should not be given unless there is a good history of maternal analgesic administration 1–3 hours prior to delivery, or two doses within 6 hours.

When it is indicated the dose is 10–20 μg/kg and it should be given intravenously for immediate response. Naloxone is short acting and so repeated doses or intramuscular treatment may be needed to reverse later depression.

Glucose administration is rarely needed as an emergency procedure during resuscitation as stress causes glycogenolysis with hyperglycaemia rather than hypoglycaemia.

Hypoglycaemia (less than 1.5 mmol/l) soon after birth, however, can occur in infants with hyperinsulinaemia (infants of diabetic mothers, infants with severe erythroblastosis or Beckwith's syndrome).

Hypoglycaemia is defined as a glucose strip test reading below 1.5 mmol/l (25 mg/dl).

After a venous sample has been withdrawn for confirmation, 3 ml/kg of 10% dextrose should be given intravenously.

On no account should 25 or 50% dextrose solutions be used in the newborn as they cause vascular damage leading to ischaemic necrosis.

AFTER CARE OF THE ASPHYXIATED BABY

The aim of care is to minimize the sequelae of asphyxia (see Table 7). The following therapies have been widely used to manage asphyxiated babies but few of them have been tested in properly controlled clinical trials.

Anti-cerebral Oedema Therapy (see also p. 222)

Fluid restriction, dexamethasone, mannitol infusions and hyperventilation may be used.

Fluid Intake

Because of renal failure, inappropriate ADH secretion and cerebral oedema, fluids should be restricted to 40–60 ml/kg/day. Fluid overload will increase cerebral oedema and hyponatraemia, and may cause seizures. Assessment of fluid needs should be made on measurements of urine output, electrolytes and osmolality of urine and plasma, blood pressure and weight. Low blood pressure and poor perfusion may be indications of hypovolaemia and should be treated with plasma, albumin or blood 10 ml/kg over 2 hours.

Metabolic Disorders

Hypoglycaemia should be detected by frequent glucose strip testing and corrected as described on p. 172. Hyperglycaemia may cause acidosis and increase cerebral oedema. Hypocalcaemia is due to depression of the parathyroids (see p. 174) and phosphate retention. Hypocalcaemia can be reduced by increasing calcium supplements to 1–2 mmol/kg/day. Hyponatraemia from inappropriate ADH secretion usually responds to fluid restriction but sodium supplementation may be needed (see p. 176). Hyperkalaemia occurs early because of renal failure and acidosis. Potassium supplements should not be given for at least 24 hours and more aggressive therapy with ion exchange resins and dialysis is sometimes needed (p. 178).

Seizures (see also p. 224)

These occur in the first 24 hours, are usually tonic but occasionally may be subtle. A loading dose of 20 mg/kg of phenobarbitone should be given and this may be followed by 10 mg/kg if necessary. Phenobarbitone should probably be given prophylactically to all babies with severe asphyxia. Should phenobarbitone fail to control seizures phenytoin is the next drug of choice.

Cardiovascular Support

Poor perfusion is often helped by volume expansion but occasionally positive inotropic support with dopamine is necessary. Echocardiography may be used to assess the degree of myocardial dysfunction (see Chapter 24). The dose of dopamine is 5 μg/kg/min which will improve myocardial contractility, renal blood flow and decrease systemic and pulmonary vascular resistances. Dopamine at a higher dose of 15 μg/kg/min will cause increase in systemic vascular resistance.

OUTCOME OF SEVERE ASPHYXIA (see also p. 222)

Outcome is difficult to predict. Many babies with low Apgar scores survive without disability. More than 95% of those with Apgar scores of 5 or less at 5 min have normal development. Only 33% of babies with this Apgar score develop encephalopathy (HIE) (p. 219). The prognosis is worsened by failure to establish spontaneous respirations within an hour of birth, persistent seizures, profound metabolic disturbance and presence of abnormal ultrasound scan (cerebral haemorrhage, later cerebral infarction and atrophy; see Chapter 24). Cerebral palsy is the only neurological deficit clearly linked to perinatal asphyxia. Although mental retardation and epilepsy may accompany cerebral palsy, there is no evidence that they are caused by perinatal asphyxia unless cerebral palsy is also present.

NURSING POINTS

1. Senior neonatal nurse to be present for high-risk deliveries
2. Bring portable incubator with ventilator, monitors, etc.
3. Bring back-up emergency box with equipment and drugs
4. Check back-up emergency box each shift and replace missing items
5. Forewarn NICU about impending delivery so that stabilization cot can be prepared
6. Talk to parents and reassure them
7. Keep any specimens that are needed, e.g. blood, amniotic fluid or gastric aspirate
8. Ensure accurate notes are taken documenting timing of events
9. Nursing care of the asphyxiated baby includes careful observation of activity, seizures, cry, sucking, urine output and fluid intake, urine testing for blood and protein (see also Chapter 16)

REFERENCES AND FURTHER READING

American Academy of Pediatrics. Committee on Fetus and Newborn (1986). Use and abuse of the Apgar score. *Pediatrics* 78: 1148.

Barrie, H. (1963). Resuscitation of the newborn. *Lancet* i: 650.

Dawes, G. S. (1968). *Fetal and Neonatal Physiology*. Chicago: Year Book Medical Publishers.

Drew, J. H. (1982). Immediate intubation at birth of the very-low-birth-weight infant. Effect on survival. *Am. J. Dis. Child* **136**: 207.

Halliday, H. L. (1988). Care of preterm babies in the first hour. *Care Crit Ill* **4**: 7.

Levene, M. I. and Evans, D. H. (1985). Medical management of raised intracranial pressure after severe birth asphyxia. *Arch. Dis. Child* **60**: 12.

Linder, N., Aranda, J. V., Tsur, M. *et al.* (1988). Need for endotracheal intubation and suction in meconium-stained neonates. *J. Pediatr.* **112**: 613.

Lissauer, T. (1981). Neonatal resuscitation. *Hosp. Update* **7**: 109.

McClure, B. G. (1979). Delivery room care of the preterm infant. *J Mat. Child Health* **4**: 466.

Nelson, K. B. and Ellenberg, J. K. (1981). Apgar scores as predictors of chronic neurological disability. *Pediatrics* **68**: 35.

Scott, H. (1976). Outcome of very severe birth asphyxia. *Arch. Dis. Child* **51**: 712.

Steiner, H. and Neligan, G. (1975). Perinatal cardiac arrest. Quality of survivors. *Arch. Dis. Child* **50**: 686.

Versmold, H. T., Kitterman, J. A., Phibbs, R. H., Gregory, G. A. and Tooley, W. H. (1981). Aortic blood pressure during the first 12 hours of life in infants with birth weights 610–4220 g. *Pediatrics* **67**: 607.5.

5. Transitional Care and Transport

Infants who are obviously ill or distressed at birth should be admitted to the special care nursery. Infants weighing less than 1800 g or of gestational age less than 35 weeks are usually admitted. There are some infants who at birth may be somewhat distressed, but with good resuscitation improve so that they require observation for a while before deciding to admit to either the nursery or the postnatal wards. This transitional care is best provided in the labour ward.

The infant having transitional care should be placed naked in an incubator so that he/she may be observed and kept warm.

Enough oxygen should be provided to abolish cyanosis. If more than 40% oxygen is required at this time, the infant should be admitted at once to the nursery.

Transitional care includes close observation of the infant with recording of vital signs (temperature, pulse rate, respiration rate). In addition, measurement of packed cell volume and glucose strip test are helpful.

Infants who have mild or moderate asphyxia (Apgar score >5 at 5 min) but are normal by 1 hour of age may be safely admitted to the postnatal wards, but their progress should be reviewed at 4 and 24 hours.

Those who continue to have respiratory distress and require oxygen to keep them pink at 1 hour of age should be admitted to the nursery. Table 11 lists the indicates for admission to special care nursery.

ADMISSION PROCEDURE

1. Forewarn nursery of impending admission: get necessary staff and equipment ready
2. Keep baby warm: servo-controlled radiant warmer or servo-controlled incubator with access
3. Give enough warmed, humidified oxygen to abolish cyanosis: start about 40%

Table 11. Indications for admission to special care nursery.

1. Birth weight <1800 g or gestational age <35 weeks
2. Babies needing $\geqslant 40\%$ oxygen to abolish cyanosis
3. Persisting respiratory distress; grunting, indrawing and tachypnoea (>60/min) after 1 hour or earlier if point 2 applies
4. Babies with major malformations requiring assessment and surgery
5. Babies that have suffered from severe birth asphyxia
   (a) Apgar scores <3 at 1 min
   <5 at 5 min
   (b) meconium found below cords
6. Infant of diabetic mother (see Table 5)
7. Severe erythroblastosis (see Chapter 13)
8. Major congenital malformations
9. Seizures

4. Attach electrodes for monitors: heart rate, respiration, transcutaneous $P\text{O}_2$ or pulse oximeter
5. Brief examination of infant: respiratory system, cardiovascular system, abdomen, central nervous system, weight, length and head circumference, gestational age. Do not remove infant from oxygen or allow to cool. Avoid excessive handling
6. Simple investigations: glucose strip test, haematocrit, blood gases, cultures and blood pressure. Chest radiograph after arterial catheter and endotracheal tube have been inserted if these are indicated (Chapter 9)

TRANSPORTATION

Ill infants born outside the hospital may need to be transported for intensive care. Table 12 suggests indications for transfer to the neonatal intensive care unit. The availability of surfactant for replacement therapy at regional centres has modified our indications for transfer of babies weighing less than 2000 g. Early transfer and treatment of these babies improves outcome. Transportation of the ill infant is not an ideal situation and, by anticipation of problems in high-risk

Table 12. Suggested indications for transfer of the newborn to a hospital with an intensive care unit.

1. Very low birth weight infant ($\leqslant$ 1500 g) unless obviously small for gestational age, i.e. > 32 weeks
2. Severe RDS at any weight:
   P_aO_2 < 8 kPa (60 mmHg) in 60% oxygen,
   early apnoea or shock,
   acidosis (pH < 7.15)
3. Moderate RDS if < 2000 g:
   P_aO_2 < 8 kPa (60 mmHg) in 40% oxygen,
   apnoea or shock,
   pH < 7.20
4. Severe meconium aspiration syndrome:
   meconium below cords at birth and any subsequent respiratory distress,
   > 40% oxygen needed, presence of complicating air leak, e.g. pneumothorax
5. Major malformations:
   cardiology investigation
   surgical condition

pregnancies, prior transport of the mother for her delivery in the perinatal centre is to be preferred. However, about 40% of preterm labours cannot be predicted antenatally and some of these babies will be born outside perinatal centres. Their immediate resuscitation and stabilization may be critical as regards outcome. Sadly, not all transfers in the UK are successful and babies refused admission to neonatal intensive care units have a higher mortality than those fortunate to be accepted.

Transportation of a sick preterm infant is a complex procedure requiring the coordination of medical and nursing staffs from the two hospitals concerned. All infants referred by paediatricians or other doctors from outlying hospitals are accepted when possible. If no cots are available it is our policy for the resident doctor taking the call to find a cot on another site if possible. No referring paediatrician should be left with an ill infant about whom there is sufficient concern to have requested admission to our nurseries. Much time can be spent on the telephone that might be better used and successful admission is not always achieved.

REQUIREMENTS FOR TRANSPORTATION

1. Suitably equipped ambulance available at all times
2. Experienced medical and nursing staff available at all times
3. Transport incubator:
   - Battery and mains
   - Adequate heat supply
   - Easy access - portholes for drips
   - Oxygen supply variable from 25–100%
   - Monitors - heart rate, respiration, transcutaneous or pulse oximeter
   - Pump for controlled fluid administration
   - Positive pressure ventilation and CPAP
4. Nursing packs:
   - Umbilical vessel catheterization
   - Endotracheal intubation
   - Pleural drains
5. Drugs (Appendix XIV)
6. Other equipment (Appendix XIV)

GENERAL RULES OF TRANSPORTATION

1. Stabilization:
   - Airway and oxygen
   - Blood gas/radiograph
   - Assisted ventilation
   - Arterial cannulation
   - Intravenous fluids, dextrose; check blood pressure
   - Temperature and correction of acidosis
2. Explanation and reassurance of mother and father. Polaroid photograph for them to keep
3. Consent for procedures (cardiac catheterization, surgical procedures)
4. Copy of all relevant notes, radiographs, specimen of mother's blood
5. Careful monitoring during transport (see above)

SOME SPECIFIC PROBLEMS

1. Significant RDS: intubate before transport (see p. 76)
2. Pneumothorax: pleural drain before transport (see p. 92)

3. Heart failure: begin digoxin and diuretics (see p. 237)
4. Seizures: LP and glucose strip test before transport and anticonvulsants if indicated (see p. 226)
5. Open lesions, e.g. myelomeningocele, omphalocele: cover with warm saline soaks and polythene bag (polybag). Gastroschisis should have intravenous fluids
6. Intestinal obstruction: nasogastric tube (intermittent drainage of oesophageal atresia) and intravenous fluids

RETURN TO REFERRAL HOSPITAL

The transfer of infants back to the hospital of birth will depend upon:

1. Resolution of the major clinical problems
2. Ability of referring hospital to continue basic support

Our experience has shown that half of all our transported infants qualify for transfer back to the peripheral hospitals after about 7–10 days. This has three main advantages:

1. Frees intensive care cots
2. Moves the infant closer to parents so that visiting becomes easier
3. Encourages referring obstetricians and paediatricians to seek intensive care again

DISCHARGE

To some extent this is determined by the development of the community services: community midwifery, health visiting, general practitioner and community paediatrics. In general, if a baby is feeding well, can maintain his body temperature in a cot and has a competent mother (and father) he can be discharged no matter what he weighs. Some babies with weights of 1600 g have been safely discharged from hospital.

Babies with continuing problems such as congenital anomalies, apnoeic attacks, bronchopulmonary dysplasia or neurological sequelae can be successfully discharged but may need additional care including tube feeding, domiciliary oxygen or apnoea monitors.

NURSING POINTS

1. Stabilization cot, warmed incubator or radiant warmer prepared for each new admission
2. Check equipment readily available: oxygen/air, headbox, ventilator, cardiorespiratory monitor, pulse oximeter, suction, low-reading thermometer, glucose stix, IV fluids, specimen bottles, charts for note taking
3. Keep baby warm; give enough oxygen to abolish cyanosis, check baby's identity; record vital signs (temperature, pulse, respiration and blood pressure); measure blood glucose (glucose strip test) and packed cell volume; take superficial swabs for culture; **THEN MINIMAL HANDLING**
4. Talk to parents; take a polaroid photograph; reassure
5. Planning discharge is important; needs communication with community nurses, explanation of all home treatments and review appointment

REFERENCES AND FURTHER READING

British Association of Perinatal Medicine Working Group (1989). Referrals for neonatal medical care in the United Kingdom over one year. *Br. Med. J.* **298**: 169.

Davies, P., Haxby, V., Herbert, S. and McNeish, A. S. (1979). When should preterm babies be sent home from neonatal units? *Lancet* **i**: 914.

Dear, P. R. F. and McLain, B. I. (1987). Establishment of an intermediate care ward for babies and mothers. *Arch. Dis. Child* **62**: 597.

Fanaroff, A. A. and Klaus, M. H. (1986). Transportation of the high-risk infant. In: *Care of the High-risk Neonate*, 3rd edn, (eds, Klaus, M. H. and Fanaroff, A. A.). Philadelphia: W. B. Saunders.

Roper, H. P., Chiswick, M. L. and Sims, D. G. (1988). Referrals to a regional neonatal intensive care unit. *Arch. Dis. Child* **63**: 403.

Whitby, C., de Cates, C. R. and Roberton, N. R. C. (1981). Infants weighing 1.8–2.5 kg: do they need neonatal unit or postnatal ward care? *Lancet* **i**: 322.

6. The Low Birth Weight Infant

DEFINITIONS

A low birth weight (LBW) infant is one whose birth weight is 2500 g or less. The cause may be (a) short gestation (preterm <37 weeks), (b) growth retardation (small-for-gestational-age (SGA) <10th percentile) or (c) both of the foregoing.

Growth charts of weight against gestation (Fig. 4) are used to determine whether an infant is appropriately grown or not. SGA babies lie below the 10th percentile of weight for gestation and large-for-gestational-age infants (LGA) lie above the 90th percentile. Infants are post-term if they are born beyond the 42nd week of pregnancy (see Chapter 7).

The two groups of LBW infants have different problems so early accurate assessment necessary. Assessment will involve:

1. Gestational age:
   Menstrual history
   Early antenatal ultrasonic scan
   Dubowitz assessment (Figs 5, 6, and Tables 13, 14)
   Neurological assessment (Robinson, 1966) (Table 15)
   Shorter external assessment (Usher *et al.*, 1966)
   (This uses five external characteristics: skin creases on soles of feet, breast size, ear development, lanugo hair and external genitalia.) Below 28 weeks, gestational age assessment using external characteristics is unreliable. Gestational age is a better predictor of outcome than birth weight for infants of over 800 g
2. Growth: plot weight, length and head circumference against gestational age (p. 358)

THE PRETERM INFANT

Characteristically the preterm infant shows:

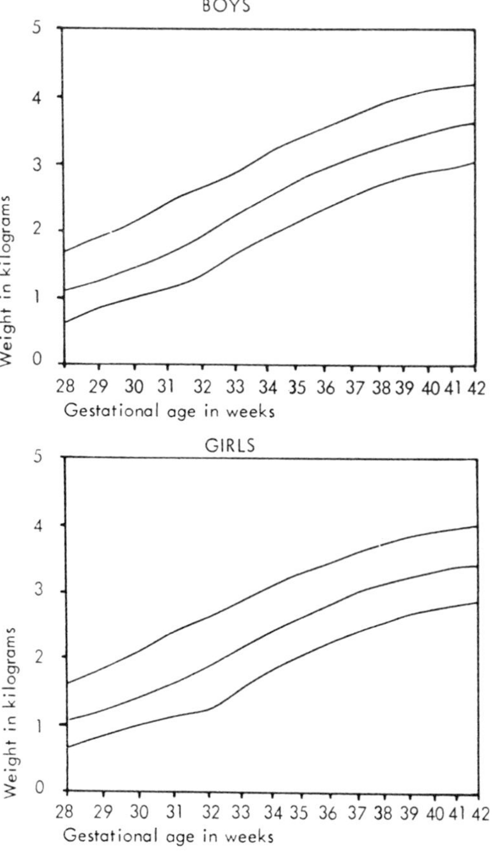

Fig. 4. Growth charts of weight against gestation for boys and girls (see also Appendix VIII). After Thompson *et al.* (1968).

1. Inactive, extended posture
2. Feeble cry
3. Irregular respirations
4. Translucent skin, thick vernix, few skin creases
5. Prominent lanugo
6. Poor breast development
7. Soft nails
8. Immature external genitalia

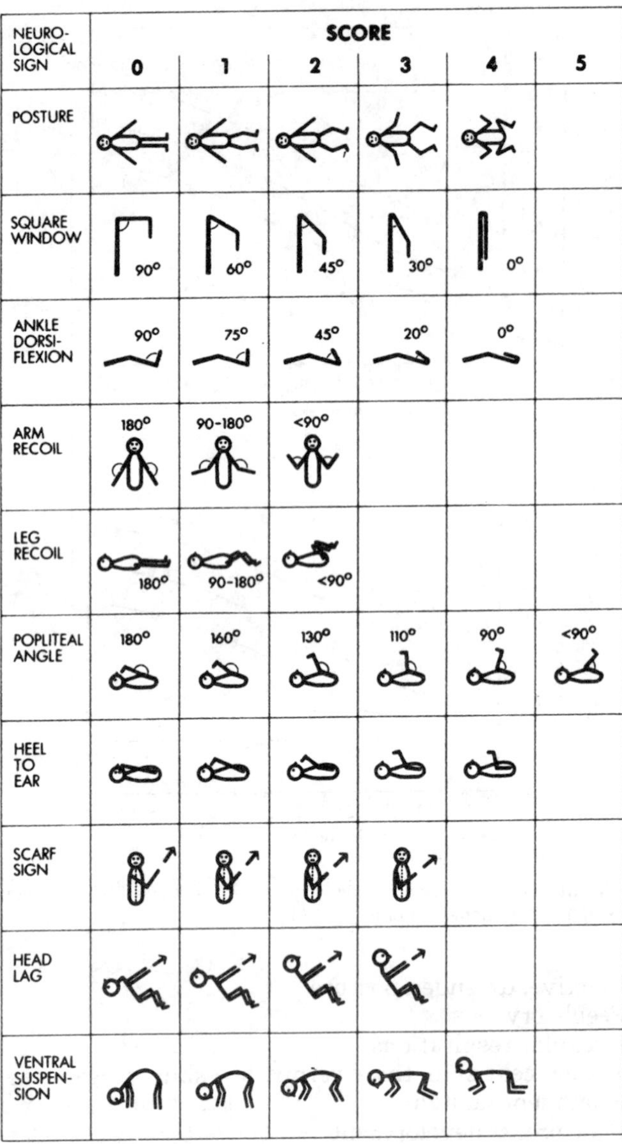

Fig. 5. Neurological criteria in the Dubowitz score. From Dubowitz *et al.* (1970) (as adapted from Amiel-Tison, 1968) with kind permission of the authors and the editor of *Journal of Pediatrics*.

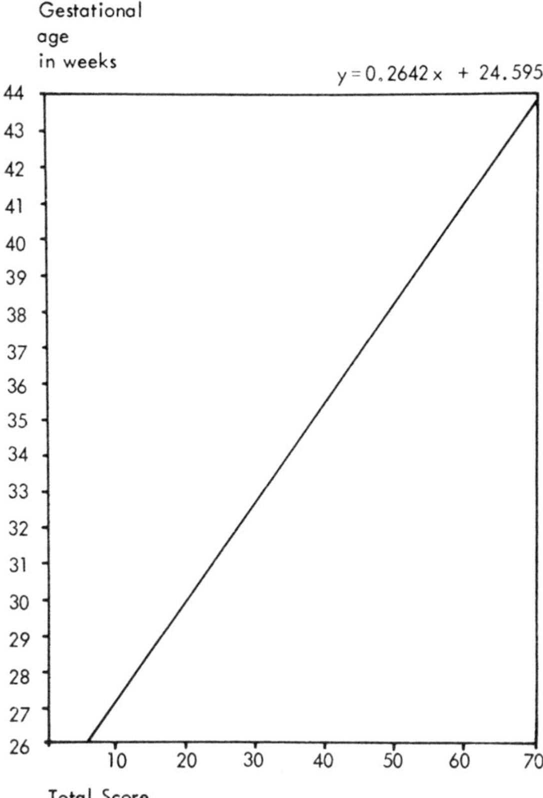

Fig. 6. Graph for reading gestational age from total score. From Dubowitz *et al.* (1970) with kind permission of the authors and the editor of *Journal of Pediatrics*.

Physiological Handicaps

Temperature instability

Difficulty in maintaining body temperature because of increased heat loss due to reduced subcutaneous fat and large surface area to body weight ratio. Also reduced heat production because of inadequate brown fat.

Table 13. Scoring of external criteria in Dubowitz score.

External sign	*Score*				
	0	1	2	3	4
Oedema	Obvious oedema hands and feet; pitting over tibia	No obvious oedema hands and feet; pitting over tibia	No oedema		
Skin texture	Very thin, gelatinous	Thin and smooth	Smooth; medium thickness. Rash or superficial peeling	Slight thickening. Superficial cracking and peeling especially hands and feet	Thick and parchment-like; superficial or deep cracking
Skin colour **(*infant not crying*)**	Dark red	Uniformly pink	Pale pink; variable over body	Pale. Only pink over ears, lips, palms or soles	
Skin opacity **(*trunk*)**	Numerous veins and venules clearly seen, especially over abdomen	Veins and tributaries seen	A few large vessels clearly seen over abdomen	A few large vessels seen indistinctly over abdomen	No blood vessels seen
Lanugo **(*over back*)**	No lanugo	Abundant: long and thick over whole back	Hair thinning especially over lower back	Small amount of lanugo and bald areas	At least half of back devoid of lanugo
Plantar creases	No skin creases	Faint red marks over anterior half of sole	Definite red marks over more than anterior half; indentations over less than anterior third	Indentations over more than anterior third	Definite deep indentations over more than anterior third

Table 13. Scoring of external criteria in Dubowitz score (continued).

External sign	*Score*				
	0	1	2	3	4
Nipple formation	Nipple barely visible; no areola	Nipple well defined; areola smooth and flat diameter <0.75 cm	Areola stippled, edge not raised; diameter <0.75 cm	Areola stippled, edge raised diameter >0.75 cm	
Breast size	No breast tissue palpable	Breast tissue on one or both sides <0.5 cm diameter	Breast tissue both sides; one or both 0.5–1.0 cm	Breast tissue both sides; one or both >1 cm	
Ear form	Pinna flat and shapeless, little or no incurving of edge	Incurving of part of edge of pinna	Partial incurving whole of upper pinna	Well-defined incurving whole of upper pinna	
Ear firmness	Pinna soft, easily folded, no recoil	Pinna soft, easily folded, slow recoil	Cartilage to edge of pinna, but soft in places, ready recoil	Pinna firm, cartilage to edge, instant recoil	
Genitalia male	Neither testis in scrotum	At least one testis high in scrotum	At least one testis right down		
Females (with hips half abducted)	Labia majora widely separated, labia minora protruding	Labia majora almost cover labia minora	Labia majora completely cover labia minora		

After Farr *et al.* (1966) and Dubowitz *et al.* (1970)

Table 14. Some notes on techniques of assessment of neurological criteria.

Posture	Observed with infant quiet and in supine position. Score 0, arms and legs extended; 1, beginning of flexion of hips and knees, arms extended; 2, stronger flexion of legs, arms extended; 3, arms slightly flexed, legs flexed and abducted; 4, full flexion of arms and legs
Square window	The hand is flexed on the forearm between the thumb and index finger of the examiner. Enough pressure is applied to get as full a flexion as possible, and the angle between the hypothenar eminence and the ventral aspect of the forearm is measured and graded according to diagram. (Care is taken not to rotate the infant's wrist while doing this manoeuvre)
Ankle dorsiflexion	The foot is dorsiflexed onto the anterior aspect of the leg, with the examiner's thumb on the sole of the foot and other fingers behind the leg. Enough pressure is applied to get as full flexion as possible, and the angle between the dorsum of the foot and the anterior aspect of the leg is measured
Arm recoil	With the infant in the supine position the forearms are first flexed for 5 s, then fully extended by pulling on the hands, and then released. The sign is fully positive if the arms return briskly to full flexion (score 2). If the arms return to incomplete flexion or the response is sluggish it is graded as score 1. If they remain extended or are only followed by random movements the score is 0
Leg recoil	With the infant supine, the hips and knees are fully flexed for 5 s, then extended by traction on the feet, and released. A maximal response is one of full flexion of the hips and knees (score 2). A partial flexion scores 1, and minimal or no movement scores 0
Popliteal angle	With the infant supine and his pelvis flat on the examining couch, the thigh is held in the knee-chest position by the examiner's left index finger and thumb supporting the knee. The leg is then extended by gentle pressure from the examiner's right index finger behind the ankle and the popliteal angle is measured
Heel-to-ear manoeuvre	With the baby supine, draw the baby's foot as near to the head as it will go without forcing it. Observe the distance between the foot and the head as well as the degree of extension at the knee. Grade according to diagram (Fig. 5). Note that the knee is left free and may draw down alongside the abdomen
Scarf sign	With the baby supine, take the infant's hand and try to put it around the neck and as far posteriorly as possible around the opposite shoulder. Assist this manoeuvre by lifting the elbow across the body. See how far the elbow will go across and grade according to illustrations. Score 0, elbow reaches opposite axillary line; 1, elbow between midline and opposite axillary line; 2, elbow reaches midline; 3, elbow will not reach midline

Table 14. Some notes on techniques of assessment of neurological criteria (continued).

Head lag	With the baby lying supine, grasp the hands (or the arms if a very small infant) and pull him slowly towards the sitting position. Observe the position of the head in relation to the trunk and grade accordingly. In a small infant, the head may initially be supported by one hand. Score 0, complete lag; 1, partial head control; 2, able to maintain head in line with body; 3, brings head anterior to body
Ventral	The infant is suspended in the prone position, with examiner's hand under the infant's chest (one hand in a small infant, two in a large infant). Observe the degree of extension of the back and the amount of flexion of the arms and legs. Also note the relation of the head to the trunk. Grade according to diagrams

If the score for an individual criterion differs on the two sides of the baby, take the mean

Table 15. Neurological assessment of gestation.

		Gestation (weeks)	
Reflex	*Response*	*Positive*	*Negative*
Pupillary light	Constriction	>28	<32
Glabellar tap	Blink	>31	<35
Wrist traction	Neck flexion	>32	<37
Neck righting	Trunk follows head rotation	>33	<38

After Robinson (1966)

Respiratory difficulties

Deficiency of surfactant leading to respiratory distress syndrome (see Chapter 10). Additional problems due to poor gag and cough reflexes, incoordinated suck and swallow resulting in increased risk of aspiration. Pliable thorax and weak respiratory musculature result in less efficient ventilation. Immaturity of respiratory centre (chemoreceptors) in the medulla may cause periodic breathing and apnoea (p. 211).

Gastrointestinal and nutritional problems

Poor sucking and swallowing reflexes especially before 34 weeks gestation.

1. Decreased intestinal motility leading to abdominal distension
2. Decreased gastric volume and increased gastric emptying times
3. Reduced digestive and absorptive activity of fats, fat-soluble vitamins and certain minerals
4. Lactase in intestinal brush border deficient before term but enzyme rapidly induced by feeding
5. Body stores of calcium, phosphorus, proteins, vitamins A, C and E, trace elements and iron are less than term infant and deficiencies may occur with growth

Hepatic immaturity

Impaired conjugation and excretion of bilirubin. Deficiency of vitamin-K-dependent clotting factors.

Renal immaturity

Inability to excrete large solute loads, and a relatively dilute urine is produced. Fluid and electrolyte balance may prove difficult and metabolic acidosis may result from accumulation of inorganic acids.

Immunological disturbances

Reduced ability to combat infection as a result of absent placental transmission of 19S immunoglobulins (IgM, IgA): Relative inability to produce antibodies. Impaired phagocytosis and reduced inflammatory response (see Chapter 13).

Neurological immaturity

Immature sucking and swallowing reflexes. Decreased intestinal motility (probably neural and hormonal). Recurrent apnoea and bradycardia (paradoxical response to hypoxia and hypercapnia). Increased susceptibility to intraventricular haemorrhage. This last problem is due to relatively unsupported but highly vascular periventricular area (the germinal plate) and perinatal stresses; for example, hypercapnia and hypertension may predispose to bleeding in this area and into the ventricles (see p. 00).

Ischaemic events may also occur, perhaps as a result of venous infarction leading to periventricular leucomalacia (PVL). Hypotensive episodes may predispose (see Chapter 16.)

THE SMALL-FOR-GESTATIONAL-AGE INFANT

There are two types exhibiting different intrauterine growth curves (Fig. 7):

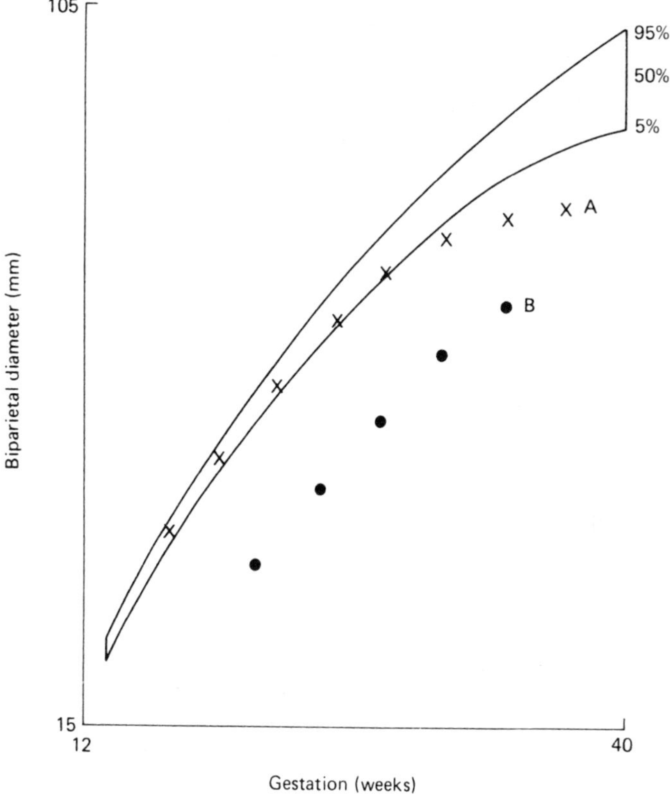

Fig. 7. Intrauterine growth curves of biparietal diameter showing the types of growth retardation. A = late onset or asymmetrical, B = early onset or symmetrical. From Campbell (1969) with kind permission of the editor of *Journal of Obstetrics and Gynaecology of the British Commonwealth*.

Asymmetrical growth retardation – due to intrauterine 'malnutrition' – shows relative sparing of length and head circumference compared with body weight. Causes include:

1. Placental insufficiency
2. Pre-eclampsia
3. Hypertension
4. Renal disease
5. Long-standing diabetes
6. Smoking
7. Altitude

Symmetrical growth retardation – due to early intrauterine infection, chromosomal abnormality, skeletal abnormality or fetal alcohol syndrome – shows reduced length and head circumference as well as body weight. Some constitutionally small babies are classed in this group.

SGA infants have higher morbidity than infants who are appropriate for gestational age, partly because of the greater incidence of congenital abnormalities and infections.

They should be assessed for congenital anomalies, intrauterine infection, perinatal asphyxia, hypoglycaemia, polycythaemia and pulmonary haemorrhage. Vitamin K should be given at birth.

MANAGEMENT OF THE LOW BIRTH WEIGHT INFANT

Preterm Infant

Asphyxia and resuscitation

Prenatal management is designed to detect and correct fetal asphyxia and to minimize trauma.

Asphyxia in the preterm infant is poorly tolerated and increases morbidity in the immediate and late postnatal period. At least one study has shown improved survival of very low birth weight infants who were electively intubated at birth for resuscitation.

An increasing proportion of immature infants are being born by elective ceasarean section, especially those that are breech presentation, but this may be traumatic if the lower uterine segment is poorly formed.

EXPERT DELIVERY AND NEONATAL RESUSCITATION IS ESPECIALLY IMPORTANT FOR THE LOW BIRTH WEIGHT INFANT

Temperature

Keep the infant warm either under radiant heater or in an incubator which is servo-controlled.

Infants should be placed in a neutral thermal environment where oxygen consumption is minimal (see Chapter 8). Alternative is a servo-controlled incubator or radiant heater to maintain skin temperature at 36.5°C. Woollen hats help to prevent heat loss.

When the preterm infant reaches about 1600–1800 g, he/she is usually able to maintain temperature out of the incubator.

Monitoring for apnoea and bradycardia

Infants of gestation <34 weeks or birth weight <1750 g have an increased risk of apnoea and bradycardia.

Heart rate and respiration rate monitoring should be performed on all these infants. Use continuous recording of heart rate and respiration with an electronic monitor for all ill infants.

For other infants use recording of ECG and respiratory trace on a simpler monitor (see Chapter 9).

Simple pressure apnoea monitors (see Fig. 36) or apnoea alarm mattresses are less informative but must be used when no other systems are available.

Fluids and nutrition

See also Chapter 11. The quantity and route of administration will depend upon the size, age and condition of the infant.

Infants <1500 g may tolerate oral feeding poorly for the first few days of life. Intravenous 5 or 10% dextrose at a rate of 80–100 ml/kg/day is used during the first 24 hours.

In the very immature infant, glycosuria or hyperglycaemia (glucose strip test > 8 mmol/1) may occur so that the concentration of dextrose should be reduced.

After 24 hours, if the infant cannot tolerate oral feeding, the intravenous dextrose is supplemented with amino acids according to parenteral nutrition routine (see Chapter 11).

For infants less than 34 weeks, tube feeding may be required because of risk of aspiration as a result of incoordinated suck and swallow. Tube feeds may be given by either intermittent or continuous orogastric intubation.

Orogastric rather than nasogastric intubation is used since the latter causes increase in airway resistance and may lead to apnoea.

The feeds should begin with quantities of 1–5 ml/hour and increase cautiously every 12 hours depending upon the amount of gastric aspirate. There may also be gastric distension and reflux. Alternatively, transpyloric (orojejunal) feeding by a silastic feeding tube may be used but increased risk of necrotizing enterocolitis has been reported. We do not routinely check for positioning of transpyloric tubes by radiography.

Intermittent feeding has some advantages over continuous feeding by encouraging normal enterohumoral responses but immature babies may tolerate the smaller quantities of milk used in continuous feeding.

For infants less than 1200 g use continuous intragastric or transpyloric infusion of milk beginning with 1 ml/hour.

Expressed breast milk is probably the best food for small or asphyxiated infants (see Chapter 11). Because of the risks of AIDS only mother's breast milk is used and donations to milk banks have generally ceased. Preterm babies fed on EBM do not grow as rapidly as babies fed on proprietary formulae but other benefits such as anti-infective properties of breast milk outweigh this disadvantage.

Fluid requirements increase daily to a maximum of 150–200 ml/kg/day depending on environmental and renal losses. Urine specific gravity measurements help to control intake.

Minimal energy and protein requirements for growth are 460 kJ/kg/day (110 kcal/kg/day) and 2–3 g/kg/day, respectively.

Oxygen requirements

Preterm infants should not be placed routinely in oxygen. Hypoxaemia is the only true indication for oxygen therapy.

When oxygen therapy is being used, the ambient oxygen level should be continuously recorded.

If central cyanosis is present, the infant may be placed initially in the minimum oxygen concentration required to abolish cyanosis.

If an infant requires oxygen 30 min after birth to maintain normal colour then it is essential that arterial oxygen tensions are measured. This may be performed by intermittent radial artery puncture, umbilical or radial arterial catheterization or transcutaneous oxygen monitoring if the infant is not shocked (see Chapter 9).

Oxygen therapy should aim to keep arterial oxygen tension in the range 7–10 kPa (60–80 mmHg) to reduce the risks of retinopathy of prematurity (retrolental fibroplasia) and to avoid hypoxic brain damage.

Small-for-Gestational-Age Infant (SGA)

Assess for congenital malformation and intrauterine infection.

About 60% of preterm SGA infants and 30% of term SGA infants will develop hypoglycaemia if not adequately managed. Infants below the third percentile are especially at risk (Appendix VIII).

Glucose strip test and packed cell volume should be measured on all SGA infants on admission. Glucose strip test readings below 1.5 mmol/l (25 mg/dl) are taken as hypoglycaemia (see p. 171).

Intravenous 10% dextrose by infusion, not as bolus, should be used to maintain blood sugar in the range 1.5–2.5 mmol/l (25–45 mg/dl).

Polycythaemia may occur and is defined as venous packed cell volume of over 65%.

Partial exchange transfusion with plasma or albumin considered for all infants with venous packed cell volume over 70%, or for symptomatic infants with packed cell volume over 65% (see pp. 110, 282).

For infants below the third percentile measure coagulation (prothrombin time and partial thromboplastin time) and give fresh frozen plasma 10 ml/kg if prothrombin time is greater than 20 sec and partial thromboplastin time greater than 70 sec.

Pulmonary haemorrhage occurs in SGA infants. Cause is unknown but is possibly due to a combination of hypoglycaemia, hypothermia, hypoxaemia and coagulation factor deficiency. It presents with respiratory distress of acute onset with blood-stained tracheal fluid. The mortality is high (see p. 147).

Long-term follow up is indicated for both the preterm and the SGA infant (Chapter 26).

NURSING POINTS

1. Temperature control and nutrition are especially important
2. Humidified incubator is better than prolonged use of radiant warmer
3. Dress infant in warm clothes as soon as condition stable
4. Feeding method depends on maturity and state of health
5. Encourage breast feeding; expressed milk

6. Full explanation of all procedures to parents. Joint meetings with senior medical staff ensures consistency of advice

REFERENCES AND FURTHER READING

Amiel-Tison, C. (1968). Neurological evaluation of the maturity of newborn infants. *Arch. Dis. Child* **43**: 89.

Campbell, S. (1969). The prediction of fetal maturity by ultrasonic measurement of the biparietal diameter. *J.Obstet. Gynaecol. Br. Commonwealth* **76**: 603.

Dornan, J. C. and Halliday, H. L. (1988). Preterm Birth. *In: Perinatal Medicine* (eds, McClure, G., Halliday, H. L. and Thompson, W.). London: Baillière Tindall.

Drew, J. H. (1982). Immediate intubation at birth of the very low birth weight infant. Effect on survival. *Am. J. Dis. Child* **136**: 207

Dubowitz, L. M., Dubowitz, V. and Goldberg, C. (1970). Clinical assessment of gestational age in the newborn infant. *J. Pediatr.* **77**: 1

Farr, V., Kerridge, D. F. and Mitchell, R. G. (1966). The value of some external characteristics in the assessment of gestational age at birth. *Dev. Med. Child Neurol.* **8**: 657.

Halliday, H. L. (1989). Care of preterm babies in the first hour. *Care Critic. Ill* **4**: 7.

Halliday, H. L., McClure, G. and Ritchie, J. W. K. (1988). Intrauterine growth retardation. In: *Perinatal Medicine* (eds, McClure, G., Halliday, H. L. and Thompson, W.). London: Baillière Tindall.

Keen, D. V. and Pearse, R. G. (1988). Weight, length, and head circumference curves for boys and girls of between 20 and 42 weeks' gestation. *Arch. Dis. Child* **63**: 1170.

McClure, B. G. (1979). Delivery room care of the preterm infant. *J. Mat. Child Hlth* **4**: 466.

Patterson, C. C. and Halliday, H. L. (1988). Prediction of outcome shortly after delivery for the very low birthweight (<1500 g) infant. *Paed. Perinatal Epid.* **2**: 221.

Robinson, R. J. (1966). Assessment of gestational age by neurological examination. *Arch. Dis. Child* **41**: 437.

Thompson, A. M., Billewicz, W. Z. and Hytten, F. E. (1968). The assessment of fetal growth. *J. Obstet. Gynaecol. Br. Commonwealth*, **75**: 903.

Usher, R. H. and McLean, F. (1969), Intrauterine growth of live-born Caucasian infants at sea level: standards obtained from measurements in 7 dimensions of infants born between 25 and 44 weeks gestation. *J. Pediatr.* **74**: 901.

Usher, R. H., McLean, F. and Scott, K. E. (1966). Judgement of fetal age. II Clinical significance of gestational age and an objective method for its assessment. *Pediatr. Clin. North Am.* **13**: 835.

7. The Big Baby

DEFINITIONS

Large for gestational age (LGA): babies whose birth weight is greater than the 90th percentile for gestational age (Appendix VIII).

Post-term (prolonged pregnancy): babies whose gestational age exceeds 42 weeks.

Postmaturity: this refers to the appearance of the baby from a prolonged pregnancy who shows signs of growth retardation. These may include dry, cracked, meconium-stained skin, alert (old man) appearance and signs of recent weight loss.

Table 16. Causes of big babies.

Constitutionally large
Maternal diabetes
Severe erythroblastosis
Other causes of hydrops (Table 17)
Prolonged pregnancy
Transposition of the great arteries
Beckwith's syndrome
Sotos', Marshall's and Weaver's syndromes

Big babies may have problems related to their size, or to prolonged pregnancy or associated with the underlying causes (Table 18).

REFERENCES AND FURTHER READING

Clifford, S. H. (1954). Postmaturity-with placental dysfunction: clinical syndrome and pathologic findings. *J. Pediatr.* **44**: 1.

Table 17. Causes of hydrops fetalis.

Hydrops fetalis may be caused by:

1. Rhesus isoimmunization
2. Homozygous α-thalassaemia
3. Fetomaternal haemorrhage (Kleihauer)
4. Cardiac failure:
   congenital heart disease
   supraventricular tachycardia
5. Hypoproteinaemia:
   congenital nephrosis
   renal vein thrombosis
   congenital hepatitis
6. Intrauterine infection:
   syphilis
   TORCH
   Parvovirus
7. Others:
   umbilical vein thrombosis
   fetal neuroblastoma
   placental chorioangioma

Table 18. Problems of big babies.

Obstetric trauma:
shoulder dystocia — Erb's palsy, fractured clavicle
fractured skull or long bones
subdural haemorrhage

Prolonged pregnancy:
birth asphyxia
meconium aspiration
hypoglycaemia
polycythaemia
coagulation defects

Others:
congenital anomalies
hypoglycaemia

Dornan, J. C., Halliday, H. L. and Reid, M. Mc. C. (1988). Post-term pregnancy. In: *Perinatal Medicine* (eds, McClure, G., Halliday, H. L. and Thompson, W.). London: Baillière Tindall.

Stevenson, D. K., Hopper, A. O., Cohen, R. S. *et al.* (1982). Macrosomia: causes and consequences. *J. Pediatr.* **100**: 515.

8. Basic Principles of Neonatal Intensive Care

Categories of neonatal care have been set out by the British Association of Perinatal Medicine (see Glossary and Appendix XVI).

The basic principles are:

ANTICIPATION, PREVENTION, DETECTION, EARLY CORRECTION AND MINIMAL DISTURBANCE

By adhering to these principles one can often avert major problems.

The aim of neonatal intensive care is to provide life support and vital-signs monitoring in a controlled, stable environment for the ill infant. This environment should be clean, warm and friendly. Parents are present in the units and every effort should be made to accommodate them and their needs.

HYGIENIC ENVIRONMENT

The hands of the medical and nursing attendants, and all equipment that is used to treat the newborn, should be scrupulously clean. Hands and forearms should be washed after removing rings and watches and rolling up sleeves. The primary wash on entering the nursery should last 5 min. Use an antiseptic solution like chlorhexidine or Betadine. After handling each infant, a secondary wash should be carried out lasting 1 min. The risk of cross-infection is related to the number of infants in the unit and the amount of handling by staff. Staff or visitors with or recovering from an infectious illness, such as respiratory infection, gastroenteritis, active herpes simplex lesions (before crusting) or boils, should be excluded from the nursery. Mothers with infected wounds or with pathogens in vaginal swab should be admitted after careful handwashing. One should avoid use of communal instruments such as stethoscopes. Each infant should have his/her stethoscope attached to the incubator. If senior medical staff insist on using their own stethoscopes, they should be wiped after each use with alcohol wipes. Infected infants should be isolated. Place infant in incubator in an area where all other infants are also in incubators.

Invasive techniques such as intravascular cannulation (see Chapter 9) should be carried out under full aseptic conditions.

All ill newborn babies should be handled minimally (see p. 294).

TEMPERATURE CONTROL

Heat production is limited because of reduced activity and absence of shivering.

Non-shivering thermogenesis relies on the oxidation of brown fat after catecholamine stimulus.

Heat losses are increased because of the newborn's large surface area to body weight ratio, and reduced subcutaneous fat for insulation.

The newborn is able to maintain body temperature over quite a narrow range and it is important to reduce energy consumption by nursing him/her in the neutral thermal environment (NTE). The NTE is defined as that range of environmental temperature over which heat production, oxygen consumption and nutritional requirements for growth are minimal provided body temperature is normal. The NTE will vary according to the maturity of the infant and whether he/she is nursed clothed in an incubator or naked under a radiant warmer.

When a radiant warmer is used the servo-control should be set to maintain skin temperature at 36.5 °C.

For incubators without a plastic heat shield use the tables of Scopes and Ahmed (1966) to determine incubator temperature (Table 19). Lower incubator temperature by 1 °C each week and at around 1800 g weight move into an open cot. Very immature infants, those below 28 weeks gestation, often need early care in humidified incubators.

Rapid lowering of environmental temperature should be avoided as this can lead to apnoea.

Infants less than 1500 g birth weight who are nursed in

Table 19. Neutral thermal environment (NTE) during first 3 days.

Birth weight (g)	*Incubator temperature* (°C)
1000	35
1500	34
2000	33.5
2500	33.2
3000	33
4000	32.5

Room temperature should be 28–29°C
After Scopes and Ahmed (1966), and Hey and Katz (1970)

incubators often need a plastic heat shield to reduce heat losses (Fig. 8). Woollen hats are also helpful as heat loss from the relatively large head is significant.

Disadvantages of servo-control include:

1. Loss of thermal instability as an indication of sepsis
2. Overheating - detachment of probe

Avoid radiant heater after 24 hours if possible because of:
1. Increased insensible water loss
2. Electrolyte upsets, increased bilirubin levels
3. Tendency to overhandle the infants
4. Draughts

Hypothermia should be avoided as it causes:

1. Increased oxygen consumption
2. Vasoconstriction and acidosis
3. Increased free fatty acid production (may displace bilirubin from albumin)
4. Hypoglycaemia
5. Coagulation disorders

Hyperthermia should also be avoided as it may cause apnoea in the immature infant. Usual cause is overheating of the environment but it may occur as a result of loss of temperature control in neonatal sepsis, brain injury or drug therapy.

Sweating does not occur in infants of less than 34 weeks so that hyperthermia will present as tachypnoea, tachycardia and

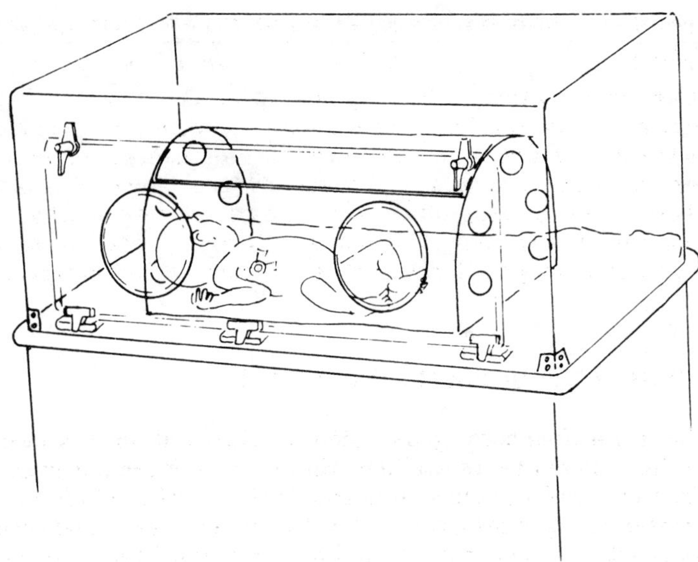

Fig. 8. Use of plastic heat shield inside an incubator to maintain temperature in a very low birth weight infant.

restlessness or apnoea. Hyperthermic babies often lie in an extended position as if 'sunbathing'.

OXYGEN THERAPY

Oxygen is a dangerous drug. In the premature newborn it has been associated with retinopathy of prematurity and pulmonary damage (bronchopulmonary dysplasia, see p. 148). Atelectasis can also occur after nitrogen washout if 100% oxygen is used to ventilate the lungs (resorption atelectasis).

The primary aim of oxygen therapy is to maintain normal arterial oxygen tensions:

Mature infant	7–10 kPa	(60–80 mmHg)
Immature infant (<1500 g)	6–9 kPa	(50–70 mmHg)

Or oxygen saturation measured by pulse oximetry:

Acute respiratory disease	88–94%
Chronic lung disease	86–92%

Record amount of oxygen as a concentration (%) not a flow in litres/min.

REMEMBER: Retinopathy of prematurity is related to high arterial oxygen tensions, not high environmental oxygen concentrations. There is *no* safe lower limit of oxygen concentration for a preterm infant. Arterial oxygen tensions of over 13 kPa (100 mmHg) may predispose to retinopathy of prematurity after only 2–4 hours exposure. Preterm infants with normal lungs will attain these tensions in 25% oxygen.

RETINOPATHY OF PREMATURITY (ROP)

The actual arterial oxygen tension and the duration of exposure to that oxygen tension which will cause ROP are not known. Try to avoid P_aO_2 values over 15 kPa (115 mmHg) at all times. In infants <34 weeks, this P_aO_2 will cause intense retinal vessel constriction which may be followed by proliferation of new

Table 20. Classification of retinopathy of prematurity.

Stage	*Acute proliferative*
0	Severe constriction of retinal vessels
I	Dilatation and tortuosity of retinal vessels with peripheral neovascularization
II	Neovascularization with retinal haemorrhages; increased vitreous haziness
III	Proliferation into vitreous; localized peripheral retinal detachment
IV	One half retina detached
V	Entire retina detached
Grade	*Chronic cicatricial*
I	Small areas of retinal pigment irregularities; small scars in retinal periphery
II	Disc distortion
III	Retinal fold
IV	Incomplete retrolental mass; partial retinal detachment
V	Complete retrolental mass; total retinal detachment

After Patz (1969)

capillaries if ischaemia of the retina has occurred. The growth of new vessels may cause fibrosis and scarring of the retina leading eventually to detachment and blindness (Table 20). This classification of Patz has recently been replaced by an international classification (Table 21). The new classification removes the term cicatricial and suggests the term retinopathy of prematurity for all stages and manifestations of the disease. The reason for this is that the major cause of visual loss and blindness in ROP is the traction detachment of the retina that

Table 21. International classification of retinopathy of prematurity.

Stage No.	*Characteristic*		
1	Demarcation line		
2	Ridge		
3	Ridge with extraretinal fibrovascular proliferation		
4	Subtotal retinal detachment (a) extrafoveal (b) retinal detachment including fovea		
5	Total retinal detachment		
	Funnel:	Anterior	Posterior
		open	open
		narrow	narrow
		open	narrow
		narrow	open

Table 22. Aetiological factors in ROP.

1. Genetic factors and gestational age
2. Multiple births
3. Congenital anomalies
4. Blood transfusions
5. Vitamin E deficiency
6. Vitamin A deficiency
7. Hypoxia and hyperoxia
8. Hypercapnia and acidosis
9. Infection
10. Drugs: indomethacin

often has exudative features. Therapeutic efforts must be aimed at preventing and repairing this detachment (see below). Remember that blood from the lower aorta (umbilical catheter) may have a lower P_aO_2 than that from the retinal arteries because of R–L shunting through the ductus arteriosus. Other aetiological factors are listed in Table 22.

All babies who have been treated with oxygen should have their eyes examined by an ophthalmologist before discharge or transfer back to referral hospital. The earliest changes of ROP are not seen until about 6 weeks after birth when all babies should be examined even if still ventilator dependent. We have an incidence of ROP which is much lower than that reported from the USA (about 4% of very low birth weight infants, cf. USA around 50%). This difference may be partly due to classification of fundal changes. There is some evidence to suggest that large prophylactic doses of vitamin E (100 mg) may be helpful (see also p. 281) but the most important recent advance has been the demonstration that cryotherapy prevents progression of ROP.

It is important to maintain constant oxygen concentrations at all times - care must be taken during suctioning or feeding to ensure that hypoxaemia does not occur. Episodes of hypoxaemia have been shown to correlate with both ROP and outcome.

Oxygen therapy may be given using a Perspex headbox, or when ventilation is supported by either continuous positive airways pressure (CPAP) or mechanical ventilation (intermittent positive pressure ventilation, IPPV), when the infant has intractable hypoxia, respiratory failure or apnoea (see Chapter 9).

MONITORING

To ensure a constant environment for the ill infant undergoing neonatal intensive care various measurements are monitored either continuously or intermittently:

1. Heart rate and variability (continuously)
2. Respiration rate and pattern (continuously)
3. Temperature: skin temperature (continuously) and core temperature (axilla is preferred) (intermittently, about 4 hourly)

4. Blood gases: arterial (intermittently, about 4 hourly) and transcutaneously or by pulse oximeter (continuously)
5. Glucose strip test/blood glucose (intermittently, about 4 hourly)
6. Electrolytes and urea (intermittently, at least once daily)
7. Calcium and magnesium (intermittently, at least once daily)
8. Bilirubin (intermittently, usually at least 12 hourly for the first 5 days)
9. Packed cell volume (intermittently, at least daily)
10. Blood pressure (6 hourly)
11. For babies having parenteral nutrition (see p. 166)

Cardiorespiratory monitors should be used to record heart rate and respiration rate continuously in all ill infants undergoing intensive care. This continuous monitoring detects and records any attacks of apnoea and bradycardia that occur in the spontaneously breathing infant. Periodic respiration will also be detected. In addition, heart rate variability is measured by these monitors. Reduced long-term variability (less than 5 beats/min) is highly predictive of the severity and outcome of respiratory distress syndrome. Persistent reduction in long-term variability is associated with increased mortality of all babies undergoing intensive care.

Normal blood gas values in the newborn are shown in Table 23. pH and $P\text{CO}_2$ are slightly lower than the normal values in adults. Figure 9 shows the change in blood gas values over the

Table 23. Normal blood gas values.

	pH	$P\text{CO}_2$ kPa (mmHg)	$P\text{O}_2$ kPa (mmHg)	*Base excess*	*Standard bicarbonate* (mmol/l)
Arterial	7.30–7.40	4.5–5 (33–38)	7–11 (60–90)	0 to −2	20–22
Capillary	7.28–7.38	4.5–5 (36–40)	5–7 (40–60)	−2 to −4	16–22
Venous	7.25–7.30	5–6.5 (40–50)	3.5–5.5 (30–45)	−4 to −6	13–20
Arterialized capillary	7.30–7.40	4.5–5 (33–38)	7 (60)	0 to −2	20–22

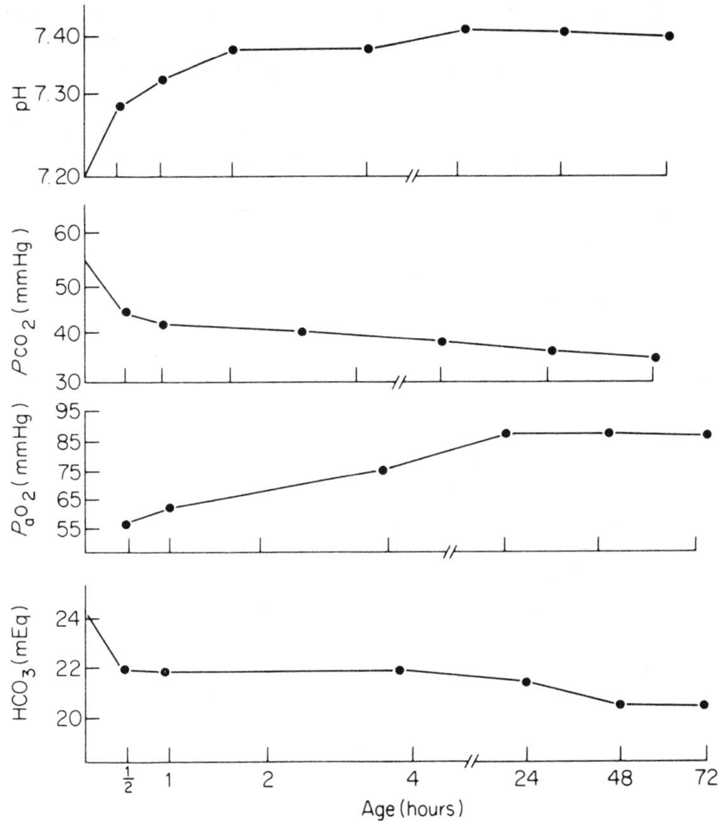

Fig. 9. Change in pH, Pco_2, P_aO_2 and bicarbonate with time following birth. After Klaus and Fanaroff (1979).

first 3 days of life. Table 24 shows typical blood gas values in situations of acidosis and alkalosis.

The causes of *respiratory acidosis* are:

1. Alveolar hypoventilation: for example RDS, respiratory depression, asphyxia, pneumonia, pneumothorax
2. Alveolar–capillary block: for example RDS, pneumonia

Table 24. Abnormal arterial blood gas values.

	pH	P_{CO_2} kPa (mmHg)	P_{O_2} kPa (mmHg)	*Base excess*	*Standard bicarbonate* (mmol/l)
Respiratory acidosis (with hypoxaemia)	7.25	7.5 (55)	5 (40)	−2	23
Metabolic acidosis	7.25	4.5 (35)	9 (70)	−11	15
Mixed acidosis (with hypoxaemia)	7.20	7 (50)	6 (45)	−7	19
Respiratory alkalosis	7.50	3.5 (28)	12 (90)	−2	22
Metabolic alkalosis	7.50	5 (38)	9 (70)	+6	30

The causes of *metabolic acidosis* are:

1. Hypoxia and shock
2. Infection
3. Patent ductus arteriosus and cardiac failure
4. Excessive protein intake, parenteral nutrition or starvation
5. Hyperchloraemia (p. 000)
6. Diarrhoea
7. Renal failure, renal tubular acidosis, amino acidurias, organic acidurias, congenital lactic acidosis

In severe respiratory distress syndrome, asphyxia and pneumonia there is usually a mixed metabolic and respiratory acidosis.

Treatment of respiratory acidosis is by improvement of ventilation with assisted ventilation.

In metabolic acidosis the underlying cause should be sought and corrected. If shock is present then a blood or plasma transfusion should be given. Bicarbonate solutions are administered to correct metabolic acidosis where the pH is below 7.25 and the base excess greater than −10, provided shock is not present (correct shock first).

The causes of *metabolic alkalosis* are:

1. Hypochloraemia (p. 179)
2. Excessive bicarbonate therapy

3. Hypokalaemia (p. 178)
4. Post-hypercapnia
5. Phosphate excess
6. Post-exchange transfusion

In neonatal intensive care respiratory alkalosis is more common than metabolic alkalosis and, if the infant is being mechanically ventilated, is an indication to reduce the amount of ventilation being provided (see Chapter 9). Marked respiratory alkalosis (pH > 7.50 and $P\text{CO}_2$ < 2.5 kPa (20 mmHg) may be hazardous as it is associated with severe reduction in cerebral blood flow and reduction in cardiac output. Under certain circumstances, e.g. treatment of cerebral oedema (p. 223 or pulmonary hypertension (p. 000), this degree of alkalosis may be beneficial.

Most blood gases are sampled from indwelling umbilical or radial arterial catheters (see Chapter 9). When arterial cannulation is contraindicated or has failed, measure arterial blood gases by intermittent arterial puncture of the radial artery as described in Chapter 9.

As an alternative in the short term an umbilical venous catheter may be passed through the ductus venosus and across the foramen ovale into the left atrium to sample 'arterial' blood, but see note of caution on p. 102.

The introduction of transcutaneous oxygen tension monitoring has been of great benefit but, because carbon dioxide tensions cannot as yet be measured reliably in this manner and tissue pH measurement is still not yet perfected, there remains a need for arterial cannulation in the ill newborn. In the future these less invasive methods of measuring blood carbon dioxide and pH may replace currently invasive techniques. In some infants with chronic respiratory disease, arterialized capillary blood is used to measure blood gases. These techniques are described in Chapter 9.

With proper warming of the heel and a free flow of blood the values for pH, $P\text{CO}_2$ and $P\text{O}_2$ obtained reflect fairly closely those of arterial blood. This comparison is shown in Table 19. Up to $P_a\text{O}_2$ 7 kPa (60 mmHg) there is a one-to-one relationship between arterial and arterialized capillary blood.

NURSING ROLE

Nurse staffing numbers are important: five nurses for each intensive care cot and 1.5 for each special care cot are recommended but rarely achieved in the UK.

Nursing goals:

1. Maintenance of constant environment
2. Non-invasive monitoring of infant's condition with minimal handling
3. Ready access to medical advice – both at a junior and senior level
4. Reassurance of parents

REFERENCES AND FURTHER READING

British Paediatric Association (1983). Minimum standards of neonatal care. *Arch. Dis. Child* **58**: 943.

British Paediatrics (1985). Categories of babies requiring neonatal care. *Arch. Dis. Child* **60**: 599.

Committee for the classification of ROP (1984). The International classification of ROP. *Pediatrics*, **74**: 127.

Cryotherapy for ROP Cooperative Group (1988). Multicenter trial of cryotherapy for ROP: preliminary results. *Pediatrics* **81**: 697.

Hey, E. N. and Katz, G. (1970). The optimal thermal environment for naked babies. *Arch. Dis. Child* **45**: 328.

Hittner, H. M., Godio, L. B., Rudolph, A. J. *et al.* (1981). Retrolental fibroplasia: efficacy of vitamin E in a double blind study of preterm infants. *N. Engl. J. Med.* **305**: 1365.

Hull, D. (1988). Thermal control in very immature infants. *Br. Med. Bull.* **44**: 971.

Kretzer, F. L. and Hittner, H. M. (1988). Retinopathy of prematurity: clinical implications of retinal development. *Arch. Dis. Child* **63**: 1151.

Lucey, J. F. and Dangman, B. (1984). A re-examination of the role of oxygen in retrolental fibroplasia. *Pediatrics* **73**: 82.

Patz, A. (1969). Retrolental fibroplasia. *Surv. Ophthalmol.* **14**: 1.

Royal College of Physicians (1988). Medical care of the newborn in England and Wales. London: RCP.

Rutter, N. (1988). The immature skin. *Br. Med. Bull.* **44**: 957.

Scopes, J. W. and Ahmed, I. (1966). Range of critical temperatures in sick and premature newborn babies. *Arch. Dis. Child* **41**: 417.

Speidel, B. D. (1978). Adverse effects of routine procedures on preterm infants. *Lancet* **i**: 864.

9. Procedures in Neonatal Intensive Care

These procedures are described with the aid of line diagrams in most cases. Never undertake a procedure unless you have observed it at least twice and performed it under supervision. In the ill infant some of these invasive procedures may be harmful even when correctly performed. Avoid tendency to overtreat, try to balance cost-to-benefit ratio in all situations before performing a procedure. If in doubt, ask.

BAG AND MASK VENTILATION

Most commonly used method of emergency assisted ventilation (Fig. 10). Two types:

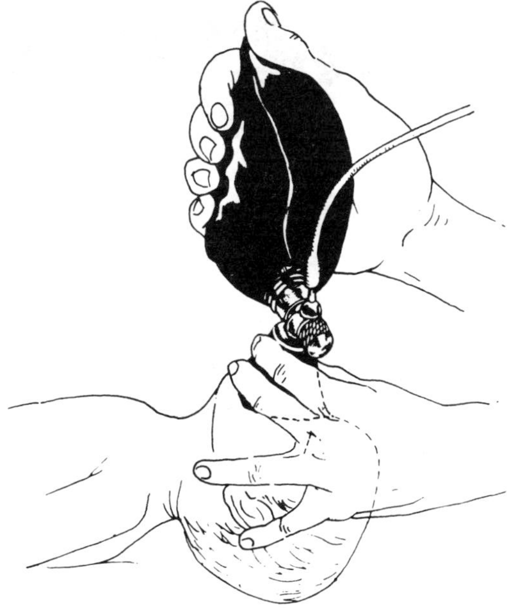

Fig. 10. Resuscitation with the anaesthetic bag and mask.

1. *Anaesthetic bag and mask*. Can generate high pressure and uses high oxygen concentrations. Therefore potential dangers to lungs (pneumothorax) and eyes (retinopathy of prematurity). This type of bag and mask is necessary for resuscitation as others generate insufficient pressures
2. *Cardiff or Ohio self-inflating bags* (Fig. 11). Low pressure, low oxygen concentration. Therefore safe, but may be ineffective. Used with babies having short apnoeic episodes

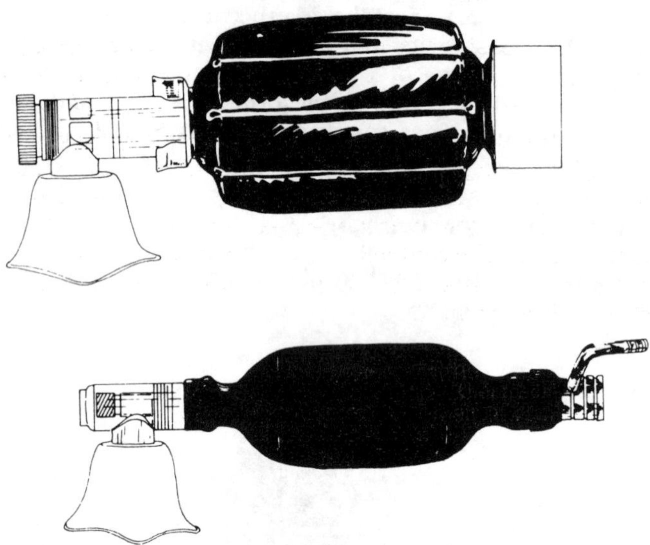

Fig. 11. Self inflating bags with masks. Top, Ohio bag; bottom, Cardiff (Penlon) bag.

Method

1. Place infant on firm surface, briefly aspirate airway
2. Choose mask of correct size
3. Place mask firmly over mouth and nose, allow 4–5 litres/min flow
4. Open blow-off valve (anaesthetic bag only)
5. Insufflate lungs, 30–40 breaths/min

This should result in:

1. Good chest wall movement
2. Good air entry on auscultation
3. Improved colour

If air entry is poor and little chest movement:

1. Insufficient pressure: tighten blow-off valve slightly
2. Airway blocked: inspect with laryngoscope and aspirate
3. Correct position of neck: avoid flexion or over-extension

If still no improvement, intubate (see below).

HEAD BOX

This is the commonest means of prolonged oxygen administration (Fig. 12). Oxygen and air mixture from wall supply is humidified and warmed in nebulizer. Be sure nebulizer has sufficient water, otherwise overheating will occur. Oxygen concentration can be controlled using blender or mixer. At least 5 litres/min flow should be allowed to prevent carbon dioxide build-up inside head box.

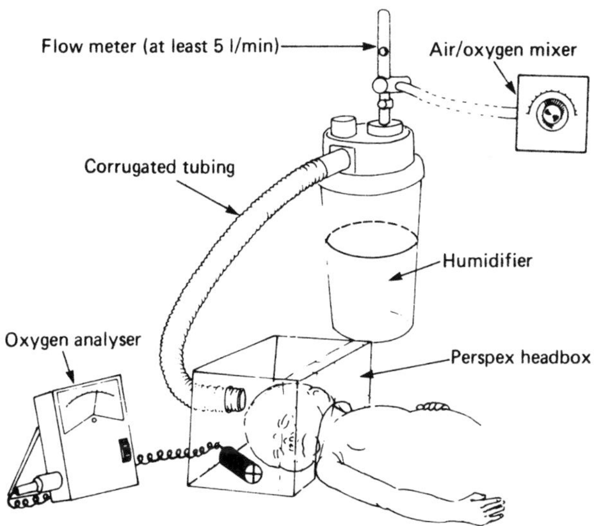

Fig. 12. Supply warmed humidified oxygen to a baby in a head box.

Ambient oxygen should be continuously monitored in the head box near the infant's face.

Do not remove box from baby for procedures like X-rays or feeding as rapid change in ambient oxygen concentration will occur and hypoxaemia and apnoea may ensue.

INTUBATION OF TRACHEA (Figs 13, 14)

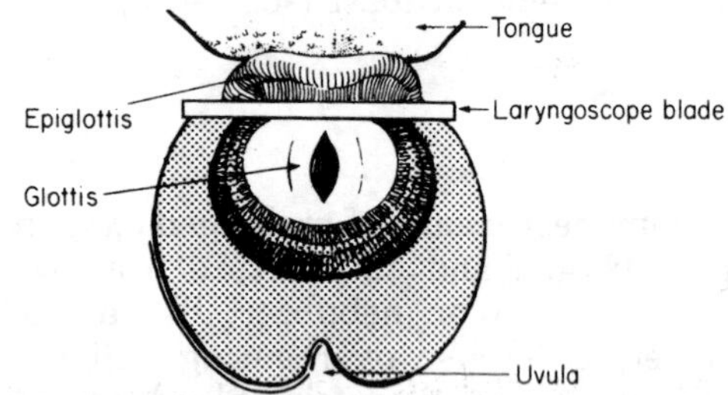

Fig. 13. Superior view of the neonatal larynx at laryngoscopy. After Barrie (1963).

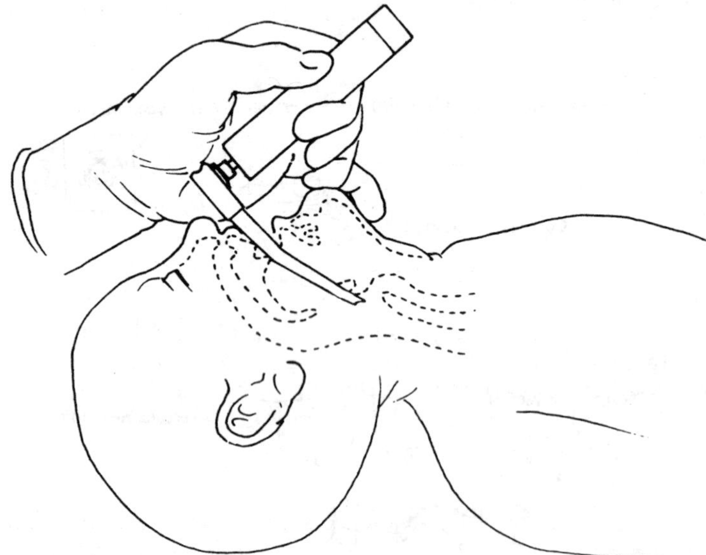

Fig. 14. Lateral view of the newborn at laryngoscopy. The laryngoscope blade gently lifts the tongue and epiglottis anteriorly to expose the glottis. After Cockburn and Drillien (1974).

Table 25. Tube sizes for neonatal intubation.

Infant's weight (g)	*Tube diameter* (mm)	*Distance from anterior nares to mid trachea* (cm)*
500–750	2.5	7.5
750–1250	2.5–3.0	8.5
1250–2000	3.0–3.5	9.5
2000–2500	3.5	10.5
2500–4000	3.5–4.0	11.0–12.0

* Allow 2 cm extra for tube fixation. Tube should be 1 cm above carina which is usually visible on X-ray
After Coldiron (1968)

Orotracheal

1. Select tube size and introducer if using straight Portex tubes (Table 25). Ensure that introducer does not protrude beyond the end of the tube. Curve distal end slightly. Alternative is to use curved, shouldered Cole's tubes, especially for resuscitation when introducer is not necessary
2. Check laryngoscope light and blade lock
3. Check suction apparatus
4. Check bag and mask, and bag and tube connector
5. Place infant on firm surface (in incubator or under radiant warmer)
6. Ventilate by bag and mask for 30 sec
7. Pass laryngoscope blade gently along right side of infant's mouth
8. Gently pull tongue and epiglottis forwards by lifting the blade - do not rotate blade to use as a lever
9. Aspirate airway if necessary
10. Pass tube about 2 cm below glottis, or if using a Cole's tube as far as the shoulder
11. Gently insufflate lungs

NOTE: Chest moves both sides, air entry good on auscultation, colour improves. If tube is too far in, it will usually pass into right main bronchus reducing air entry and chest movement on the left.

IF YOU FAIL, STOP. REMEMBER THERE ARE OTHERS WHO CAN HELP. CONTINUE WITH BAG AND MASK VENTILATION UNTIL HELP ARRIVES

Nasotracheal

More difficult but better fixation possible; use for long-term ventilation. Some units use orotracheal intubation and fixation for long-term ventilation:

1. Select and cut tube to right length (Table 25)
2. Lightly smear the tip with clear lubricating jelly to ease passage through nose
3. Pass tube through nostril; keep tip angled medially and along floor of nose to avoid trauma
4. Pass laryngoscope as for orotracheal intubation
5. Tube is passed until it can be seen behind soft palate
6. Further manipulation is the same as for endotracheal intubation except Magill's forceps may be needed to place tip of tube into glottis. Often this is unnecessary as gagging allows tube to be passed forward into the glottis

FIXATION OF NASOTRACHEAL TUBE FOR LONG-TERM VENTILATION (Fig. 15)

1. Paint tube protruding from nose with benzoin compound tincture
2. Paint infant's upper lip, cheek and central forehead with same to ensure proper adherence of tape
3. Wind thin pieces of tape around tube and attach free end to upper lip and cheek
4. Always confirm tube position radiographically if intubation has been performed for long-term ventilation

Tube end should be 1 cm above carina which is usually visible on radiograph.

Alternative methods of endotracheal tube fixation include:

1. Oral plate
2. Plastic support
3. Cotton tapes
4. Strong elastoplast

APPLICATION OF CPAP AND IPPV

Continuous positive airways pressure (CPAP) is used to treat RDS (p. 133), apnoeic attacks (p. 215) and heart failure in PDA (p. 240). The effects of CPAP are to increase functional residual capacity (FRC) and cause more regular breathing. Work of breathing is usually lessened (mask) but may be increased (nasal prongs). Compliance, minute volume and tidal volume are decreased, R-L shunting is reduced and P_aO_2 rises. Sometimes P_aCO_2 is increased, especially if pressures above 8–10 cmH_2O are used. In infants with RDS, CPAP increases central venous pressure and decreases pulse pressure. Peripheral blood flow may also be reduced by CPAP. CPAP may be applied by at least four different methods:

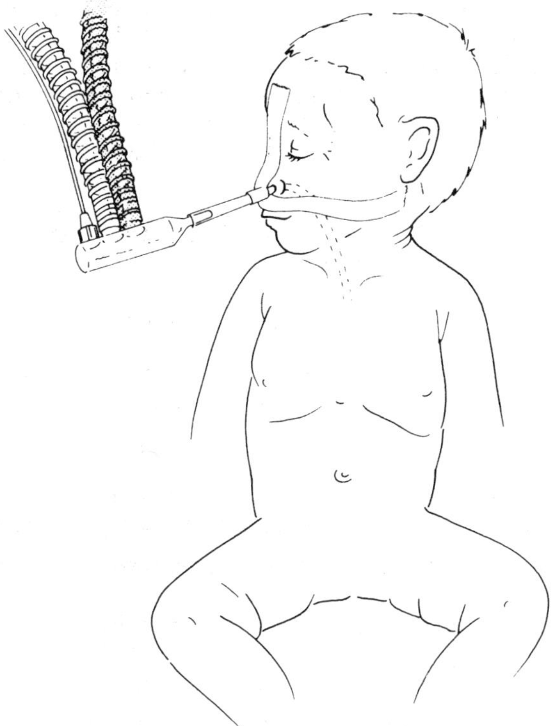

Fig. 15. Taping a nasotracheal tube in position to allow the baby's head to be turned from side to side and to minimize nasal trauma.

1. Endotracheal tube (Fig. 15)
2. Bennett face mask (Fig. 16)
3. Nasal prongs
4. Nasopharyngeal tube
5. Face chamber
6. Gregory box (now obsolete)

The advantages of mask/nasal prong CPAP are:

1. Easy to apply
2. Good for low and medium pressure CPAP

Its disadvantages are:

1. Difficult to achieve pressure > 8 cmH_2O
2. Mask may cause cerebellar haemorrhage if elastic strap is used: now avoided by using Netelast
3. Abdominal distension unless gastric tube is used
4. Difficult to suction mouth and airway
5. Unstable in large, active baby

The advantages of endotracheal CPAP are:

1. Stable system
2. Good pressure range easily attained
3. Can switch over to IPPV instantly

Its disadvantages are:

1. Complications of intubation
2. Risk of tube blocking or kinking
3. Infection
4. If nasotracheal tubes are used, nasal damage may occur

Complications of CPAP

1. Prongs – nasal trauma
2. Mask – facial swelling, corneal abrasion, airway obstruction, deformation of head
3. All types – inaccessibility, problems with feeding, increased incidence of pneumothorax, need for mechanical ventilation in 30–50% of babies, parental concern (especially if face is hidden)

CPAP should only be undertaken in nurseries where IPPV can be applied easily when failures occur.

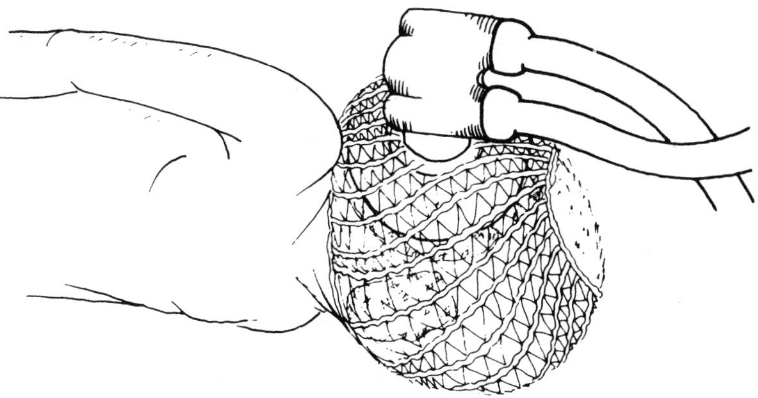

Fig. 16. Application of Bennett face mask for CPAP using elastic stockinette (Netelast). Always use free draining orogastric tube to decompress stomach. Cotton wool pads are used to protect ears and eyes.

Method

Select type of CPAP to be applied: mask or nasal prong for infants with apnoea or mild to moderate RDS, endotracheal tube CPAP for severe RDS.

The CPAP circuit is shown in Fig. 17. Ensure that the system will blow off at 10–15 cmH_2O, especially when endotracheal tube is used.

MECHANICAL VENTILATION

Mechanical ventilation is used to treat respiratory failure (p. 134) and intractable apnoeic attacks (p. 216).

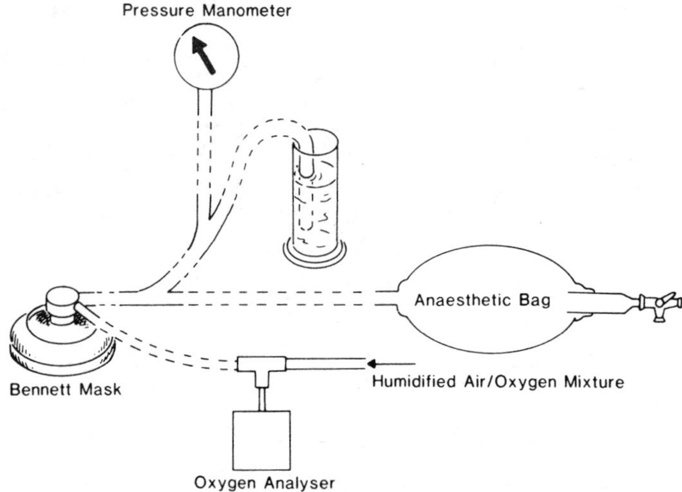

Fig. 17. Schematic circuit for continuous positive airways pressure (CPAP).

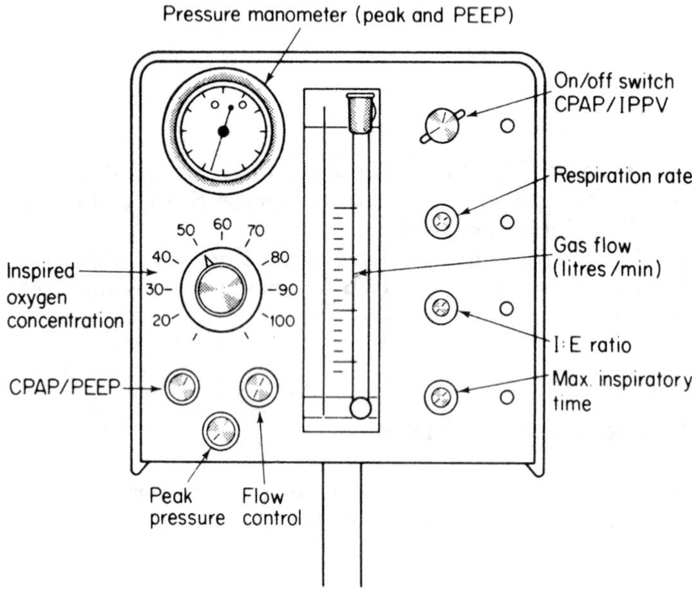

Fig. 18. Face of Bourns' BP 200 ventilator.

Ventilators

There are many types of ventilators, but three commonly used are:

1. Bourns' BP 200 (Fig. 18)
2. Draeger Baby Log (Fig. 19)
3. Sechrist (Fig. 20)

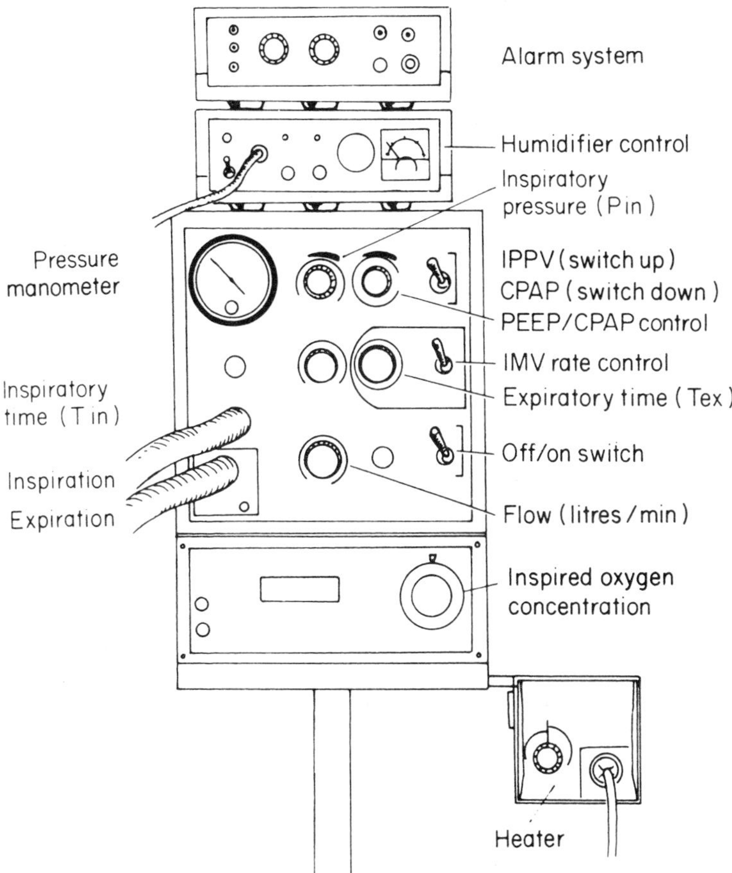

Fig. 19. Face of Draeger Baby Log ventilator.

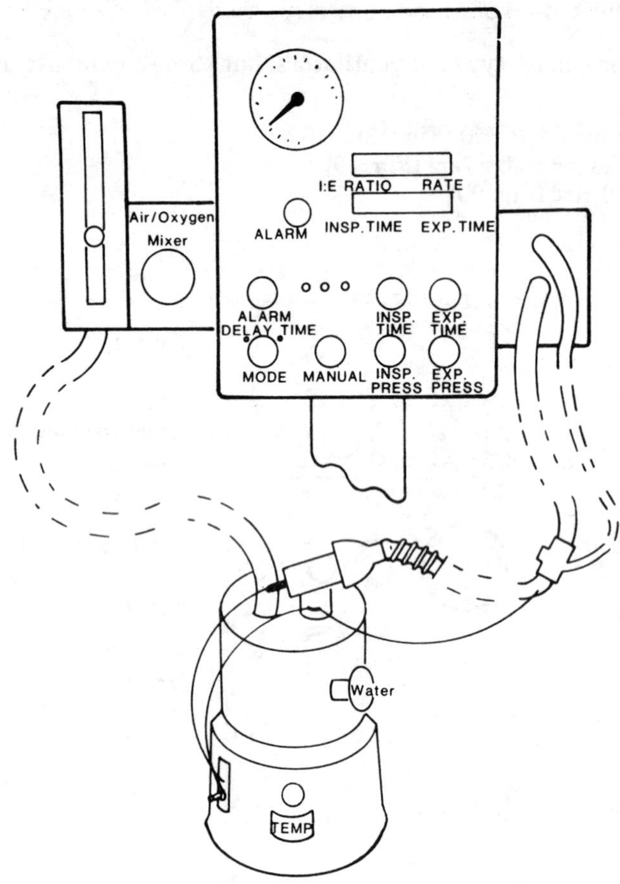

Fig. 20. Face of Sechrist ventilator showing system of humidification.

The Vickers ventilator or Sechrist may be used for transports. The Bourns', Draeger and Sechrist are pressure-limited ventilators with the following variables:

1. Inspired oxygen concentration: select 5% higher than before ventilation
2. Gas flow rate: start with about 7 litres/min
3. Peak airway pressure: see below for settings

4. Post end-expiratory pressure (PEEP): see below for settings
5. Ventilation rate: see below for settings. The rate is dialled directly on the Bourns' but calculated from graph of inspiratory and expiratory times on the side of the Draeger Baby Log. For example, with inspiratory time 0.5 sec and expiratory time 1 sec, frequency will be $60 \div (0.5 + 1) = 40$ breaths/min
6. Inspiratory to expiratory ration (I:E) can be set initially between 2:1 and 1:3. For the Bourns', dial in as Fig. 18 shows. For the Draeger Baby Log, for example, with inspiratory time of 0.5 sec and expiratory time 1 sec, I:E ratio becomes 1:2.

The circuit diagrams for these ventilators are given in Appendices II and III (pp. 345, 346). The Sechrist ventilator (Fig. 20) has certain advantages:

1. Compact and easily portable
2. Easy to obtain high rate
3. I:E ratios calculated and displayed

Mechanical ventilation may be needed to treat:

1. Normal lungs, e.g. hyperventilation in cerebral oedema, immaturity, apnoea and sepsis
2. Lung disease, e.g. respiratory distress syndrome and meconium aspiration syndrome

Immature babies' problems are different from bigger babies and are managed differently.

Ventilation of the baby < 1200 g with RDS

It is important to assess the severity of the lung disease as soon as possible. This may be done by determining the pressure needed to manually ventilate the lungs, the amount of oxygen needed to maintain normal oxygen saturation and the appearances of the chest radiograph.

1. If the lung disease is mild and IPPV is needed for apnoea or extreme immaturity, then the aim is to maintain adequate gas exchange without overdistending the lungs or adversely affecting the circulation:

Peak pressure, 10–15 cmH_2O or lower if chest moves
PEEP, 2–3 cmH_2O
Rate, 10–40 breaths/min depending upon baby's own respiratory effort and asynchrony of breathing
Inspiratory time, 0.4–0.6 sec

2. If lung disease is severe (non-compliant lungs), the aim is to expand the lungs early with the lowest pressures possible. Surfactant replacement is most beneficial in these babies (see Chapter 10). Small babies generally prefer high rates:
   Peak pressure, 15–25 cmH_2O lower or higher if needed
   PEEP, 3–5 cmH_2O
   Rate, 60–120 breaths/min depends upon synchrony of breathing unless muscle relaxants given
   Inspiratory time, 0.3–0.6 sec to keep I:E ratio about 1:1

Wean by first lowering peak pressure to keep P_aCO_2 levels in normal range (Table 23) and chest moving. Then lower rates, keeping inspiratory times constant at about 0.4–0.5 sec to prevent air trapping. Inspired oxygen concentrations should be adjusted to keep P_aO_2 levels and oxygen saturation in normal range (p. 68).

Ventilation of the Bigger Baby

Underlying disease is not always RDS and may be meconium aspiration syndrome (MAS) or post-asphyxia for example.

1. If the lung disease is mild, e.g. the baby needing hyperventilation after asphyxia, low pressures and moderate rates are often all that are required as for the baby < 1200 g
2. For severe lung disease (severe RDS or MAS) low rate ventilation with long inspiratory times may be used:
   Peak pressure, 20–30 cmH_2O as needed
   PEEP 3–6 cmH_2O
   Rate, 30–40 breaths/min
   Inspiratory time, 0.8–1.2 sec to keep I:E ratio 1.5:1 to 2:1

Muscle relaxants are often needed with these settings to prevent the baby 'fighting' the ventilator.

An alternative method for ventilating these babies uses faster rates. This may be particularly beneficial in the baby with pulmonary interstitial emphysema:

Peak pressure, 20–30 cmH_2O
PEEP, 3–4 cmH_2O
Rate, 60–80 breaths/min
Inspiratory time, 0.4–0.5 sec

If oxygenation is still unsatisfactory the rate may be increased by shortening the expiratory time to keep I:E ratio about 1:1. If still unsatisfactory, muscle relaxants and increased peak pressures may be needed.

Recent developments include very high frequency ventilation, which is of three types:

1. High frequency positive pressure ventilation (rates from 60–200 breaths/min) uses conventional ventilators, e.g. Sechrist
2. High frequency jet ventilation (120–600 breaths/min)
3. High frequency oscillation (400–2400 breaths/min)

These techniques have recently been subjected to controlled trials which show that for most babies they are not superior to conventional mechanical ventilation so that their use should be strictly limited to research centres.

The effectiveness of mechanical ventilation is judged by:

1. Observing chest wall movements
2. Auscultation of breath sounds over both lungs
3. Arterial blood gas analysis checked 20 min after ventilation starts

Aims are to keep P_aCO_2 in the range of 5–6 kPa (40–50 mmHg) so the pH remains above 7.25 and P_aO_2 should be in the range 7–10 kPa (60–80 mmHg). If P_aCO_2 is not falling and pH remains < 7.25, ventilation needs to be increased. Peak pressure can be raised. If hypoxaemia is not corrected then one of three things may be done:

1. Increase oxygen concentration
2. Increase PEEP
3. Increase I:E ratio

Care of Endotracheal Tube

Endotracheal tubes should be suctioned as indicated by the baby's condition. Infants with pneumonia may need suctioning each hour, but those with respiratory distress syndrome may not need suctioning more frequently than 4 hourly. Suctioning is a skilled procedure usually carried out by the nursing staff; an experienced nurse and an assistant are needed. Aseptic technique should be used and suctioning should not last longer than 10 sec at each attempt. It is helpful to bag ventilate the baby before suctioning and to use 0.5 ml sterile saline to lubricate the endotracheal tube. The nurse should observe baby closely as endotracheal tube is sucked out (Table 26). If cyanosis, or transcutaneous $P\text{O}_2$ (Tc$P\text{O}_2$) < 5.5 kPa (40 mmHg), or pulse oximeter shows oxygen saturation $< 75\%$, or heart rate < 100 beats/min then the procedure must be stopped at once and the baby bag ventilated. Chest physiotherapy can also cause deterioration and the above methods of monitoring should apply.

SHOULD INFANT DETERIORATE ON VENTILATOR SEE INSTRUCTIONS ON p. 138

WEANING from the ventilator is made easier by use of intermittent mandatory ventilation (IMV). This allows the ventilation rate to be reduced and the infant to breathe as he/she wishes between each ventilation. Weaning can usually be attempted when $P_a\text{CO}_2$ is less than 6.5 kPa (50 mmHg), pH greater than 7.3 and $P_a\text{O}_2$ greater than 7 kPa (60 mmHg) in less than 50% oxygen with peak pressures less than 20 cmH_2O.

Table 26. Suctioning of endotracheal tube.

1. Measure length of suction catheter against length of endotracheal tube
2. Pre-oxygenate baby for 10 sec
3. Disconnect and pass catheter until resistance is just felt, then withdraw 2 mm before occluding side hole of suction catheter
4. Gently suction airways for no more than 10 sec
5. If using saline, be sure to bag-up between attempts at suctioning
6. If cyanosis, Tc$P\text{O}_2$ $<$ 5.5 kPa (40 mmHg), or O_2 sat. $<75\%$ or heart rate <100 then stop and bag up

When starting to wean make small changes reducing peak pressure first by 1–2 cm H_2O. Reduce inspired oxygen concentration by 3–5% at a time and ventilator rate by about 5 breaths/min. When lowering ventilation rate remember to adjust I:E ratio so that inspiratory time remains at about 0.4–0.5 sec. Always check blood gases within 30–60 min of each ventilator change to ensure that P_aCO_2 is not rising.

Endotracheal CPAP can usually be employed when less than 40% oxygen is required and peak airway pressure is under 20 cm H_2O.

Extubation is usually attempted only after a successful period of some hours on endotracheal CPAP. An exception to this rule is the very immature infant who has been ventilated through a 2.5 mm tube, since he/she may find breathing difficult due to the high resistance in this narrow tube. Infants with 2.5 mm endotracheal tubes are extubated when they can tolerate IMV of 10 breaths/min.

Difficulty in weaning may be due to a number of problems:

1. Pneumonia: culture secretions, change antibiotics if appropriate, chest physiotherapy (see below), regular, efficient suctioning
2. Post-extubation collapse and retained secretions: gentle chest physiotherapy and perhaps CPAP
3. PDA: fluid restriction and diuretics. Echocardiography and consider indomethacin or ligation (p. 240)
4. Apnoea: may be due to hypocapnia or hypoxaemia. Keep haematocrit over 45%, consider aminophylline or prolonged CPAP (p. 215)
5. Early BPD: difficult to diagnose, fluid restriction and diuretics. Perhaps physiotherapy and CPAP. Consider dexamethasone if no evidence of infection (p. 150)
6. Subglottic oedema or stenosis: laryngoscopy or bronchoscopy, dexamethasone before extubation or racemic epinephrine afterwards, very occasionally needs tracheostomy (p. 153)
7. Malnutrition/debilitation: increase calorie intake, intravenous feeding including fats. Increase oral intake by using transpyloric tube (see Chapter 10)

If weaning has failed, wait 7–10 days, improve the baby's general condition and try again.

Extubation

If laryngeal oedema is likely after prolonged intubation or previous failure, try intravenous dexamethasone 2 mg about half to 1 hour before extubation.

The upper airway should first be well suctioned and then with a clean catheter the tube should be suctioned as it is withdrawn. The end of the endotracheal tube is cut off into sterile container and sent for culture. Some extubated infants are placed on mask or nasal prong CPAP to lessen the likelihood of atelectasis. Half an hour after extubation arterial blood gases should be sampled and at 4 hours do chest radiography routinely to look for collapse. Physiotherapy and gentle suctioning of upper airways are helpful after extubation. Infants are not fed for at least 8 hours after extubation and then only small amounts by orogastric tube, unless a transpyloric tube is in position, when feeding can resume after 1–2 hours.

Risks of Mechanical Ventilation

Acute risks include:

1. Tube problems:
   - Trauma to nose, palate, larynx and trachea
   - Infection
   - Displacement
   - Blockage
   - Kinking
2. Circuit tubing problems:
   - Gas leaks
   - Water obstruction or inhalation
   - Kinking
3. Humidifier:
   - Overheating
   - Gas leaks
   - Infections, e.g. *Pseudomonas*
4. Gas supply:
   - Failure
   - Wrong air/oxygen mix

5. Ventilator:
   Failure
   Raised pressure: pneumothorax, interstitial emphysema

Chronic risks include:

1. Airway
   Trauma with deformities of nose
   Subglottic stenosis
   Tracheal ulceration
   Palatal groove
   Abnormal dentition
2. Lungs:
   Bronchopulmonary dysplasia
   Post-extubation collapse
   Bronchial granuloma causing emphysema

CHEST PHYSIOTHERAPY

This can be a 'two-edged sword'; very helpful if performed efficiently and gently in the correct baby at the appropriate time but potentially harmful if not. Table 27 gives guidelines for use of physiotherapy in a NICU.

Table 27. Chest physiotherapy in the NICU.

1. Should be ordered by a consultant or registrar
2. Each order expires after 3 days and must be renewed if necessary
3. Babies likely to benefit include:
   (a) post-extubation atelectasis
   (b) meconium aspiration syndrome
   (c) pneumonia, if localized or lobar
   (d) exudative phase of bronchopulmonary dysplasia
4. Unlikely to benefit and may harm babies who have been intubated for:
   (a) apnoea
   (b) respiratory distress syndrome
   (c) pneumothorax
   (d) pulmonary hypertension

These babies need very gentle routine endotracheal tube care (see p. 88)

TRANSILLUMINATION OF THE CHEST

This technique is used to make an immediate diagnosis of pneumothorax in big babies. If an infant receiving mechanical ventilation suddenly deteriorates the chest may be transilluminated using a cold-light source (fibreoptic Minilight) in a semi-darkened room (Fig. 21). There will be hyperlucency on the affected side. This may not differentiate large from small pneumothorax so chest radiograph may be needed for confirmation. Very preterm infants may appear to transilluminate with no pneumothorax.

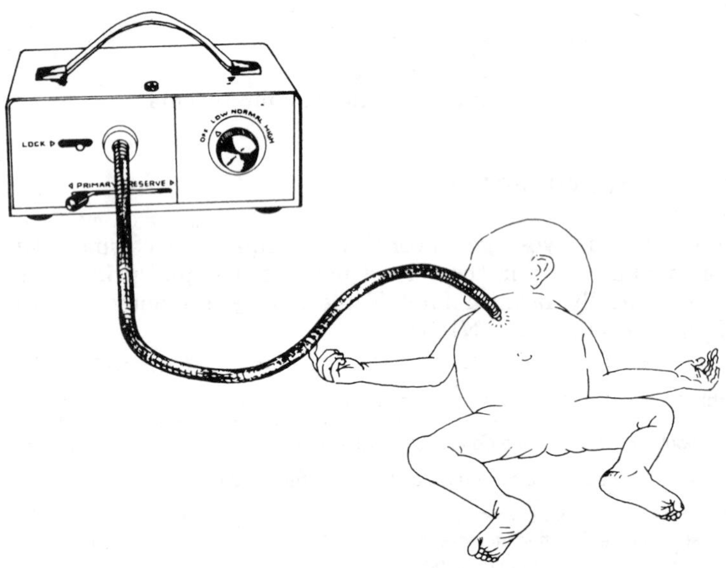

Fig. 21. Transillumination of the chest with fibreoptic light (Minilight) to diagnose pneumothorax.

DRAINAGE OF A PNEUMOTHORAX

Immediate aspiration of a tension pneumothorax in a deteriorating infant (cyanosis, tachypnoea, circulatory failure, hypotension) is advisable even before radiographic confirmation. This may be performed with a 21 gauge scalp vein needle connected to a three-way stop-cock and 20 ml syringe (Fig. 22).

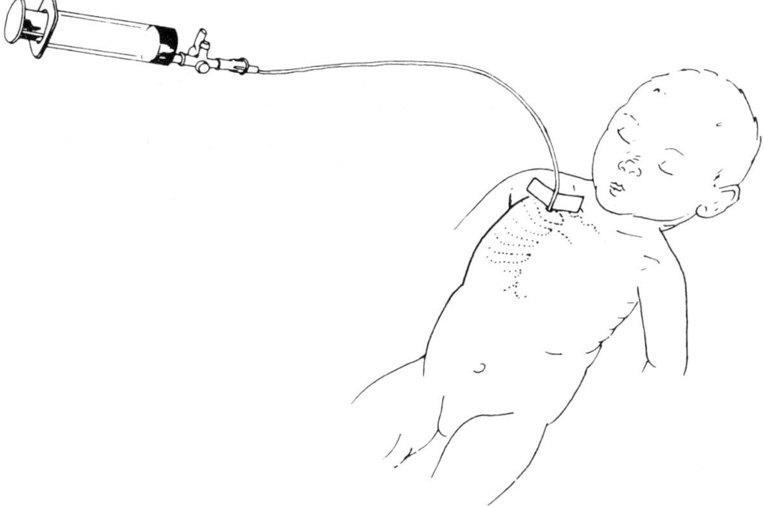

Fig. 22. Emergency drainage of pneumothorax using a scalp vein needle, three-way tap and 20 ml syringe. The needle is inserted through the second intercostal space anteriorly in the mid-clavicular line.

After cleaning the skin with alcohol and povidone–iodine the needle may be inserted through the second intercostal space in the mid-clavicular line on the affected side. Air should be easily aspirated into the syringe, which can be emptied by turning off the three-way tap.

This procedure should be followed in almost all cases by insertion of a more permanent pleural drain (see below). This is a specialized skill, especially in the preterm infant, so observe the procedure a few times before attempting it. If experienced help is not immediately available it is safer to continue drainage by aspiration through the scalp vein needle.

Permanent Drainage (Figs. 23, 24)

There are two sites for insertion of the catheter:

1. Full-term: second intercostal space anteriorly, mid-clavicular line

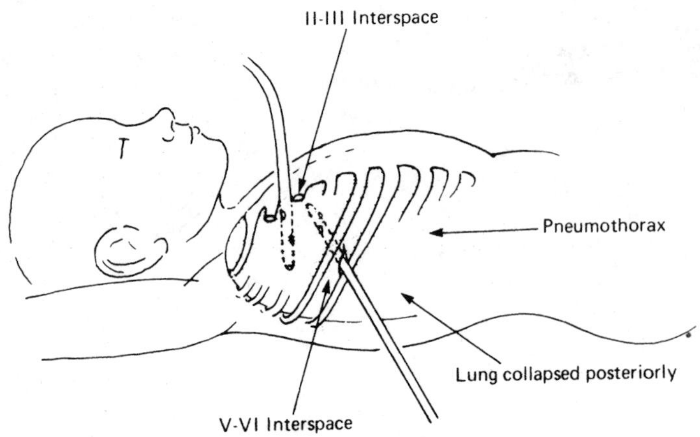

Fig. 23. Sites for insertion of pleural drains in neonatal pneumothorax. Only one drain is usually necessary (see text).

2. Preterm: fourth to sixth intercostal space, anterior axillary line because anteroposterior (AP) diameter of chest is insufficient in preterm infants to allow adequate drainage

The technique is as follows:

1. Prepare skin with full aseptic technique and infiltrate skin with 1% lignocaine as a local anaesthetic
2. Use 10–12F pleural catheter with trocar (small babies may need 8F)
3. Make small incision in skin with a fine scalpel and gently separate intercostal muscle fibres with curved artery forceps
4. Clamp tube and trocar with artery forceps 1 cm from tip, i.e. at side hole. This prevents over-penetration of chest
5. When approaching laterally rather than anteriorly the baby should be positioned on his side and the trocar aimed towards the angle of Louis
6. Push and twist tube and trocar gently through incision into pleural space as far as clamp allows (1 cm)
7. Remove trocar and connect tube to underwater seal
8. Manipulate tube gently so that tip lies anteriorly in thoracic cavity (Fig. 23)
9. Secure tube with purse-string suture and apply

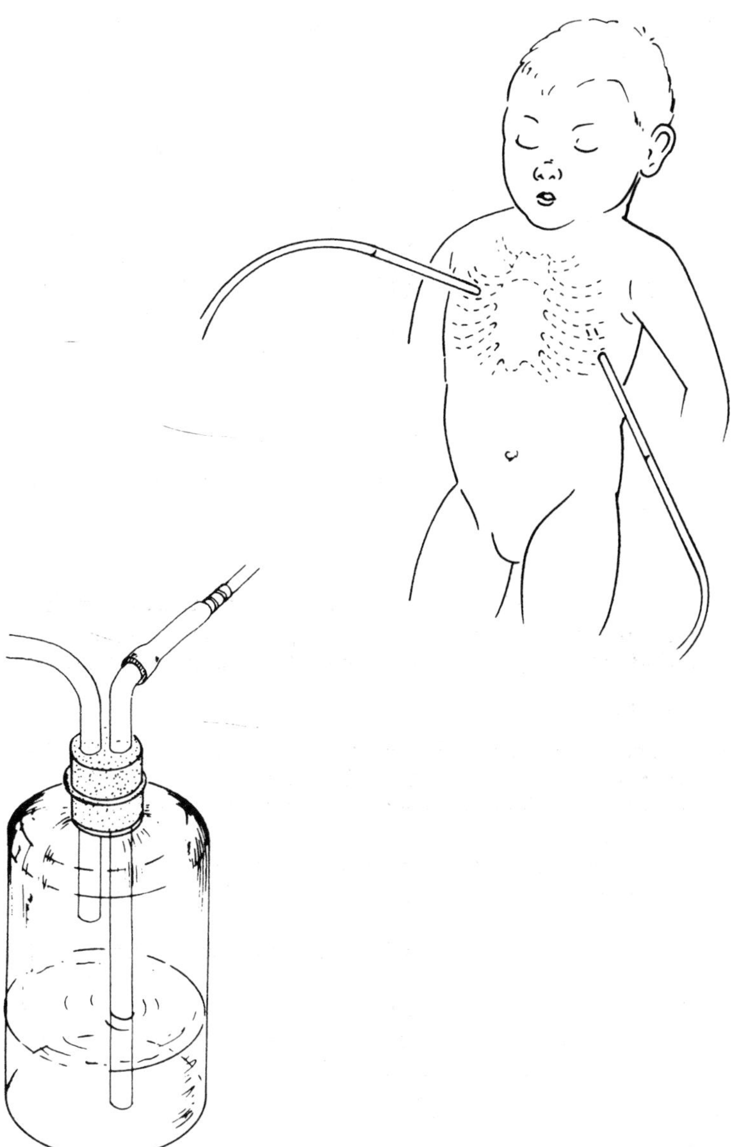

Fig. 24. Sites for insertion of pleural drains and connection to underwater seal. Make sure pleural drain is connected to long limb of underwater seal bottle which is placed below the infant.

povidone–iodine cream to puncture site covered by gauze dressing

10. Tape tube securely to the chest wall using split zinc oxide tape
11. Chest radiography (AP and lateral films) to check tube position and resolution of pneumothorax

The pleural drain is connected to an underwater seal bottle as shown in Fig. 24. Suction on the open limb of this bottle at -10 to -20 cmH_2O is helpful, and should be done in spontaneously breathing infants.

Removal of chest drain when respiratory distress has resolved. When no bubbling off for 24 hours, clamp the tube and remove a further 12–24 hours later if no deterioration. The purse-string suture should be tightened and adhesive plaster dressing with collodion used. Chest radiography 2–4 hours after drain removal.

ARTERIAL CATHETERIZATION

Arterial catheters (umbilical, radial or posterior tibial) are inserted so that blood gases may be monitored in babies who require more than 40% oxygen and in the initial management of most infants less than 1000 g birth weight. Continuous measurement of arterial oxygen tension may be made using indwelling oxygen electrodes, e.g. Searle.

Use smaller (3.5F or 4F) catheters for infants less than 1200 g and larger (5F) for other infants.

Insertion of an arterial catheter must be performed under full aseptic conditions (mask, gown and gloves).

The anterior abdominal wall and cord stump should be gently cleansed with a dilute antiseptic solution (e.g. Savlon, povidone–iodine); avoid alcoholic solutions, especially under radiant warmers, as these can cause skin burns.

Before cutting the umbilical cord tie a piece of ribbon gauze around the base to control venous bleeding from the cut end (Fig. 25). The cord should be cut at least 1 cm above the abdominal wall. The arteries may be identified as small thick-walled and spiralling vessels in comparison to the larger thin-walled veins.

Hold umbilical stump between finger and thumb or if too short then use toothed forceps.

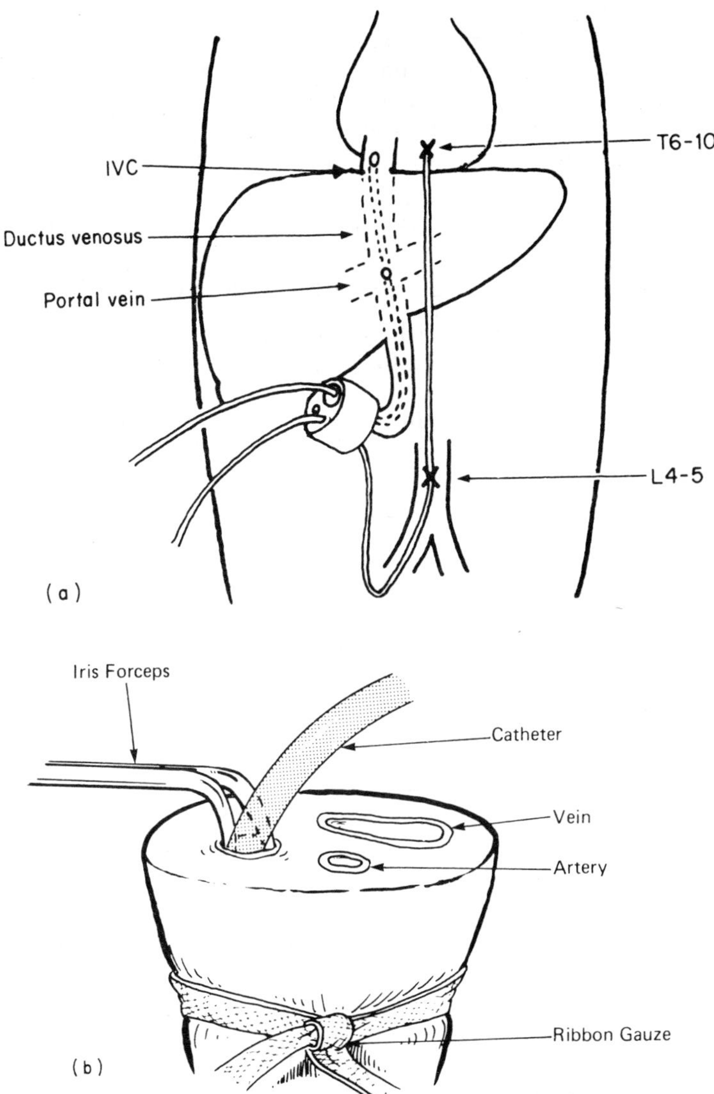

Fig. 25. (a) Sites for umbilical catheter placement. X, arterial; O, venous. (b) Umbilical stump showing catheterization of the artery after dilatation with iris forceps. Note the ribbon gauze tied around the base of the stump to prevent bleeding from the umbilical vein.

The mouth of one of the arteries should be dilated using straight or curved iris forceps.

The saline-filled catheter may then be gently inserted into the artery and passed into the aorta (Fig. 25). Do not push hard as tip of cannula may penetrate arterial wall.

There are two commonly used positions for catheter placement:

1. Lower aorta, below the renal arteries (radiograph at L4–L5).
2. Upper aorta, above the diaphragm (radiographs of T6–T10)

In general, use the high catheter position for infants less than 1500 g and the low position for bigger babies.

Table 28 is used to calculate the length of catheter that should be inserted to obtain correct placement in the aorta.

Table 28. Umbilical artery catheter positions.

Shoulder–umbilicus length (cm)	*Umbilicus–lower aorta length* (cm)	*Umbilicus–upper aorta length* (cm)
8	4	10
10	5–6	12
12	6–7	15
14	8	18
16	10	20
18	10–11	22

After Dunn (1966)

Immediately after insertion, the legs and buttocks should be checked for pallor or blueness and the femoral pulses palpated. The catheter may then be stitched to the cord stump and taped in 'goal-post' fashion as shown in Fig. 26.

Radiograph should be taken to confirm catheter position; ultrasound may also be used. If a catheter is in too far (above T5) then it should be withdrawn to below T6. If below T10 then it must either be withdrawn to the lower aorta (L4–L5) or totally replaced under aseptic conditions. Catheters that have been placed below L5 or those passing down the iliac artery should be replaced. Under no circumstances should a non-sterile catheter be advanced into the umbilical artery. After

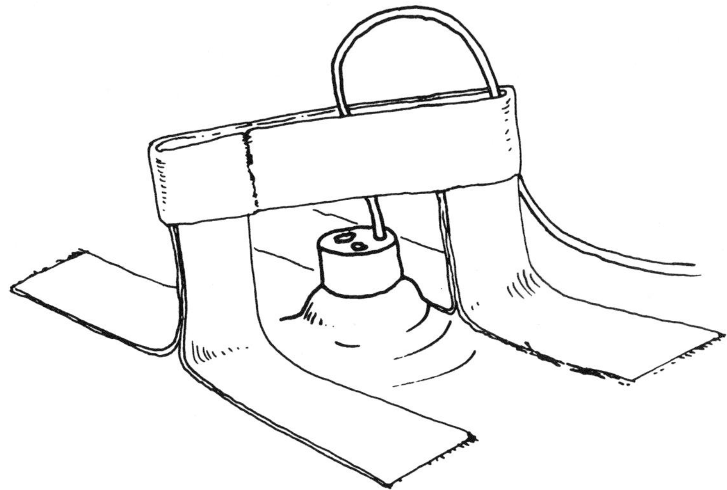

Fig. 26. Taping of umbilical vessel catheters ('goal posts').

insertion, the catheter and three-way tap are connected to an infusion pump delivering 0.9% saline (watch sodium intake in babies less than 28 weeks for first 3 days) at 1 ml/hour to keep catheter open. Use peripheral vein to infuse dextrose solutions, electrolytes and antibiotics. Figure 25 illustrates these two sites for catheter placement in the aorta (marked X).

To take a sample of blood for blood gas analysis three syringes are required to reduce contamination of the catheter. Technique is as follows:

1. First a 2 ml syringe is used to aspirate the infusing solution and a further 1.5 ml of blood from the aorta
2. The tap should then be closed and the first syringe removed but not discarded
3. Remove 0.4 ml of arterial blood for analysis into 1 ml syringe, heparinized by wetting its inside with heparin of 1000 units/ml strength
4. If the sample is not to be analysed within 10 min, it should be put on ice
5. The first syringe is then reattached and the 1.5 ml blood plus 0.5 ml of infusate replaced
6. The third syringe of 5 ml capacity contains heparinized saline (1 unit/ml) and is used to flush the catheter using a

tapping motion on the plunger. No blood should remain within the catheter at the finish of this procedure

7. After sampling ensure that all fittings are tight and that the three-way tap is turned to allow flow of infusate into baby

Removal of Arterial Catheter

Arterial catheters are removed when infants require less than 40% oxygen. The catheter should be removed in one movement and firm pressure applied over the umbilicus and lower abdomen to control bleeding. The tip of the catheter is cut off into a sterile bottle and sent for culture. Up to 5 min of pressure on the lower abdomen is usually required to control bleeding. Thereafter a nurse should observe the cord stump for a further 5 min to check for further blood loss. Do not cover stump after removal of catheter.

Complications of Arterial Cannulation

1. Leg and gluteal blanching and cyanosis; if prolonged may lead to necrosis
2. Major artery thrombosis: aorta, renal, mesenteric
3. Emboli: clot or air
4. Infection
5. Haemorrhage

If leg or foot becomes pale and ischaemic, arterial catheter must be removed at once. If the toes become blue but not pale, arm the other foot with saline soaks to cause reflex vasodilation. If no improvement or progression to pale foot, catheter must be removed. After a while the other umbilical artery may be catheterized.

VENOUS CATHETERIZATION

Venous Sampling

Use any prominent superficial vein, e.g. antecubital, temporal or back of hand. If silastic catheter (long line) for parenteral

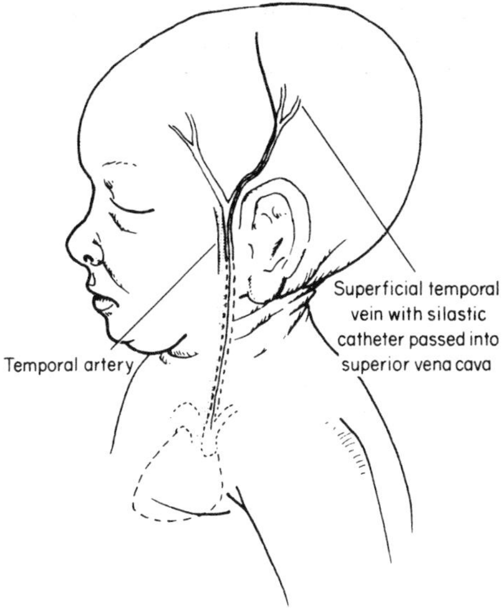

Fig. 27. Superficial temporal artery and vein. The artery lies anterior to the vein and may be used for intermittent arterial blood gas sampling. A silastic catheter is inserted into the vein and advanced to the superior vena cava.

nutrition is likely to be required, do not use the temporal vein (see Fig. 27).

Venous Infusions

Use veins in the following order of preference: scalp, forearm or antecubital fossa, back of the hand or wrist, leg veins or after cut-down. Careful observation and immobilization should avoid subcutaneous infiltration which may cause necrosis. Dextrose of 10% or stronger, Vamin, calcium salts and some antibiotics are quite irritating and great care should be taken. Intravenous feeding should use peripheral veins (see Fig. 27 and p. 162). The dextrose, amino acid, electrolyte and vitamin solution should be prescribed daily and made up under aseptic conditions. These are connected under aseptic conditions to the intravenous catheter via a Millipore filter (0.22 μm). The Intralipid is connected via a Y-connector beyond the filter and as close to the vein as possible (Fig. 28).

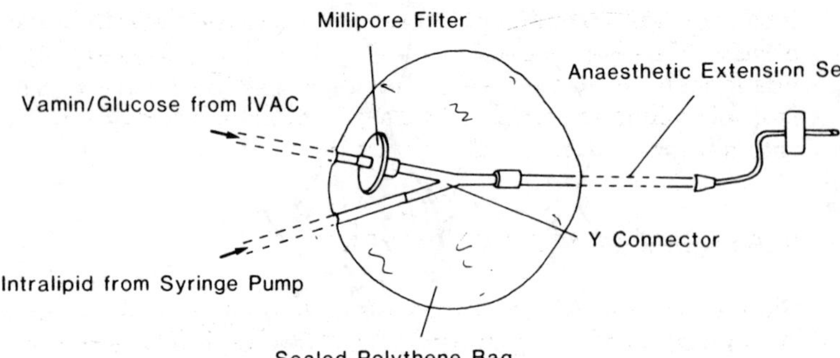

Fig. 28. Circuit for intravenous feeding showing how the amino acid and fat solutions are mixed close to the patient.

Venous catheters may be either central or peripheral.

Umbilical venous catheterization is rarely justified but may be needed in the following circumstances:

1. For resuscitation in the labour ward
2. For exchange transfusion
3. For blood gas sampling under conditions where arterial catheterization has failed

Use full aseptic technique as for arterial cannulation.

A 5F catheter is used and should be placed via the ductus venosus into the inferior vena cava if this is possible. In practice only about 60% of venous catheters will pass through the ductus venosus; others remain in the liver or in the portal circulation. The catheter tip should be placed at either of the two sites shown in Fig. 25, that is either in the inferior vena cava or in the portal sinus (marked o).

Complications of Umbilical Venous Catheters

1. Infection
2. Thrombosis of portal vein
3. Pulmonary emboli
4. Air embolus

In order to provide 'arterial' blood for analysis, an umbilical venous catheter may be advanced from the inferior vena cava into the right atrium and across the foramen ovale to the left atrium. This is potentially dangerous and should probably be abandoned as a method of monitoring blood gases. Only isotonic saline should be infused through such a catheter at a rate not greater than 1–2 ml/hour.

PERIPHERAL SILASTIC CATHETERS

Silastic catheters for intravenous feeding are sometimes used. A 19 gauge needle is inserted in the superficial temporal vein. A fine silastic catheter (0.635 mm (0.025 inch) outside diameter) is passed through this needle and advanced via jugular vein to superior vena cava under strict aseptic conditions (Fig. 27). The needle is then slipped back along the catheter and removed. A blunt size 21 gauge needle is then attached to the free end of the catheter and tied on with fine silk. These catheters now come pre-packed.

All catheter positions should be confirmed by radiography. Silastic catheters need to be filled with radio-opaque dye for this.

INTERMITTENT ARTERIAL SAMPLING

Radial or temporal artery is preferred site for intermittent sampling, though latter should not be used for permanent catheterization as cerebral infarction has occurred.

The brachial artery is an end-artery and as such percutaneous puncture is more hazardous. The median nerve runs close to this artery in the antecubital fossa and median nerve palsies have been reported in the newborn after sampling in this area. Avoid femoral artery puncture as this can damage underlying hip joint.

Palpate *radial artery* at wrist. In the preterm infant, the vessel may be visible as a blue streak and can be outlined by transillumination. Also confirm presence of ulnar artery by palpation. Technique is then as follows:

1. Use 23 or 25 gauge needle attached to 1 ml syringe which has been lightly coated with heparin (1000 units/ml)
2. Insert needle at angle of 45° to skin surface just proximal to first wrist skin crease (Fig. 29)

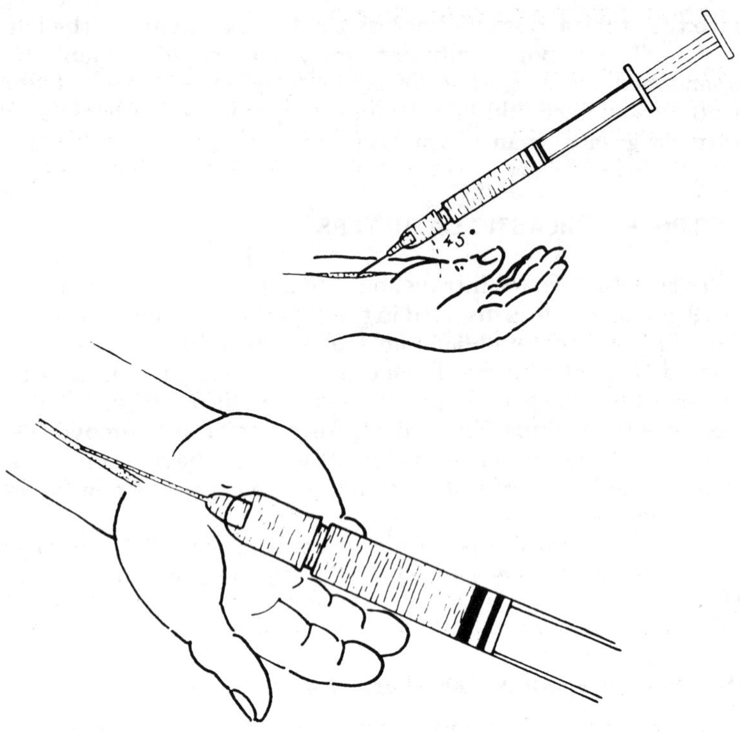

Fig. 29. Site for intermittent radial artery sampling for blood gases.

3. Aspirate 0.4 ml blood
4. Remove needle and cap sample
5. Occlude with firm pressure for 5 min to prevent haematoma formation

Use local anaesthetic to infiltrate skin around site of puncture, especially if baby is likely to be distressed, e.g. older babies with chronic lung disease.

Temporal artery sampling is similar and the vessel may be found running anteriorly to the external ear (Fig. 27).

RADIAL ARTERY CATHETERIZATION

The radial artery may be catheterized using a 22 gauge intravenous cannula connected to a T-connector. This has the advantages of accessibility for longer after birth and measurement of pre-ductus oxygen tensions if right radial artery is used.

Technique (Fig. 30)

1. Use right radial artery if possible
2. Hold infant's hand supine
3. Palpate radial and ulnar arteries and observe effect of occlusion of former. Fibreoptic light may help to outline vessels (p. 92).
4. Use 22 or 23 gauge intravenous cannula and puncture artery as for intermittent sampling (see above)
5. When blood appears in flash point, advance cannula while holding the guiding needle stable
6. Remove needle and attach T-connector as shown in Fig. 30
7. Keep cannula patent by infusion of heparinized saline at 1–2 ml/hour
8. Sample as for umbilical artery catheter (p. 99)

The dorsalis pedis artery (running between first and second metatarsals) and the posterior tibial artery (behind the medial malleolus) may also be used for intermittent sampling or catheterization.

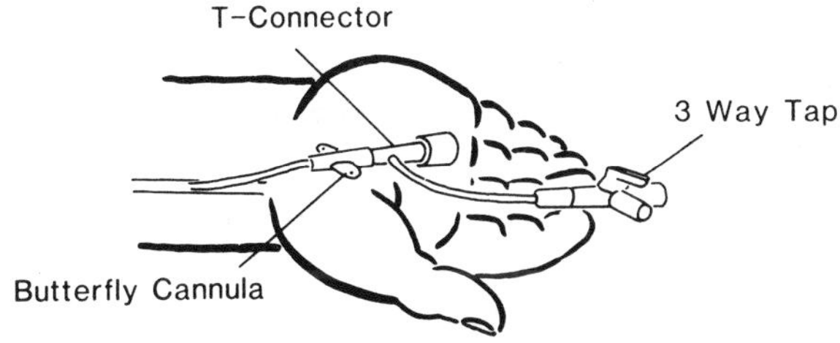

Fig. 30. Catheterization of the radial artery.

THE HEEL STAB

Capillary blood drawn from a heel stab (or prick) may be used for blood gases, electrolytes, calcium, glucose, packed cell volume and even blood culture.

If heel is warmed to 40°C for 3 min and *free-flowing blood* is obtained, measurements of pH, $P\text{CO}_2$ and $P\text{O}_2$ up to 7 kPa (60 mmHg) correlate with arterial samples (Table 23).

The medial part of the heel should be used for the stab (Fig. 31) and a thin layer of petroleum jelly smeared there before puncture makes it easier to collect the blood. Use a disposable sterile lancet and insert to a maximum depth of 2 mm. Osteomyelitis of os calcis has been reported after deep incision. Other complications are tissue atrophy and inclusion dermoids which can lead to painful feet. Do not squeeze blood out as this leads to erroneous results from haemolysis.

Arterialized capillary blood for blood gas analysis should be

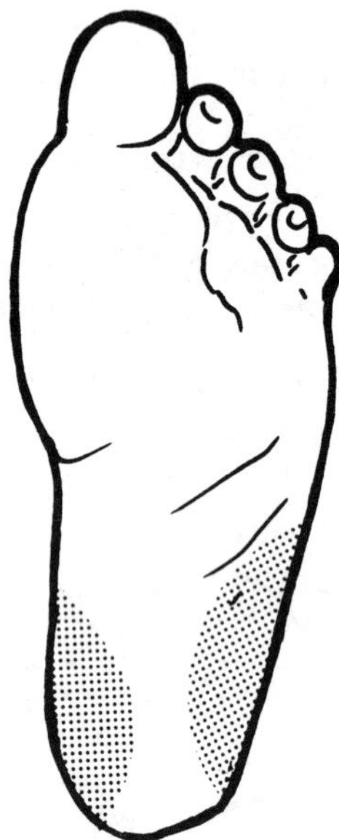

Fig. 31. Site for heel stab (shaded area). The lancet should be used to pierce the medial aspect of the heel to a depth of 1–2 mm to obtain capillary blood.

collected into heparinized capillary tubes and analysed immediately. Blood for electrolytes, calcium and bilirubin may be collected into plastic microtubes which are capped before sending to the laboratory.

CARDIAC MESSAGE

Both thumbs are placed over the middle to lower thirds of the sternum as shown in Fig. 32. The sternum should then be depressed 1.5–2.5 cm about 100 times/min.

After every third depression the lungs should be ventilated. Efficient external cardiac massage can only provide 50% of normal cardiac output.

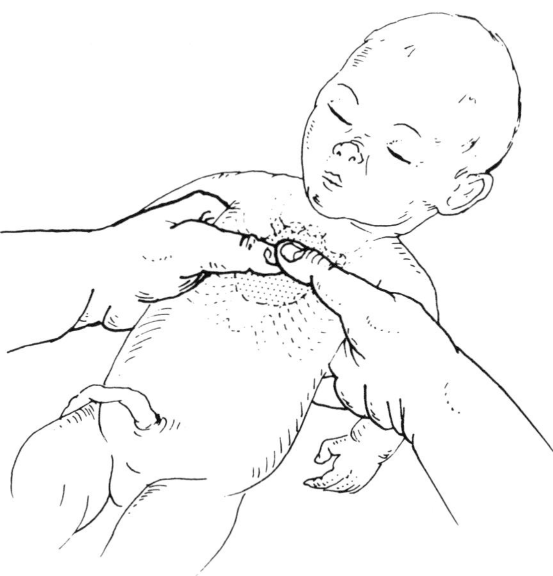

Fig. 32. Neonatal cardiac massage. Thumbs should be placed over the middle third of the sternum.

EXCHANGE TRANSFUSION

Indications are:

1. Blood group incompatibility, especially rhesus
2. Hyperbilirubinaemia from other causes
3. Sepsis, sclerema or DIC (see p. 286)
4. Drug intoxication due to diazepam, magnesium sulphate, mepivicaine

Blood should be ABO compatible, CMV, HIV, HBV and rhesus negative. Should be less than 48 hours old because of risk of hyperkalaemia. Citrate phosphate dextrose (CPD) blood is better than acid citrate dextrose (ACD) blood because it has a higher pH and more 2,3-diphosphoglycerate.

Use semi-packed cells (remove 100 ml plasma from pack) except for exchange for hyperbilirubinaemia when whole blood is used. Buffer donor blood with 10 ml of 5 or 8.4% sodium bicarbonate per 500 ml if pH is < 7.1. Volume of exchange 180 ml/kg. Use equal amounts in and out unless central venous pressure is initially high when a deficit of 10–20 ml should be allowed.

Two techniques can be used. The *isovolumetric* method causes less circulatory disturbance as both umbilical artery and vein are catheterized. The *single venous catheter* technique is easier to use but circulatory disturbance is more common. Full aseptic technique in both techniques. Vessel(s) catheterized and position checked by radiography (see p. 97).

The *isovolumetric* technique is:

1. Cannulate both umbilical artery and umbilical vein
2. Connect three-way tap and 10 ml syringe to arterial catheter. This is used for withdrawing blood
3. Donor blood passes to heating coil in a water bath and then to three-way tap attached to umbilical venous catheter
4. Connect another three-way tap to venous catheter for giving blood. Attach blood pack via giving set through warmer to the three-way tap and 10 ml syringe (Fig. 33)
5. Blood may then be simultaneously withdrawn and given by two operators. Use 10–20 ml cycles taking 2–3 min/cycle

In the *single vessel* technique (Fig. 34) umbilical vein is used for withdrawal and giving blood. A 10 ml syringe with two three-way taps is attached to the catheter. Remove blood from

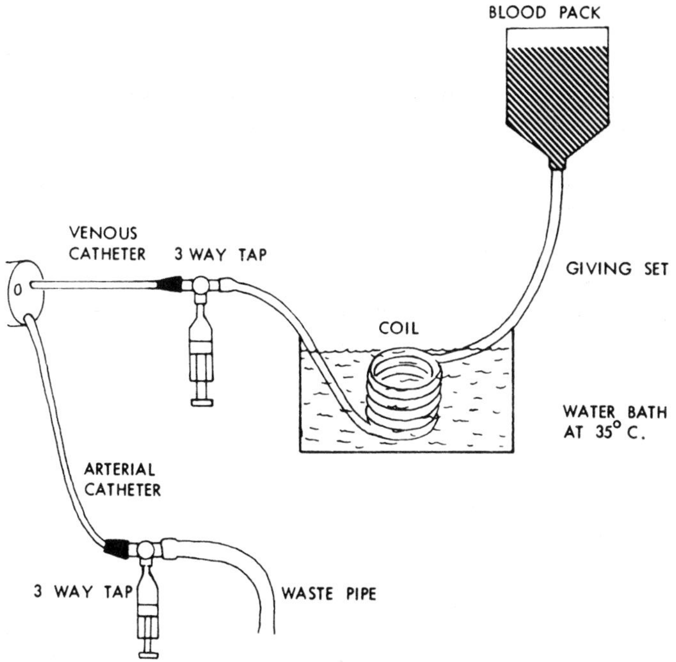

Fig. 33. Circuit for isovolumetric exchange transfusion.

baby to syringe and discard this blood to waste pipe attached to a closed Uribag system. Fill syringe with donor blood and transfer this blood to infant. Repeat, taking 1 min/cycle for 5 ml in preterm and 2 min/cycle for 10 ml term infant.

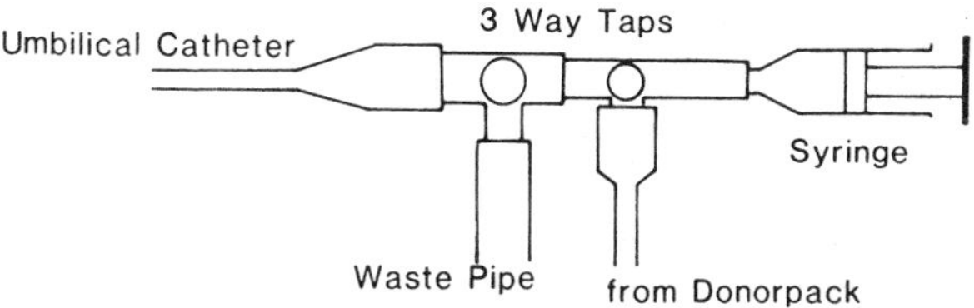

Fig. 34. Set-up for single vessel (venous) exchange transfusion.

Observe:

1. Continuous cardiorespiratory monitoring with ECG trace in all infants
2. Clinical signs of deterioration are cyanosis, pallor, tachypnoea, apnoea, abdominal distension, vomiting and bloody diarrhoea. If these occur the procedure should be stopped and the cause determined.

Complications of exchange transfusion are:

1. Metabolic acidosis
2. Hypothermia
3. Circulatory overload
4. Electrolyte disturbances: hyperkalaemia, hypernatraemia and hypocalcaemia
5. Acute dilatation of the stomach
6. Ischaemia of the intestine, perforation or necrotizing enterocolitis
7. Air embolism
8. Cardiac arrhythmias
9. Infection
10. Hypoglycaemia
11. Thrombocytopenia

At the end of an exchange transfusion blood should be sent to the laboratory for analysis of haemoglobin, total and direct bilirubin, electrolytes, calcium, glucose, blood culture and for cross-matching in the event of another exchange. Venous catheters should always be removed after exchange transfusion and arterial catheters often need replacement as they may become blocked.

Cut-off catheter tips are sent for culture. No routine antibiotic cover for exchange transfusion.

PLASMA EXCHANGE FOR POLYCYTHAEMIA

Indications are polycythaemia with venous packed cell volume $> 70\%$ or $> 65\%$ if symptoms present (see pp. 57, 282). Use peripheral vein for giving blood and radial artery for removal if possible; if not then use umbilical vein. Same techniques as for exchange transfusion; volume needed usually 20 ml/kg (p. 284).

Use plasma or 5% salt-poor albumin as donor solution. Remove catheter at end of exchange.

HEART AND RESPIRATION MONITORING

The *Corometrics* monitor (Fig. 35) picks up ECG trace from two chest leads and a lead on the right leg. The ECG is displayed on a very small oscilloscope and heart rate is shown both digitally and as a continuous trace. Newer models store these traces in memory in a small microprocessor. Both long- and short-term heart rate variability are calculated every 512 beats. Respiration rate is also shown as a continuous paper trace. *Roche-Kontron* monitors display heart rate and respiration rate both digitally and as continuous traces on an oscilloscope. Similar monitors manufactured by Life Trace. High and low alarms can be set for each of these monitors. Generally, use heart rate limits of 100–200 beats/min and apnoea alarm at 10 sec of apnoea.

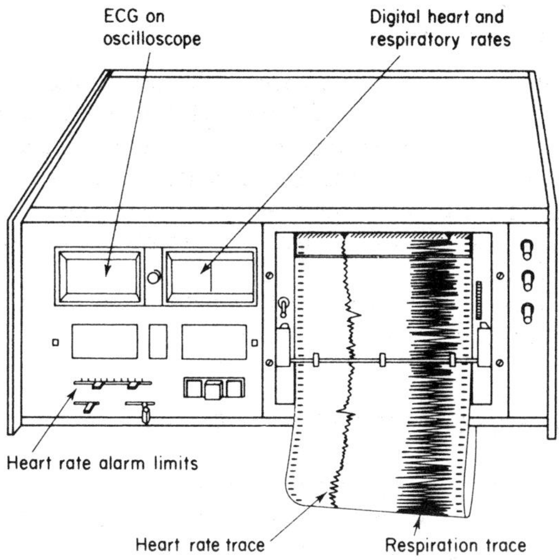

Fig. 35. The Corometrics 512 neonatal monitor measures heart rate and respiration rate, respiratory pattern and heart rate variability.

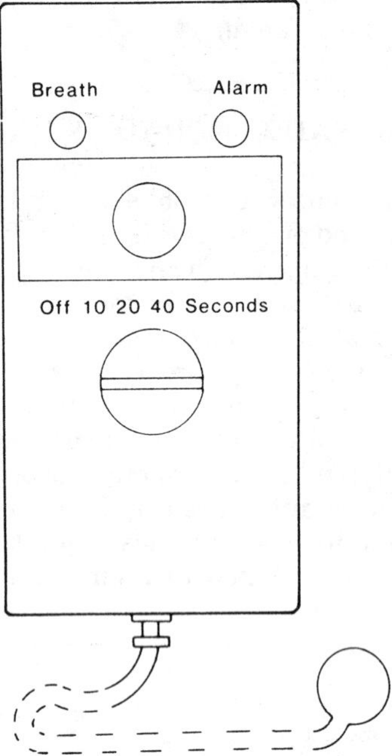

Fig. 36. Pye apnoea monitor. The plastic pad is taped to the upper abdomen near the xiphisternum.

Last resorts for apnoea monitoring are the *apnoea mattress* or Pye monitor (Fig. 36) which detect infant movement. These are unreliable as heart beat or seizures may cause sufficient compression of sensor to prevent alarm occurring when respiration has ceased. They may fail to detect distinctive apnoea.

All babies less than 34 weeks (1750 g) and all ill babies need monitoring until stable.

For discussion of home monitoring of babies with recurrent apnoea or siblings of SIDS, see p. 341.

TRANSCUTANEOUS OXYGEN MONITORING

A heated electrode measures oxygen tension across the skin; Roche (Fig. 37a), Draeger–Hellige or Radiometer monitors are

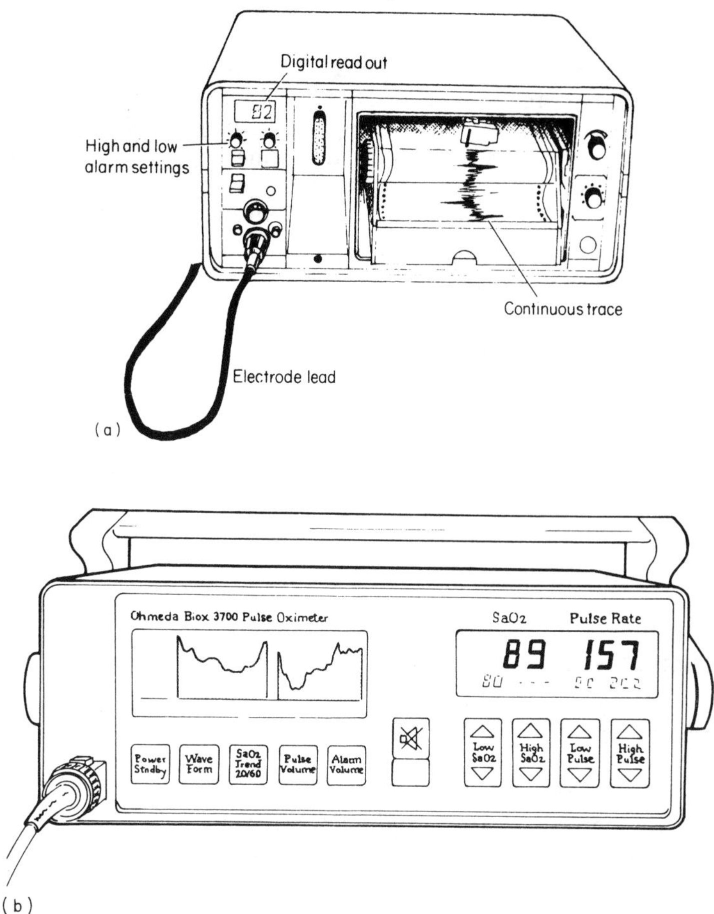

Fig. 37. (a) Transcutaneous oxygen monitor (Roche). (b) Pulse oximeter (Ohmeda).

commonly used. Calibrate according to user manuals. Needs *in vivo* calibration against arterial blood sample. Dangers of underestimating central P_aO_2 in shocked babies and of skin burns when temperature of 44 °C is used. Oedema and sclerma may lead to erroneous readings. Electrodes should be re-sited every 4–6 hours to avoid skin burns.

PULSE OXIMETRY (Fig. 37b)

The pulse oximeter calculates oxygen saturation by measuring oxyhaemoglobin as a proportion of total functional haemoglobin. As a ratio is measured rather than an absolute value no external calibration is needed. The oximeter probe consists of a light emitter and a light sensor placed on opposite sides of the foot or hand. Advantages over transcutaneous monitors:

1. Easy to use; no calibration or warm up period
2. Fast response time
3. Easily portable
4. Simultaneous heart rate measurement
5. Less affected by peripheral oedema or poor perfusion
6. Causes no skin burns

Disadvantages:

1. Susceptible to patient movement
2. Frequent alarm calls
3. Accuracy and standards for babies not determined
4. Altered slightly by jaundice and phototherapy

LUMBAR PUNCTURE (SPINAL TAP)

Indications include:

1. Suspected meningitis (sepsis work-up in ill infant)
2. Unexplained apnoea
3. Suspected subarachnoid haemorrhage
4. Treatment of post-haemorrhagic hydrocephalus
5. Unexplained seizures
6. Congenital syphilis

Needs good technique, especially in ill infant. Have an experienced nurse hold the baby (Fig. 38). Avoid neck flexion as this leads to hypoxaemia. Very ill infants need airway control first, sometimes with intubation. Full aseptic technique. Use needle with stylet to prevent a core of skin leading to a dermoid cyst in later life. Use lumbar space L4–L5 opposite iliac crest. Gently insert needle in direction of umbilicus until subarachnoid space is penetrated (slight give in needle, about 1 cm from skin in term infant, 0.5–0.75 cm in preterm). Remove stylet and allow CSF to drip out. Collect about 12 drops in each of three or four

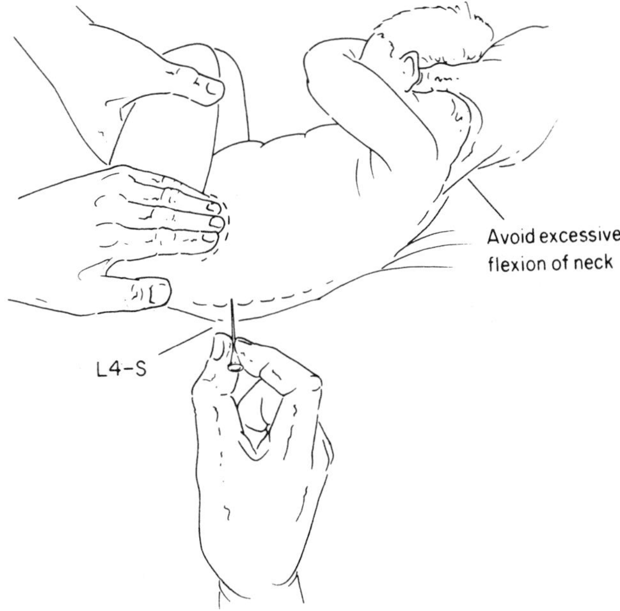

Fig. 38. Technique of lumbar puncture in the newborn.

bottles; less if the infant deteriorates. Inspect for colour and turbidity. If turbid and meningitis is suspected clinically, intrathecal gentamicin may be given (p. 201). Use small adhesive plaster with collodion to cover skin.

Samples sent for analysis:

1. Bacteriology: culture, Gram stain, cell count, counter-immune electrophoresis
2. Biochemistry: glucose, protein
3. Neurochemistry: haemoglobin and bilirubin by spectrophotometry
4. Virology, serology

VENTRICULAR TAP

Transillumination or ultrasound scan of the head (p. 324) may suggest dilatation of the ventricles.

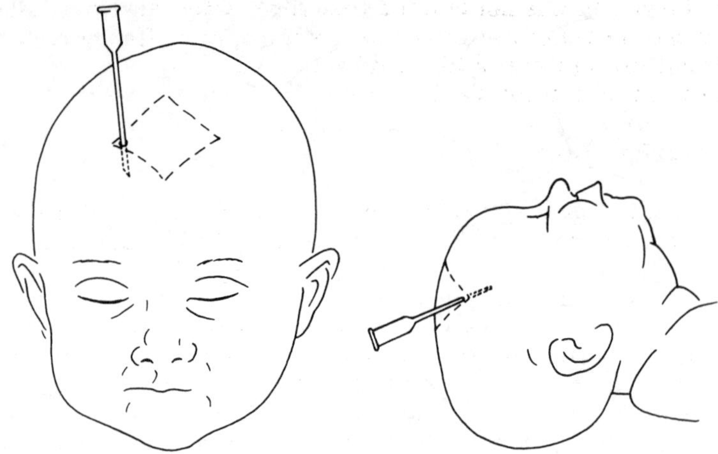

Fig. 39. Line of insertion of lumbar puncture needle with stylet and when performing ventricular tap.

Ventricular tap may be used to diagnose ventriculitis or intraventricular haemorrhage or to perform an air ventriculogram, though CAT scanning and ultrasound have generally replaced this invasive technique. Antibiotics are sometimes given by this route (p. 201).

The decision to perform ventricular tap should be taken by a consultant as complications like porencephalic cysts can occur. Figure 39 shows the angle of insertion of the needle in ventricular tap. Ultrasound scanning is now used to guide the needle towards the lateral ventricle.

Full aseptic technique should be used after shaving the scalp. A lumbar puncture needle with stylet is gently inserted at the lateral angle of the anterior fontanelle and angled towards the inner corner of the eye on the same side. Once the skin has been pierced, the stylet may be removed and the needle gently advanced until CSF wells up the needle (about 1–2 cm if the ventricles are dilated, or 3–4 cm in term babies with normal sized ventricles).

CSF from the ventricles should be collected by allowing it to drip into a sterile bottle.

ON NO ACCOUNT SHOULD A SYRINGE BE ATTACHED TO THE NEEDLE TO ASPIRATE THE FLUID

If the ventricle is not entered first time, withdraw the needle along line of insertion and try again at slightly different angle. Use ultrasound scan for guidance.

SUBDURAL TAP

This may be indicated for unexplained seizures, especially those that are unilateral and follow birth trauma. Ultrasound and CT scanning have largely replaced this technique for diagnosis of subdural haematoma (see Chapter 24).

The tap is performed with a short wide-bore needle (Pitkin needle) which is inserted through the lateral angle of the anterior fontanelle and aimed laterally into the subdural space (about 0.5 cm). If blood is present it should be gently aspirated with a syringe. Repeated taps may be needed as subdural effusions can re-accumulate.

BLADDER TAP (SUPRAPUBIC ASPIRATION)

Indications for bladder tap are as follows:

1. Inconclusive cultures of clean voided specimens (clean catch or Uribag)
2. Suspicion of septicaemia in any ill infant
3. To determine the effectiveness of treatment of urinary infection
4. The presence of vulvovaginitis, urethritis or balanitis when urinary tract infection is suspected

Contraindications of suprapubic aspiration are:

1. Recent urination or empty bladder
2. Abdominal distension with dilated loops of bowel
3. Bleeding disorder

Procedure is performed as illustrated in Fig. 40:

1. A wide area of skin over the lower abdomen is aseptically prepared as described previously
2. Using ultrasound guidance a number 21 sterile disposable needle attached to a 10 ml syringe is used to puncture the skin 0.5–1.0 cm above the symphysis pubis in the midline

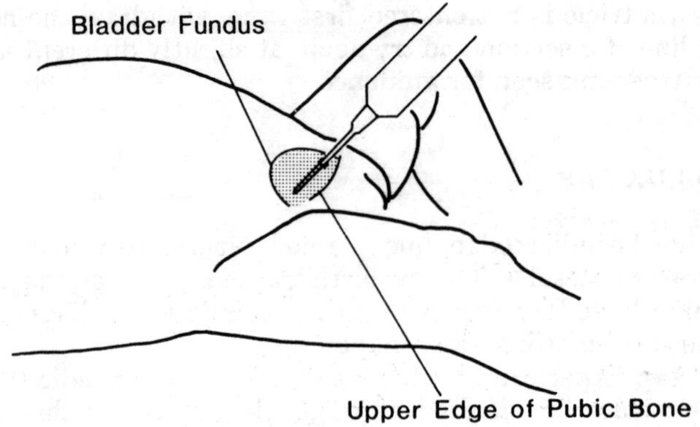

Fig. 40. Suprapubic aspiration or bladder tap in the newborn. The needle should be aimed slightly superiorly in the midline and 0.5 cm above the upper edge of the public bone.

3. The needle should be advanced gently towards the fundus of the bladder, angled upwards at 30° from the perpendicular
4. As the needle is slowly advanced, gentle suction should be maintained on the syringe until urine appears in it. It should not be necessary to introduce the needle further than 2.5 cm below the skin surface

BLOOD CULTURE

Full aseptic technique should be used. Do not draw blood for culture from any indwelling catheter. Use peripheral vein. Do not use femoral vein as it is impossible to clean the groin area effectively and is dangerous. Osteomyelitis of pelvis has occurred. Capillary blood cultures are more likely to be contaminated with skin bacteria but can be used if there is difficulty obtaining venous blood. Put blood in two bottles for aerobic and anaerobic culture.

THORACOCENTESIS

See also pneumothorax drainage (p. 92). Use the lower site (Fig. 23) for insertion of 19 or 21 gauge cannula connected to a three-way tap and 10 ml syringe.

PERICARDIOCENTESIS

Used for cardiac tamponade due to pneumopericardium (see p. 144). Often sudden deterioration on ventilator with pallor and shock. May occur with or without pneumothoraces. **INFORM CONSULTANT AT ONCE.**

Technique (see Fig. 41)

Use a 21 gauge cannula connected to a three-way tap and 10 ml syringe. Insert under the ribs to the left of the xiphisternum and advance up and to the left at 45° to the vertical and 45° from the midline. Keep gentle traction on the plunger of the syringe and at about 1 cm depth the pericardium should be entered and air withdrawn. The cannula may be left in position and allowed to drain under water.

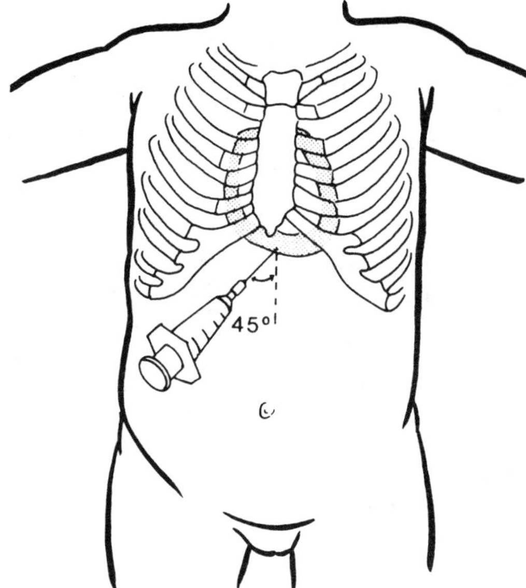

Fig. 41. Pericardiocentesis for pneumopericardium. The needle is inserted beneath the xiphisternum at 45° to the horizontal and the needle aimed 45° towards the left shoulder. Cautiously advance the needle keeping gentle suction on the syringe.

PARACENTESIS ABDOMINIS

Used to remove ascites especially in hydrops at birth (p. 187). Carefully find position of liver and spleen which are usually enlarged. Needle then advanced carefully into the right iliac fossa avoiding the liver and spleen. Fluid can be withdrawn as for thoracocentesis. Use local anaesthetic and nick the skin, muscle and peritoneum with a scalpel before inserting needle and cannula.

CARDIOVERSION (see p. 246)

NURSING THE BABY ON A VENTILATOR

1. Ensure that the endotracheal tube is firmly secured
2. Note position of the tube and check hourly for signs of displacement
3. Keep tube patent by suctioning as needed: usually 3–6 hourly using aseptic technique
4. After suctioning send aspirate to laboratory for culture twice weekly
5. Ensure that warmed, humidified gases are being given to prevent heat loss and drying of airways
6. Nurse baby semi-prone to avoid lung compression
7. Avoid traction on tube by supporting tubing and connectors. This helps to prevent trauma to larynx and vagal stimulation which may cause bradycardia
8. Change baby's position every 3 hours making sure that tubing does not kink by carefully re-positioning it
9. Record oxygen concentration, ventilator pressures and rate, and humidity temperature every hour
10. Increased surveillance is needed if muscle relaxants have been given: accidental disconnection or extubation can be very serious. Paralysed babies need gentle passive exercises of limbs
11. Avoid over-handling
12. Careful explanation of all care to parents

NURSING ROLE IN LUMBAR PUNCTURE

1. Basic pack with styletted spinal needle, local anaesthetic, lotions, collodion, universal containers and gowns, masks and gloves
2. Attach cardiorespiratory monitor and pulse oximeter if baby ill or unstable
3. Have oxygen, resuscitation masks, laryngoscope and endotracheal tubes, suction ready for ill babies
4. Hold baby gently but firmly in left lateral position with right hand on occiput and left hand around the baby's thighs; avoid flexion of head
5. Observe baby's colour and activity during procedure
6. Second nurse collects 12 drops of CSF in each of three sterile sample containers
7. Baby should lie flat for at least 1 hour after procedure with minimal handling
8. Keep parents informed

REFERENCES AND FURTHER READING

Coldiron, J. S. (1968). Estimation of nasotracheal tube length in neonates. *Pediatrics* **41**: 823

Dear, P. R. F. (1987). Monitoring oxygen in the newborn: saturation or partial pressure. *Arch. Dis. Child* **62**: 879.

Dunn, P. M. (1966). Localization of the umbilical catheter by post-mortem measurement. *Arch. Dis. Child* **41**: 69.

Goldsmith, J. P. and Karotkin, E. H. (1988). *Assisted Ventilation of the Neonate*, 2nd edn. Philadelphia: W. B. Saunders.

Greenough, A. and Greenall, F. (1988). Observation of spontaneous respiratory interaction with artificial ventilation. *Arch. Dis. Child* **63**: 168.

Halliday, H. L. (1989). When to do a lumbar puncture in a neonate. *Arch. Dis. Child* **64**: 313.

Levin, D. L., Morriss, S. C. and Moore, S. S. (1989). *A Practical Guide to Pediatric Intensive Care*, 2nd edn. St Louis: C. V. Mosby.

Milner, A. D. and Hoskyns, E. W. (1989). High frequency positive pressure ventilation in neonates. *Arch. Dis. Child* **64**: 1.

Ramsden, C. A., Reynolds E. O. R., Morley, C. T. *et al.* (1987). Ventilator settings for newborn infants. *Arch. Dis. Child* **62**: 529.

Southall, D. P., Bignall, S., Stebbins, V. A. *et al.* (1987). Pulse oximeter and transcutaneous arterial oxygen measurements in neonatal and paediatric intensive care. *Arch. Dis. Child* **62**: 882.

Tarnow-Mordi, W. (1988). How to ventilate premature babies. *Care Critic. Ill* **4**: 26.

Tarnow-Mordi, W. and Wilkinson, A. (1986). Mechanical ventilation of the newborn. *Br. Med. J.* **292**: 575.

The HIFI Study Group (1989). High-frequency oscillatory ventilation compared with conventional mechanical ventilation in the treatment of respiratory failure in preterm infants. *N. Engl. J. Med.* **320**: 88.

10. Respiratory Problems

In the newborn, respiration differs from the adult in being more rapid, more shallow and more irregular (Table 29). This is due to lower pulmonary compliance and proportionately increased work of breathing. Despite the extra work of breathing, however, $P\text{CO}_2$ and bicarbonate levels are lower than in adults (Table 23). Chemical control of ventilation is discussed in Chapter 15.

Table 29. Normal values for pulmonary function.

	Infant		
	Preterm	*Term*	*Adult*
Respiratory rate (breaths/min)	40–50	40	15
Tidal volume (ml/kg)	6	7	7
Minute ventilation (ml/kg/min)	200–300	200–280	90–110
Dead space (ml/kg)	2.5	2	2.2
Alveolar ventilation (ml/kg/min)	120	120	60
Total lung capacity (ml/kg)	60	60	80
Functional residual capacity (ml/kg)	25	30	30
Thoracic gas volume (ml/kg)	45	40	30
Vital capacity (ml/kg)	35	35	60
Lung compliance (ml/cmH_2O)	0.5–4	5	200
Airway resistance (cmH_2O/l/sec)	60	30	1.6
Work of breathing (g cm/min)	1500	1500	25 000
CO diffusion capacity (mlCO/min/mmHg)	0.3	1–3	20

Respiratory problems are the commonest cause of serious neonatal illness and death. Accurate diagnosis and management are imperative. Usually present with a combination of grunting, tachypnoea (respiratory rate >60 breaths/min), nasal flaring, sternal retractions, cyanosis.

Table 30. Causes of neonatal respiratory distress.

1. Respiratory distress syndrome (RDS)
2. Transient tachypnoea of the newborn (TTN)
3. Aspiration pneumonia (meconium, secretions or milk)
4. Pulmonary air leak: pneumothorax, interstitial emphysema, pneumomediastinum and pneumopericardium
5. Congenital pneumonia (especially group B streptococcal)
6. Congenital lobar emphysema
7. Pulmonary hypoplasia ± renal agenesis (Potter's syndrome)
8. Pulmonary haemorrhage
9. Chronic lung disease: bronchopulmonary dysplasia, Wilson–Mikity syndrome
10. Cardiac failure: congenital heart disease, PDA, supraventricular tachycardia, severe anaemia
11. Pulmonary hypertension or persistent fetal circulation
12. Metabolic acidosis (any aetiology, see p. 70)
13. Cerebral irritation: asphyxia, haemorrhage, meningitis
14. Diaphragmatic hernia
15. Airway obstruction: choanal atresia, Pierre Robin syndrome
16. Tracheo-oesophageal fistula
17. Drugs: aminophylline, narcotic analgesia in labour, diazepam
18. Over-heating or hypothermia
19. Cystic fibrosis
20. Chest wall disorders: thoracic dystrophy, myasthenia gravis

Table 30 lists some of the causes of respiratory distress; in practice the first five conditions are the commonest and account for almost 90%. Table 31 compares history, clinical findings and investigation in these common respiratory disorders of the newborn.

INITIAL ASSESSMENT

1. *History, antenatal*:
   Gestational age
   Intrauterine growth retardation (see p. 53)

Rhesus incompatibility
Maternal diabetes
Membranes ruptured before delivery
Steroids given
Vaginal culture
Maternal antibiotics
Multiple pregnancy
Antepartum haemorrhage
Previous baby with RDS

2. *Labour*:
   Normal
   Analgesics
   Fetal distress: meconium staining
3. *Resuscitation*:
   Apgar score
   Intubation
4. *Physical examination*:
   Estimated gestational age
   Pink or blue
   Active

If baby is large (>2500 g), pink and active, wait and see but beware of streptococcal pneumonia and meconium aspiration. Otherwise two questions must be asked:

1. Has the baby got respiratory distress?
2. What is the cause of respiratory distress?

Table 30 and Fig. 42 show causes of respiratory distress but a chest radiograph is necessary to confirm diagnosis.

INITIAL MANAGEMENT

Place infant in prewarmed incubator.

Give oxygen by means of head box (see p. 75) to abolish cyanosis but remember that cyanosis may be a late sign of hypoxaemia in the newborn. Figure 43 shows the haemoglobin–oxygen dissociation curves for adult and fetal haemoglobin. With a shift to the left in fetal haemoglobin, cyanosis may not become apparent until P_aO_2 is less than 5 kPa (40 mmHg). Also, if polycythaemia is present, a baby may appear cyanosed when P_aO_2 is normal. Arterial blood gas tensions must be measured if infant needs $> 30\%$ oxygen.

Table 31. Differential diagnosis of respiratory distress.

	RDS	*PHT*	*GBS*	*TTN*	*MAS*
Gestation	Usually preterm	Often term	Preterm or term	More often term	Usually post-term
Perinatal history	APH, IDM, rhesus, immature L/S ratio	Asphyxia, aspirin in pregnancy	Uterine inertia, asphyxia, PROM	IDM, C/S, asphyxia	Asphyxia, IUGR
Clinical features	Grunting prominent, gradual deterioration	Cyanosis, prominent, sudden deterioration	Shock prominent, early apnoea, pulmonary haemorrhage	RR >60, mild distress	Meconium staining, over-inflated chest, progressive deterioration
Effect of oxygen	Improvement	Cyanosis unchanged	May improve	Improvement	May improve
Blood gases	Hypoxaemia, raised $P\text{CO}_2$, mixed acidosis	Marked hypoxaemia, low or normal $P\text{CO}_2$, metabolic acidosis, (R) radial/aorta difference	Hypoxaemia, metabolic or mixed acidosis	Mild hypoxaemia, low or normal $P\text{CO}_2$, mild metabolic acidosis	Hypoxaemia, metabolic acidosis
Chest X-ray	Under-inflation, reticulogranular mottling, air bronchogram	Over-inflation, clear lung-fields, cardiomegaly	Coarse infiltrates, collapse or mimic RDS	Over-inflation, streaking, ↑ pulm. vasc., pulm. oedema, SI cardiomegaly	Coarse infiltrates, over-inflation ± pneumothorax
Echocardiogram	RPEP/RVET ↑ or normal, LPEP/LVET normal	RPEP/RVET ↑ ↑, LPEP/LVET often ↑	RPEP/RVET may ↑, LPEP/LVET normal or ↑	RPEP/RVET normal or ↑, LPEP/LVET ↑	RPEP/RVET normal or ↑, LPEP/LVET normal or ↑

Table 31. Differential diagnosis of respiratory distress (continued).

	RDS	*PHT*	*GBS*	*TTN*	*MAS*
Treatment	CPAP helpful, IPPV, surfactant replacement	CPAP unhelpful, mechanical hyperventilation or tolazoline	Penicillin, blood transfusion, ± mechanical ventilation	Oxygen, IPPV (rarely)	Airway suction at birth, may need IPPV, CPAP unhelpful
Outcome (mortality)	< 5%	~ 20%	~ 40%	0%	~ 30%

RDS = respiratory distress syndrome
PHT = pulmonary hypertension (persistent fetal circulation)
GBS = group B streptococcal pneumonia
TTN = transient tachypnoea of the newborn
MAS = meconium aspiration syndrome
APH = antepartum haemorrhage
IDM = infant of diabetic mother
PROM = premature rupture of membranes
C/S = caesarean section
IUGR = intrauterine growth retardation
L/S = lecithin/sphingomyelin
RR = respiratory rate
RPEP/RVET = ratio of right ventricular pre-ejection period to ejection time correlates with pulmonary vascular resistance
LPEP/LVET = ratio of left ventricular pre-ejection period to ejection time correlates with myocardial contractility

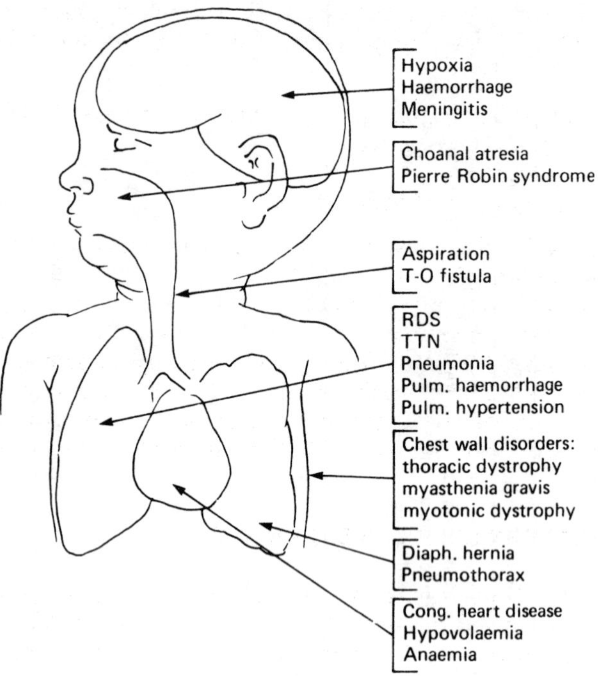

Fig. 42. Causes of respiratory distress.

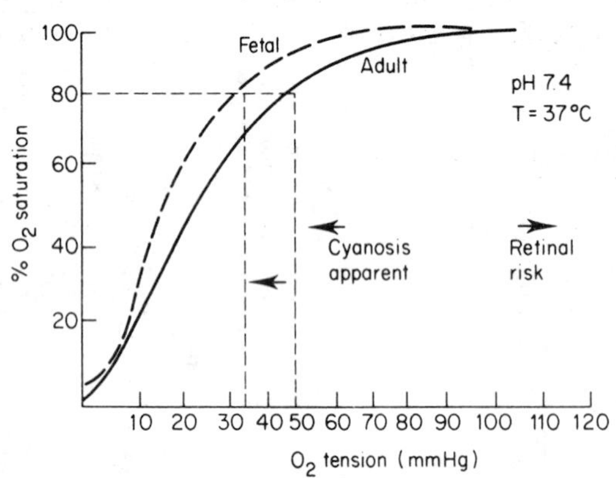

Fig. 43. The haemoglobin–oxygen dissociation curves for fetal and adult haemoglobin. Cyanosis may appear late in hypoxaemia in the newborn. After Klaus and Fanaroff (1979).

Other factors causing a leftward shift in haemoglobin–oxygen dissociation curve (increased affinity of haemoglobin for oxygen) are:

1. Reduced hydrogen ion concentration (increased pH)
2. Reduced temperature
3. Reduced P_aCO_2
4. Reduced 2,3-diphosphoglycerate

Increases in all these factors shift the curve to the right (decreased affinity).

If $>30\%$ oxygen is required and infant < 1.5 kg, insert arterial catheter and take a chest radiograph. If >1.5 kg, wait approximately 30 min to see if there is any improvement. If there is none and oxygen requirement $>40\%$, insert arterial catheter and take radiograph. Chest radiograph is important to confirm clinical diagnosis and ascertain catheter position.

RESPIRATORY DISTRESS SYNDROME

Respiratory distress syndrome (RDS) or hyaline membrane disease is caused by surfactant deficiency and affects mainly the preterm infant. The incidence of RDS varies with gestational age (Table 32); these rates will be lowered by maternal steroid treatment. Surfactant is produced by alveolar Type II cells and, by reducing alveolar surface tension, prevents alveolar collapse in expiration. The major components of

Table 32. Incidence of RDS by gestational age.

Gestation (weeks)	*Babies with RDS* (%)
26	90
28	80
30	70
32	55
34	25
36	12
38	3
40	<1–2

surfactant are phosphatidyl choline (lecithin), phosphatidyl glycerol (PG) and phosphatidyl inositol (PI). Most of the phosphatidyl choline is in the form of dipalmitoyl phosphatidyl choline (DPPC) (or dipalmitoyl lecithin) which comprises 60% of surfactant. Several of the components of surfactant must be present for it to lower surface tension as DPPC alone is ineffective. The presence of PG seems to be important (see Table 35). Surfactant is produced from 22 to 24 weeks gestation onwards at first by a pathway which is extremely sensitive to changes in temperature and pH. By 35 weeks gestation, mature surfactant is produced by a second pathway which is more resistant to alterations of pH and hypoxia. Deficiency of surfactant will lead to alveolar collapse, reduced lung volume, decreased lung compliance and ventilation/perfusion abnormalities. Figure 44 compares the compliance of the normal lung with that of an infant with RDS. In RDS there is low compliance or stiff lungs. High pressures are needed to expand the lungs. In severe RDS, pulmonary hypertension with R–L shunting will also occur.

Radiologically, the areas of collapse appear as diffuse reticulogranular mottling and air in the major bronchi is contrasted against the white background as air bronchograms (see p. 311). Hypoxaemia from ventilation/perfusion abnormalities leads to metabolic acidosis due to cellular anaerobic glycolysis with

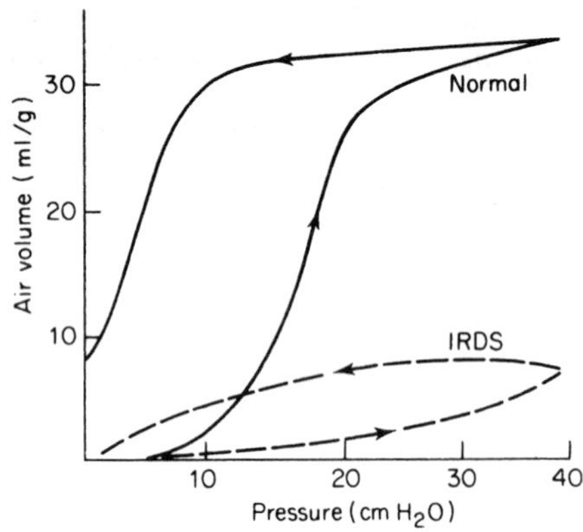

Fig. 44. Pressure–volume curves for normal infant and one with severe RDS. Compliance can be calculated as volume change per unit of pressure change (ml/cmH_2O). After Klaus and Fanaroff (1979).

lactic acid production. Respiratory acidosis is also present because of alveolar hypoventilation. The combination of acidosis and hypoxaemia reduces myocardial contractility, cardiac output and arterial blood pressure. Perfusion of kidneys, gastrointestinal tract and other non-vital organs is also reduced. Oedema and electrolyte disturbances occur.

For these reasons, the management of RDS is complex and involves more than just support of ventilation. If, however, one can correct the underlying hypoxaemia and acidosis, many of the other complications of RDS can be ameliorated.

In uncomplicated RDS, surfactant is produced after about 48 hours. The natural progression of RDS is of worsening for 36–48 hours, then stabilization for 24 hours before improvement occurs after about 72 hours. By the end of 7 days, the baby with mild or moderate RDS should be recovered. An improvement in renal function with increased urine output amounting to a diuresis often heralds improvement in pulmonary function.

Management

May be predicted by measurement of lecithin/sphingomyelin area ratio (LSAR) in amniotic fluid, tracheal aspirate or gastric aspirate. LSAR <2 associated with RDS (Table 33). For shake test see Appendix IX and Table 34. Detection of the presence of phosphatidyl glycerol (PG) improves the prediction of pulmonary maturity (Table 35). At any LSAR, presence of PG predicts low incidence of RDS (0.6%) and absence predicts a high incidence (83%).

Table 33. Incidence of RDS and death by LSAR.

LSAR	*RDS* (%)	*Died from RDS* (%)
>2.5	0.9*	0
>2.0	2.2*	0.1
1.5–2.0	40	4
<1.5	73	14

* Most were IDM, asphyxia or severe rhesus

Table 34. Incidence of RDS after shake test.*

Shake test	*RDS* (%)
+ve (3 or more tubes)	0.65
Intermediate (1–2 tubes)	15
−ve (no tubes)	39

* For method see Appendix IX

Table 35. Pulmonary maturity by LSAR and PG presence.

LSAR	*RDS* (%)	*RDS if PG present* (%)	*RDS if PG absent* (%)
≥2.0	0	0	0
<2.0	23	3.4	86
All	4.8	0.6	83

Risk of RDS is increased by:

1. History of RDS in siblings
2. Maternal diabetes or rhesus isoimmunization
3. Male sex
4. Second twin
5. Elective caesarean section
6. Birth asphyxia
7. Antepartum haemorrhage

Risk of RDS is reduced by:

1. Prenatal steroids
2. Prolonged rupture of membranes (2 days to 1 week)
3. Pre-eclampsia (probably not true)
4. Growth retardation
5. Heroin addiction

Diagnosis based on clinical picture of tachypnoea, grunting, nasal flaring and confirmed by chest radiograph. Early use of CPAP and IPPV improves the radiographic appearances of RDS by expanding collapsed alveoli.

REMEMBER: A successful outcome to this potentially fatal disease requires meticulous attention to detail.

IF IN DOUBT - ASK

Place baby in incubator at neutral thermal environment or under radiant warmer (p. 62).

If infant > 1500 g, > 32 weeks gestation and does not require > 30% oxygen; reassess half-hourly. If infant is clinically improving, continue assessment until infant is well. Use radial artery blood sampling and/or transcutaneous Po_2 monitor and/or pulse oximeter.

If there is clinical deterioration with increased grunting, retractions and O_2 requirement, or if infant < 1500 g, < 32 weeks and requires > 30% oxygen, place in head box and insert arterial catheter.

Initial Investigation

1. Blood gases, pH, chest radiograph
2. Haemoglobin, packed cell volume, glucose stix
3. Blood pressure by Doppler or flush method or transducer (see p. 243).
4. Blood culture, white cell count, IgM
5. Gastric aspirate; Gram stain and culture

Penicillin should be given to all babies with respiratory distress until cultures taken at birth prove negative. Indications of babies at increased risk include:

1. Vaginal swab has grown streptococci
2. Gastric aspirate shows polymorphs and Gram-positive organisms
3. Any atypical features seen in infant (p. 145)

Further Management

Monitoring: attach cardiorespirograph and transcutaneous oxygen monitor (or pulse oximeter), place ambient oxygen analyser close to infant's face.

Continuous positive airways pressure (CPAP) is used when P_aO_2 is < 8 kPa (60 mmHg) in 60% oxygen in babies > 1500 g. Use endotracheal, mask or nasal prong CPAP as discussed on p. 79. Start with pressure of 6–8 cmH_2O and check frequent arterial blood gas samples until improvement occurs or respiratory failure develops.

Respiratory failure is present when any one of the following occur on *two* consecutive blood gas analyses 20 min apart.

1. P_aO_2 <6 kPa (50 mmHg) in 100% oxygen on CPAP of 6–8 cmH_2O
2. pH <7.20 (often associated with P_aCO_2 over 10 kPa (75 mmHg))
3. Intractable apnoea

Mechanical ventilation is used under these circumstances or as initial management of very immature babies. Nasotracheal is preferred to orotracheal intubation as the tube is more firmly anchored and less liable to slip out or kink. Occasionally damage to anterior naris or nasal septum can occur; this is less likely if the tube is left long (see Fig. 15). The endotracheal tube is anchored by taping as shown in Fig. 15. Initial ventilator settings and further management are described in Chapter 9.

Surfactant replacement therapy has been shown to reduce mortality and complications such as pneumothorax and pulmonary interstitial emphysema in babies with severe RDS (see below). Other drugs have a very limited place in management except in the infant with very severe RDS and R–L shunting, secondary to pulmonary hypertension. This is an analogous situation to that found in persistent fetal circulation (see p. 151).

The R–L shunt may be calculated using Fig. 45. Alternatively, pre-ductus (right radial) and post-ductus (umbilical) arterial oxygen tensions may be measured to calculate the shunt. Pulmonary vasodilating drugs are used when P_aO_2 is below 5 kPa (40 mmHg), despite maximum ventilation with 100% oxygen. Tolazoline is used in a dose of 1–2 mg/kg as an intravenous bolus and, if effective, then as an infusion of 1–2 mg/kg/hour. Dangers are hypotension (correct by volume expansion) and gastric bleeding (see p. 152). Dopamine is often given with tolazoline to prevent hypotension (p. 153).

In some infants who breath asynchronously with the ventilator ('fight'), faster rates (70–100 breaths/min) often work. If this fails, muscle relaxation may be used; curare (dose 0.3 mg/kg as needed) has the advantage of having a pulmonary

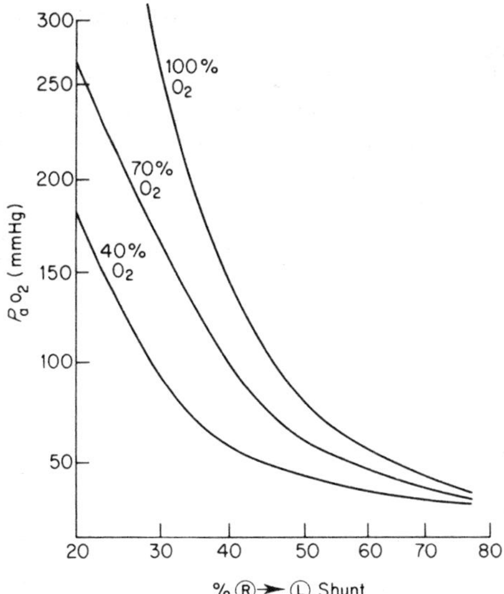

Fig. 45. Calculation of R–L shunt in 40, 70 and 100% oxygen. After Klaus and Fanaroff (1979).

vasodilating action (histamine action) but side-effects are hypotension and reduced cardiac output. Pancuronium is a shorter acting muscle relaxant said to have fewer cardiovascular side-effects (dose 0.05 mg/kg). Muscle relaxants may also lessen the risks of pneumothorax and bronchopulmonary dysplasia.

Weaning from the ventilator is described in Chapter 9 (see p. 88). Gentle chest physiotherapy is begun soon after endotracheal extubation unless the infant does not tolerate handling. A padded electric toothbrush provides gentle vibration to the thorax and may help to remove pulmonary secretions.

Correction of Acidosis

Only metabolic acidosis should be treated with alkaline solutions; the correct treatment of respiratory acidosis is assisted ventilation. Furthermore, if metabolic acidosis has an underlying cause, e.g. hypovolaemia or sepsis, then this should first be corrected.

If unexplained metabolic acidosis is present (pH less than 7.25 and P_aCO_2 less than 6 kPa (45 mmHg)) then bicarbonate should be infused slowly. Use sodium bicarbonate 8.4% diluted 4:1 with 5 or 10% dextrose in a dose of 1 mmol/kg. Note that 1 ml of 8.4% bicarbonate contains 1 mmol. Repeated or excessive use of bicarbonate in RDS is both ineffective and dangerous, especially in the very immature infant.

Correction of Hypovolaemia, Hypotension

If packed cell volume <45% or blood pressure low (see p. 32), give 10 ml/kg of whole blood, plasma or 5% salt-free albumin.

Fluids, Electrolytes, Nutrition

Preterm infants with RDS tolerate oral feeding poorly and this may lead to:

1. Increased oxygen consumption and lowered oxygen tensions
2. Abdominal distension and regurgitation
3. Necrotizing enterocolitis

For these reasons all but bigger babies require intravenous fluids, at least initially.

Fluid intake in severe RDS should be reduced because of decreased urinary output from decreased renal perfusion and increased capillary permeability. Account must be taken of increased insensible water losses under radiant heaters or phototherapy.

Start with 5 or 10% dextrose at 60–80 ml/kg/day. If infusion required for >24 hours, electrolyte supplementation (watch sodium and potassium intakes in very immature babies for first 2–3 days) and amino acids will be required (see Chapter 11).

Upon recovery, feeding can be started orally. Umbilical arterial lines should first be removed. Orogastric or transpyloric feeding are used (see Chapter 11).

Observation

All infants on assisted ventilation should be continuously supervised by a trained nurse. Any clinical deterioration will be reported immediately.

THE BEST MONITOR IS THE NAKED EYE

Other Measurements

1. *Continuous*:
   - Heart rate and variability
   - Respiratory rate
   - Transcutaneous PO_2 or pulse oximeter
   - Temperature (servo-control)
   - Blood pressure (transducer or Dinamap)
2. *4 hourly (minimum)*:
   - Blood gases and pH
   - Glucose strip test
3. *12 hourly*:
   - Bilirubin if clinical jaundice
   - Electrolytes
   - Calcium
   - Urine output and specific gravity
4. *24 hourly*:
   - Urinary output
   - Haemoglobin or packed cell volume
   - Weight

Sudden deterioration in RDS when spontaneously breathing may be caused by:

1. Pneumothorax
2. Intraventricular haemorrhage
3. Infection
4. Airway problems, aspiration
5. Apnoea

Inspect airway and suction if secretions present. Ventilation by bag and mask. Transilluminate chest.

If rapid improvement from bagging and transillumination negative, observe closely. Check blood gases for respiratory failure. If transillumination positive, treat as pneumothorax (see Chapter 9).

If little or delayed improvement, consider:

1. Infection
2. Intraventricular haemorrhage
3. Need for assisted ventilation

Rapid Deterioration on Assisted Ventilation

First check that ventilator is working; pressure needle moving and chest wall being lifted, then disconnect from ventilator and bag by hand.

If *improvement*: ventilator problem or disconnection.

If *no improvement*:

1. Tube blocked or displaced
2. Pneumothorax, interstitial emphysema
3. Infection
4. Intraventricular haemorrhage

If gradual deterioration, think of infection, patent ductus arteriosus or slowly progressive pulmonary interstitial emphysema.

Long-term Complications

1. Patent ductus arteriosus (p. 239)
2. Bronchopulmonary dysplasia (p. 148)
3. Retinopathy of prematurity (p. 65)
4. Neurological and developmental problems, intraventricular haemorrhage (see Chapters 16 and 26)

Future Developments

Will include improved methods of prevention of preterm labour, drugs to induce endogenous surfactant production and use of exogenous surfactant preparations to treat established RDS. Ritodrine, a β-mimetric drug, has been extensively used to prevent or delay preterm labour, but its benefits remain doubtful. Contraindications preclude its use in about 50% of women in preterm labour. Corticosteroids will accelerate fetal pulmonary maturation, but their impact has not been dramatic, partly because obstetricians have not been entirely convinced by the evidence from the controlled trials. Recent studies suggest that natural rather than artificial surfactant administered soon after birth to infants at risk reduces the incidence and severity of RDS.

SURFACTANT REPLACEMENT

Artificial surfactant comprising dipalmitoyl phosphatidyl choline (DPPC) and phosphatidyl glycerol (PG) has been shown to be effective in preventing RDS and reducing complications if given to preterm babies at birth. Our own experience has been with a natural surfactant prepared from pig lungs by chloroform–methanol extraction and liquid-gel chromatography. This surfactant (Curosurf) contains 99% phospholipids and only 1% protein (Table 36). Babies with severe RDS (mechanical ventilation with >60% oxygen) show dramatic improvement in oxygen needs immediately after intratracheal instillation of 200 mg/kg of Curosurf; F_iO_2 falling from 0.8 to 0.3 within a few minutes. In addition to this acute improvement, survival rate is increased and complications of pneumothorax and pulmonary interstitial emphysema reduced.

Instillation of the surfactant must ensure an even distribution into each lung segment; the baby is turned from side to side during administration. Once the baby is re-connected to the ventilator inspired oxygen concentrations can be rapidly lowered with the aid of a pulse oximeter. If high ventilator rates (>60 breaths/min) are being used it is usually possible to lower peak pressure soon afterwards. Movement of the chest wall

Table 36. Composition of natural porcine surfactant (Curosurf).

Phospholipids	99%
Phosphatidylcholine	76%
Phosphatidylglycerol	4%
Phosphatidylinositol	4%
Protein	1%

remains the best guide to pressure requirements, but simple methods to measure pulmonary compliance may soon be developed for use at the cotside. Blood pressure should also be carefully monitored after surfactant replacement and any hypotension corrected by infusion of colloid. The only likely complication of surfactant replacement is an increased incidence of PDA but this is easily detected by Doppler echocardiography and managed with intravenous indomethacin (see p. 240).

Long-term follow-up studies do not show an increase in handicaps in survivors of this treatment but some questions remain to be answered: the optimal surfactant preparation, its dose, whether repeat doses are needed, which infants respond best and which do not. Nevertheless, surfactant replacement for RDS is probably the single greatest advance in neonatal medicine for decades.

TRANSIENT TACHYPNOEA OF THE NEWBORN (TTN)

Relatively common respiratory disorder of both preterm and term infants. The cause may be delayed resorption of lung fluid and predisposing factors are:

1. Perinatal asphyxia
2. Elective caesarean section
3. Maternal diabetes (or potential diabetes)
4. Excessive maternal analgesia
5. Oxytocin and excess hypotonic fluids in labour
6. Neonatal polycythaemia

Each of these conditions is associated with increased production of lung fluid or delay in its removal via trachea, pulmonary lymphatics or veins. Transient left ventricular failure may also be involved in pathogenesis.

Clinically, the disorder mimics mild RDS with tachypnoea predominant (up to 120 breaths/min) and minimal grunting or indrawing (classical TTN).

Radiographs show increased pulmonary vascular markings, mild cardiomegaly, hyperinflation of the lungs and fluid in costophrenic angles and horizontal fissure, resembling those of pulmonary oedema (see p. 311).

In some infants with radiographic findings of TTN there may

be very marked hyperinflation and pulmonary hypertension with R–L shunting (severe type). These infants are usually very ill and resemble those with persistent fetal circulation (see p. 151). Echocardiography is helpful in distinguishing these two types of TTN (see Table 31).

Classical TTN is a short-lived illness with less than 40% oxygen needed to maintain normal arterial blood gases. Tachypnoea generally abates by 2–3 days.

In infants who are distressed or have respiratory rates over 80 breaths/min, withhold oral feeds and provide fluids and calories intravenously. Exclude infection as streptococcal pneumonia can present insidiously like TTN. Heart disease can also present in this way, e.g. total anomalous pulmonary venous drainage or anomalous left coronary artery.

In severe disease, oxygen therapy and ventilation are needed as in RDS.

ASPIRATION PNEUMONIA

Two distinct entities:

1. Meconium aspiration occurs predominantly in the post-term infant
2. Aspiration of milk or upper airways secretion, which is more common in the preterm infant

Meconium Aspiration

Meconium staining of amniotic fluid in 10% of infants at term. More common in post-term and SGA. Associated with intra-uterine hypoxia. If it occurs in preterm infants, intrauterine infection may be cause (listeriosis). Intubate the trachea of any infant born after thick meconium staining of liquor and gently aspirate any meconium below the cords. If baby is vigorous at birth intubation is not necessary. Avoid lung lavage as this liquefies the meconium and helps drive it distally.

Efficient resuscitation with suction of the trachea in the meconium-stained infant significantly improves outcome. Associated asphyxia often determines the outcome.

Massive meconium aspiration may lead to a very severe illness by two mechanisms:

1. Plugging of the small airways with hyperinflation as a result of ball-valve mechanism. Atelectasis with ventilation/perfusion imbalance and profound hypoxaemia may occur
2. Meconium pneumonitis from chemical irritation, which may be delayed

Secondary infection may also occur since meconium is able to support a variety of bacterial growth *in vitro*. Associated asphyxia will alter cerebral, myocardial, pulmonary and renal function and may help determine the outcome.

Management

Any infant with significant meconium below the cords must be admitted to the nursery irrespective of clinical condition immediately after resuscitation. Chest radiography should be performed.

Deterioration of these infants may occur slowly as the meconium tracks distally in the respiratory tract. Pneumothorax occurs in about 15% of infants.

In the nursery initial management comprises:

1. Observation
2. Humidified oxygen
3. Gentle chest physiotherapy

If chest radiograph confirms the presence of meconium aspiration, (see p. 312) oxygen will usually be required to maintain normal blood gases.

If there has been severe asphyxia or there is acute hyperinflation of the lungs, pulmonary hypertension may occur.

Metabolic acidosis should be treated with dilute bicarbonate solutions. Marked hypoxaemia with pulmonary hypertension can be treated by inducing respiratory alkalosis using high-rate mechanical ventilation (see p. 86). If this fails to maintain P_aO_2 above 5 kPa (40 mmHg) use tolazoline (p. 152).

Antibiotics should be given in cases of massive meconium aspiration.

Even with this aggressive management, the mortality is about 30% (see Table 26).

Bronchopulmonary dysplasia may occur in infants who survive.

Late Onset Aspiration

Usually a thriving preterm infant who suddenly becomes apnoeic during or soon after feeding. At resuscitation milk can usually be seen in the hypopharynx or below cords.

Chest radiograph usually shows collapse or consolidation, especially of right upper lobe. Milk should be aspirated from the airway with a suction catheter. The infant should then be bagged with 40% oxygen until spontaneous breathing recurs.

The infant should be carefully monitored for a few days following this episode, and because of the risk of superimposed or underlying infection start antibiotic therapy after a full sepsis work-up (see Table 62). Recurrent attacks of apnoea with or without aspiration may be caused by gastro-oesophageal reflux. Barium swallow may be indicated. Up to 70% of babies intubated for mechanical ventilation have recurrent bouts of aspiration. Transpyloric feeding may reduce this complication.

Aspiration of secretions, amniotic fluid or blood may occur around birth giving clinical pictures similar to meconium aspiration, RDS or pulmonary hypertension.

PNEUMOTHORAX

Asymptomatic pneumothorax probably occurs in about 1% of all newborns and does not need treatment. Symptomatic pneumothorax usually occurs as a complication of:

1. RDS or its treatment
2. Meconium aspiration
3. Over-zealous resuscitation
4. Pulmonary hypoplasia, e.g. Potter's syndrome
5. Post-thoracotomy
6. TTN, aspiration pneumonia or other causes of low compliance
7. Staphylococcal pneumonia (rare cause)

The incidence of pneumothorax in infants with RDS treated with assisted ventilation varies from 15 to 30%. In 10% the pneumothorax will be bilateral.

Alveolar rupture allows air to track along the broncho-vascular space to the mediastinum and thence into the pleural space. The usual consequence is a tension pneumothorax and the primary pneumomediastinum is not always radiologically apparent.

Tension pneumothorax is an acute emergency causing sudden deterioration. Clinically there may be shift of the mediastinum (apex beat) away from and reduced breath sounds on the affected side. There may be asymmetry of chest wall movement. Sudden collapse with hypotension and poor perfusion may occur in association with tachycardia or bradycardia.

In RDS the lungs are less compliant so that major shift of the mediastinum may not occur and a small pneumothorax on radiograph may cause marked deterioration with worsening of blood gases.

Transillumination of the chest with a fibreoptic light often shows hyperlucency of the affected side (see p. 92).

Anteroposterior (AP) and cross-table lateral chest radiographs should be taken since collapsed lung may be pushed back against posterior chest wall and the AP film may underestimate the extent of the pneumothorax (see pp. 94, 312).

Treatment

Immediate aspiration of air followed by the insertion of a pleural drain connected to an underwater seal (see Chapter 9). Always check position of pleural drain by radiography. Once an air leak has occurred in the newborn, air may spread from the mediastinum to reach the peritoneal cavity (pneumoperitoneum) or the pericardial cavity (pneumopericardium), or into the neck causing subcutaneous emphysema (uncommon in the newborn). Occasionally, air will rupture into a pulmonary blood vessel causing generalized arterial air (pneumatosis arterialis) with sudden death.

Pneumopericardium is usually a very serious condition and often requires drainage. Presents with reduced cardiac output and decreased heart sounds; diagnosis should be confirmed radiologically (see p. 312). Pericardial drainage is a very skilled procedure and the consultant on call must always be notified (see also p. 119).

Pulmonary interstitial emphysema (PIE) may occur in infants with severe RDS needing mechanical ventilation. Appearance may herald pneumothorax and sudden deterioration. High-rate ventilation with lower peak pressures may help but bronchopulmonary dysplasia is a long-term complication of survivors. Short periods of manual ventilation at high rates (120 breaths/min) may be effective in reducing the amount of PIE. It has been suggested that pleural drains be inserted cautiously to create pneumothoraces and improve pulmonary compliance.

CONGENITAL PNEUMONIA

The clinical and radiological picture may be similar to RDS.

Predisposing factors in congenital pneumonia are:

1. Prolonged rupture of the membranes
2. Maternal illness with fever or foul-smelling liquor
3. Maternal colonization with group B streptococci
4. Birth asphyxia with aspiration of infected material

Infection may be ascending, transplacental or following aspiration. The organisms most commonly isolated are β-haemolytic streptococci, coliforms, *Listeria monocytogenes, Bacteroides* and occasionally *Staphylococcus* or *Pseudomonas.*

Early onset group B *β-haemolytic streptococcal* pneumonia is becoming an increasingly important cause of neonatal illness in the UK. From 10 to 30% of pregnant women will carry this organism in the genital tract or rectum. Infants born to these mothers usually become colonized but only 1% of them will develop serious illness. Serious sepsis in three per 1000 births with a mortality rate of 30–50%.

Group B β-haemolytic streptococcal pneumonia may be very difficult to distinguish from RDS. One or more of the following findings may help:

1. Early onset of apnoea
2. Shock/hypotension
3. Metabolic acidosis
4. Pulmonary infiltrates on radiographs
5. Blood-stained tracheal aspirate
6. Neutropenia
7. Streptococci on Gram stain of gastric aspirate
8. Positive blood and gastric aspirate culture for streptococci

Because there is doubt, all infants with respiratory distress should be treated initially with penicillin in high dose (see

p. 133). If cultures prove negative, the antibiotic may be stopped after 2–3 days.

If the diagnosis is confirmed then a combination of penicillin and aminoglycoside (gentamicin, netilmicin or amikacin) is effective since these antibiotics have a synergistic action against streptococci.

Hypotension is common in congenital sepsis and should be treated with blood or plasma transfusion (10–15 ml/kg). Transfusions with fresh blood are also helpful by providing opsonins to improve the newborn's white cell function. If there is neutropenia, granulocyte or buffy coat transfusions may help.

Mechanical ventilation may be required (Chapter 9).

The overall mortality for this condition remains high (30–50%) despite early and apparently adequate treatment. The reasons for this may be:

1. Intrauterine onset of infection
2. Delay in diagnosis (confusion with RDS)
3. Immature infants are often affected
4. Affected infants may have immunological deficiencies

Incidence of infection may be reduced by giving ampicillin (2–4 g) to high-risk mothers (i.e. colonized mothers in preterm labour).

Early onset listeriosis has a similar clinical picture and high mortality; it is now more commonly seen in the UK partly as a result of imports of soft cheeses made from unpasteurized milks. *Listeria monocytogenes* grows well in low temperatures so that these cheeses should not be kept in the refrigerator.

Maternal 'flu-like' illness is a usual antecedent and the infection of the fetus is probably transplacental, though it is known that the newborn may become infected after aspirating contaminated amniotic fluid during birth.

Meconium staining in premature labour is often found and at birth the infant may have a maculopapular and petechial rash and hepatosplenomegaly. Leucopenia and thrombocytopenia are common and Gram-positive coccobacilli may be seen on smear of gastric aspirate.

Treatment with ampicillin and gentamicin is effective but the outcome is poor despite early treatment because of severe pulmonary involvement and coexisting meningitis. There is a

50% neonatal mortality and about 50% of survivors have significant handicaps.

Anaerobic organisms may also cause congenital pneumonia. Recently, *Bacteroides fragilis* has been isolated from some infants who have been born after prolonged rupture of the membranes. There is usually foul-smelling amniotic fluid and the infants are also malodorous. Though the mother may have a fever and rigors, the infant usually has a relatively benign course, with mild pneumonia, jaundice, hypocalcaemia and lethargy. Ampicillin and gentamicin in combination have been used to treat this condition, though the organism is resistant *in vitro*. Clindamycin, metronidazole or chloramphenicol are occasionally required.

PULMONARY HYPOPLASIA

Now the commonest pulmonary abnormality found at neonatal autopsy. May be caused by:

1. Oligohydramnios (renal agenesis, urinary tract obstruction, prolonged rupture of membranes)
2. Lung compression (diaphragmatic hernia, lung cysts, pleural effusions, erythroblastosis)
3. Absent fetal breathing (anencephaly, neuromuscular disorders)

For a description of Potter's syndrome see p. 306.

Presentation as asphyxia at birth, difficulty in resuscitation or respiratory distress from birth. Often develop pneumothoraces and respiratory failure. The lungs are very stiff and difficult to inflate and chest radiograph shows small lungs with a bell-shaped thorax. Sometimes mechanical ventilation with high pressures is successful in 'opening up' the lungs but surfactant replacement is unsuccessful. There is a high mortality and at autopsy the lung to body weight ratio is low, usually < 0.01. Confirmation of the diagnosis requires more sophisticated autopsy analysis with radial alveolar counts.

PULMONARY HAEMORRHAGE

The incidence of this condition is decreasing and is now most commonly seen in streptococcal pneumonia. About 5% of infants weighing less than 1500 g develop pulmonary haemorrhage. Other predisposing factors are:

1. Small for gestational age infant
2. Perinatal asphyxia
3. Hypothermia and acidosis
4. Severe erythroblastosis and exchange transfusion
5. Hypoglycaemia
6. Cardiac failure, especially left ventricular
7. Oxygen toxicity
8. Coagulation disorder

Underlying sepsis, acidosis and hypothermia should also be treated. The underlying problem may be disordered coagulation, though left ventricular failure has also been suggested as a cause.

Treatment consists of support of respiration and correction of coagulation disorder. Vitamin K and fresh blood transfusions should be given. It is possible to reduce the pulmonary bleeding by increasing peak and end-expiratory pressures to cause tamponade to pulmonary capillaries. It may be necessary to use pressures of 40–45 cmH_2O or greater to treat pulmonary haemorrhage successfully. Fresh blood or plasma transfusions help to correct the coagulation disorder.

BRONCHOPULMONARY DYSPLASIA (BPD)

The incidence of this chronic respiratory disorder is increasing (8% in infants <1500 g, or 20% of babies treated with IPPV).

Predisposing factors are:

1. Need for oxygen concentrations over 60% for 5 days or more
2. Positive pressure ventilation
3. Endotracheal intubation
4. Infection
5. Pulmonary interstitial emphysema
6. Patent ductus arteriosus and high fluid intake

With greater use of mechanical ventilation, infants who would have died are now surviving to develop bronchopulmonary dysplasia. Oxygen free radicals have been suggested as important aetiological factors. Clinically, affected babies have continued respiratory distress, 'wheezing', cyanosis and right heart failure. Prolonged ventilator dependency is a frequent presentation in the very low birth weight infant. Radiologically, four stages have been described but in severe cases there is pulmonary streaking, patchy over-inflation and emphysematous cysts (see p. 313). Bronchopulmonary dysplasia usually improves spontaneously as new alveoli may be generated for at least the first 7 years of life. There is a normal increase in alveolar number from 30 million at birth to 300 million at 7 years. Vitamin E in large doses (100 mg/day) has been used to prevent BPD but benefit is not proven (see also p. 281).

Treatment is largely symptomatic. Oxygen should be administered to keep arterial oxygen tension above 7 kPa (55 mmHg). Levels lower than this are associated with pulmonary vasoconstriction and right heart failure. During the exudative phase of bronchopulmonary dysplasia, physiotherapy with gentle suctioning of the airways is helpful. Good nutrition is essential for adequate lung growth and repair. Give vitamin E 10 mg daily in addition to usual vitamin supplements (p. 161). Diuretics and fluid restriction may be indicated in the presence

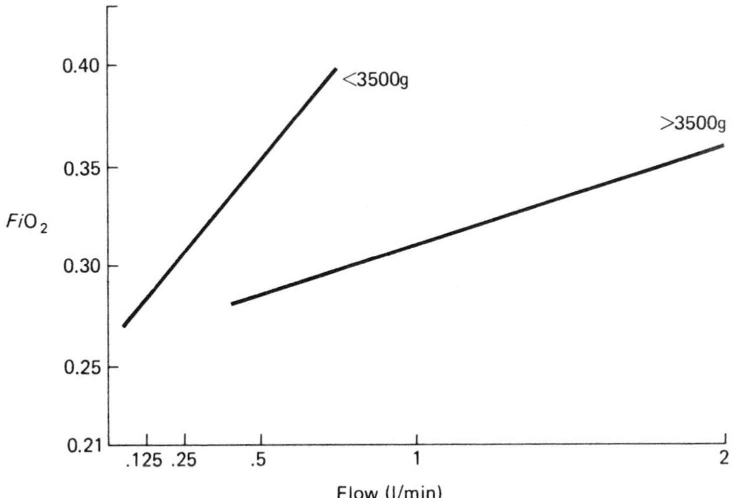

Fig. 46. Flow rates for nasal catheter for oxygen concentrations in infants with bronchopulmonary dysplasia. From Fan and Voyles (1983) with kind permission of the publishers C. V. Mosby.

of cor pulmonale. High-energy milks may help reduce fluid intake (see Table 40). Steroids have been used (dexamethasone, 0.5 mg/kg/day for 5–7 days) in an attempt to wean ventilator-dependent babies. Some acute improvement is found but long-term outlook is uncertain. Steroids may increase the risk of sepsis and gastric haemorrhage.

Most infants recover gradually, but some continue to have symptoms throughout infancy with frequent infections and hospital admissions. Domiciliary oxygen treatment allows earlier discharge from hospital and should reduce risks of developmental delay and costs. Oxygen may be given by nasal catheter (feeding tube) at very low flow rates (Fig. 46). This figure may be used to calculate flow rate to obtain the necessary inspired oxygen concentration but pulse oximeters help and may be used for home monitoring.

WILSON–MIKITY SYNDROME

This is a chronic pulmonary condition of the preterm infant that resembles bronchopulmonary dysplasia. Usually, however, there is no preceding severe RDS or need for IPPV and at about 7–10 days of age a gradually progressive form of respiratory distress develops.

There is indrawing of the chest, rising respiratory rate and slowly increasing oxygen need to about 30%. $P\text{CO}_2$ rises but there is a metabolic compensation and raised bicarbonate. Chest radiograph shows streaky infiltrates, increasing densities with cystic changes and later over-inflation.

This chronic condition tends to improve after 4–8 weeks.

Aetiology is uncertain though there are many theories: fluid retention from either excessive administration or chronic patent ductus arteriosus, mineral and vitamin deficiency (rickets), recurrent aspiration, chronic deficiency of surfactant causing alveolar instability (chronic pulmonary insufficiency of the premature, CPIP), and instability of the chest wall in the very immature infant.

Treatment should be aimed at maintaining normal blood gases with added oxygen and continuous positive airways pressure to stabilize the alveoli if necessary. Fluid restriction and diuretics may be helpful but adequate intake of protein, calories, trace elements and vitamins should be ensured.

In most cases the disease is self-limiting but some infants progress to terminal respiratory failure with worsening emphysema.

PERSISTENT FETAL CIRCULATION (PULMONARY HYPERTENSION)

With persistent pulmonary hypertension there is R–L shunting of blood across the ductus arteriosus and foramen ovale. After the first few hours of life this is abnormal and persistent fetal circulation (PFC) is said to be present (see p. 234). Pulmonary hypertension in the newborn is poorly understood but may be of primary or secondary type.

Primary type. The pulmonary capillaries and arterioles are thickened. This has been associated with constriction of the ductus arteriosus *in utero* from maternal ingestion of aspirin or indomethacin. Chronic intrauterine hypoxia has the same effect (we have seen an infant with persistent fetal circulation whose mother had Eisenmenger syndrome).

Secondary type. The causes of secondary pulmonary hypertension are:

1. Severe asphyxia: hypoxaemia, acidosis
2. Severe RDS
3. Severe meconium aspiration
4. Severe form of TTN
5. Diaphragmatic hernia
6. Some forms of bacterial pneumonia, e.g. listeriosis, group B streptococcus
7. Bronchopulmonary dysplasia
8. Pneumothorax
9. Polycythaemia, hypoglycaemia, hypocalcaemia

In secondary pulmonary hypertension the chest radiograph has the appearance of the underlying condition. In primary pulmonary hypertension lung fields are clear, with hyperinflation and cardiomegaly.

The diagnosis of pulmonary hypertension is often difficult. The infant presents with respiratory distress and cyanosis, the liver may be enlarged and hypoxaemia is usually profound, suggesting cyanotic heart disease. Myocardial dysfunction is often associated with PFC secondary to hypoxia, acidosis or hypoglycaemia.

Differential arterial blood gas sampling will reveal R–L shunt across the ductus arteriosus. The $P\text{O}_2$ of blood from the lower aorta (post-ductus) will be lower than that of the right radial artery (pre-ductus). The size of R–L shunt may be calculated from the values in Fig. 45 (see p. 135). In severe pulmonary hypertension there may be a large shunt across the foramen ovale which masks the shunt across the ductus. Echocardiography provides a useful non-invasive method of assessing pulmonary pressure (see Appendix VI).

Therapy first to correct underlying problem.

Hypoxaemia and acidosis are treated by hyperventilation (described in Chapter 9) and bicarbonate infusions. Condition often dramatically improves once alkalosis is achieved (pH over 7.45). Muscle relaxants (curare) may be needed to achieve this alkalosis. Curare dose of 0.3 mg/kg repeated as necessary. Hypoglycaemia and polycythaemia should be corrected by dextrose infusion and partial plasma exchange.

Tolazoline (Priscol) is a pulmonary vasodilating drug (α-adrenergic blocker). The dose is 1–2 mg/kg as a bolus followed by 1–2 mg/kg/hour if there is satisfactory response. The drug should be infused in isotonic saline or 5% dextrose through a scalp vein. Tolazoline also dilates the systemic circulation and may cause hypotension. Also has a histamine-like action and may cause gastrointestinal bleeding. Hypotension may be prevented by plasma volume expansion with blood, plasma or albumin and tolazoline should not be given if bleeding disorder present. The response is measured by blood gas analysis 10 min after the bolus dose (pulse oximeter) or by echocardiography. Cutaneous flush is usually seen in responding infants.

Infants with pulmonary hypertension may suddenly improve with $P_a\text{O}_2$ increasing from 5 to 20 kPa (40 to 150 mmHg). Do not enthusiastically lower ventilation or oxygen concentration. Caution is required because these infants may 'flip-flop'; this is a sudden fall in $P_a\text{O}_2$ upon reduction of ventilation or oxygen concentration and is thought to be due to increased reactivity of pulmonary circulation to oxygen and hydrogen ion concentrations. Once initial improvement is seen, parameters of ventilation (rate, pressure or both) and oxygen concentration should be cautiously lowered using the rule of twos, e.g. oxygen concentration lowered by 2%, peak pressure by a maximum of 2 cmH_2O, etc. Dopamine can be used to treat PFC associated with myocardial dysfunction and hypotension. Dose 5–10 μg/kg/min as infusion (see p. 349).

UPPER AIRWAY OBSTRUCTION

May cause problems soon after birth (p. 28).

Choanal Atresia

Uncommon, but as newborns are obligate nose breathers, respiratory distress from birth relieved only by crying. Insert a small oropharyngeal airway. Occasionally, endotracheal intubation is needed. Surgery should be electively performed by an experienced ENT surgeon.

Pierre Robin Syndrome

Triad of micrognathia, midline cleft palate and glossoptosis. May present with acute airway obstruction as tongue falls back. Insert a small oropharyngeal airway to push tongue forward. Intubation can be difficult. Surgery at a later date by an experienced maxillofacial surgeon.

Congenital Laryngeal Stridor

Usually due to laryngomalacia but occasionally to laryngeal webs or cysts, and vascular rings. Should have laryngoscopy to exclude the latter. If laryngomalacia, spontaneous improvement usually occurs. Very occasionally tracheostomy is needed.

Subglottic Stenosis

May be congenital or acquired. Latter due to prolonged endotracheal intubation, especially if tube is too big. Incidence of 1% of ventilated babies needing tracheostomy. Recently, minor surgery to split the cricoid cartilage has been advocated as an alternative to tracheostomy. Dilatation of narrowed segment at intervals by an experienced ENT surgeon.

NURSING POINTS

1. Care of the ventilated baby (see Chapter 9)
2. Remember that muscle relaxation makes tube care and over-handling hazardous. Increased vigilance for these babies
3. Babies with persistent fetal circulation need minimal handling and avoidance of invasive procedures like tube suctioning if possible
4. Big babies with meconium aspiration syndrome may appear deceptively well before they deteriorate. They need careful observations and minimal handling
5. Babies with early onset streptococcal pneumonia may be well at birth and later develop tachypnoea before collapsing. Watch out for these babies in transitional care nurseries and postnatal wards
6. Babies at risk for pneumothorax (p. 143), especially those on a ventilator with pulmonary interstitial emphysema or needing high peak pressures should be carefully monitored. Syringe with three-way tap and scalp vein needle (19 or 21 guage) should be readily available to drain chest in an emergency (p. 92)

REFERENCES AND FURTHER READING

Avery, M. E., Fletcher, B. D. and Williams, R. G. (1981). *The Lung and its Disorders in the Newborn Infant*, 4th edn. Philadelphia: W. B. Saunders.

Brooks, J. G., Bustanente, S. A., Koops, B. L. *et al.* (1977). Selective bronchial intubation for the treatment of localised PIE in newborn infants. *J. Pediatr.* **91**: 648.

Collaborative European Multicentre Study Group (1988). Surfactant replacement therapy in severe neonatal respiratory distress syndrome; an international randomized clinical trial. *Pediatrics* **82**: 683.

Fan, L. L. and Voyles, J. B. (1983). Determination of inspired oxygen delivered by nasal cannula in infants with chronic lung disease. *J. Pediatr.* **103**: 923.

Fujiwara, T., Maeta, H., Chida, S. *et al.* (1980). Artificial surfactant therapy in hyaline membrane disease. *Lancet* **i**: 55.

Goodwin, S. R., Graves, S. A. and Haberkern, C. M. (1985). Aspiration in intubated premature infants. *Pediatrics* **75**: 85.

Halliday, H. L. (1980). Measurement of ventricular systolic time intervals in the normal and ill newborn by M-mode echocardiography. In: *Fetal and Neonatal Physiological Measurements* (ed., Rolfe, P.). London: Pitman Medical.

Halliday, H. L. and Hirata, T. (1979). Perinatal listeriosis - a review of twelve patients. *Am. J. Obstet. Gynecol.* **133**: 405.

Halliday, H. L., Hirata, T. and Brady, J. P. (1980). Effects of inspired oxygen on echocardiographic assessment of pulmonary vascular resistance and myocardial contractility in bronchopulmonary dysplasia. *Pediatrics* **65**: 536.

Halliday, H. L., McClure, G. and Reid, M. Mc. C. (1981). Transient tachypnoea of the newborn: two distinct clinical entities? *Arch. Dis. Child* **56**: 322.

Harvey, D., Parkinson, C. E. and Campbell, S. (1975). Risk of respiratory distress syndrome. *Lancet* i: 42.

Howie, R. N. and Liggins, G. C. (1977). Clinical trial of antepartum betamethasone therapy for prevention of respiratory distress in preterm infants. In: *Preterm Labour* (eds, Anderson *et al.*). London: RCOG.

Lupton, B. A., Halliday, H. L., Thomas, P. S., McClure, B. G. and Reid, M. Mc. C. (1987). Chronic lung disease in a neonatal intensive care unit: eight year's experience. *Ir. Med. J.* **80**: 254.

Macklin, C. C. (1939). Transport of air along sheaths of pulmonic blood vessels from alveoli to mediastinum. *Arch. Intern. Med.* **64**: 913.

McCord, F. B., Curstedt, T., Halliday, H. L. *et al.* (1988). Surfactant treatment and the incidence of intraventricular haemorrhage in severe respiratory distress syndrome. *Arch. Dis. Child* **63**: 10.

Ramsey, G. (1985). Nursing the sick neonate. *Care Critic. Ill* **6**: 7.

Roberton, N. R. C. (1983). The care of neonates with respiratory failure. In: *Recent Advances in Perinatal Medicine*, No. 1 (ed., Chiswick, M. L.). Edinburgh: Churchill Livingstone.

Ten Centre Study Group (1987). Ten centre trial of artificial surfactant (artificial lung expanding compound) in very premature babies. *Br. Med. J.* **294**: 991.

Thibeault, D. W., Beatty, E. C., Hall, R. T. *et al.* (1985). Neonatal pulmonary hypoplasia with premature rupture of fetal membranes and oligohydramnios. *J. Pediatr.* **107**: 273.

Whittle, M. J., Wilson, A. I., Whitfield, C. R. *et al.* (1982). Amniotic fluid phosphatidyl glycerol and the lecithin/sphingomyelin ratio in the assessment of fetal lung maturity. *Br. J. Obstet. Gynaecol.* **89**: 727.

11. Fluids and Nutrition

The fluid requirements of the newborn increase during the first week of life (Table 37). Intake should be balanced against losses, both renal and insensible. Insensible water losses are very high for the preterm infant (up to 50 ml/kg/day) and are further increased by use of radiant warmers and phototherapy.

Intravenous fluids are usually required in the following circumstances:

1. Very low birth weight infant
2. Severe RDS
3. Surgical conditions
4. Hypoglycaemia
5. Infants with other serious disease, e.g. septicaemia

Ten per cent dextrose in water is usual starting fluid. After 24 hours, electrolytes should be added unless very immature baby who may develop hypernatraemia (p. 296). There is no obligatory sodium requirement in the first 24 hours as GFR is low and urine volume small (30 ml/kg) (see Chapter 19). For these infants it is important to monitor serum electrolytes every 8–12 hours and increase fluid intake. Sodium needs remain low for

Table 37. Fluid and energy requirements.

	Volume (ml/kg)		*Energy*	
Day	*Incubator*	*Radiant warmer*	kcal/kg	kJ/kg
1	50–80	80–100	40–50	167–209
2	80–100	100–120	50–70	209–293
3	100–120	120–140	70–90	293–376
4	120–150	140–160	90–110	376–460
5	150	160–180	110–120*	460–502

* Energy needs are made up as follows:

resting expenditure	50 (209)	specific dynamic action	8 (33)
intermittent activity	15 (63)	faecal loss	12 (50)
occasional stress	10 (42)	growth allowance	25 (104)

the first 3 days because of isotonic loss of sodium and water; after this 4–6 mmol/kg/day may be needed although some babies with very immature renal tubular sodium conservation may need 8–12 mmol/kg/day. Also, some very immature infants do not tolerate 10% dextrose and develop hyperglycaemia, glycosuria and dehydration. Glucose strip test measurements and urine testing should be performed on all preterm infants having intravenous fluids. If glucose strip test reads over 8 mmol/l (150 mg/dl) or glycosuria (over +) occurs then 5% dextrose should be substituted.

Fluid retention may occur in sick babies causing oedema. Excessive fluid intake or bicarbonate boluses may be responsible but infants with poor renal function due to RDS or asphyxia or those with inappropriate ADH secretion (p. 175) are also at risk. Preterm infants often have hypoalbuminaemia which may exacerbate the peripheral oedema. Excessive fluid intake has been incriminated in the pathogenesis of persistent ductus arteriosus (PDA), bronchopulmonary dysplasia (BPD), pulmonary haemorrhage and necrotizing enterocolitis (NEC). Treatment by fluid restriction to 50–60 ml/kg/day and diuretic (frusemide, 1 mg/kg) is usually effective.

Approximate daily requirements of electrolytes are listed in Table 38. These recommendations for minimal needs are rough guides so always check serum electrolytes, weight and urine output, and specific gravity each day before ordering fluids. Normal urinary output given in Table 92 (see p. 256). In calculating fluid intake take note of electrolytes and water from other sources: sodium and chloride in catheter-flushing solutions, sodium bicarbonate therapy and electrolytes in amino acid

Table 38. Daily requirements of minerals.

Sodium	2–4 mmol/kg
Chloride	2–4 mmol/kg
Potassium*	1–3 mmol/kg
Calcium	2–3 mmol/kg
Magnesium	0.25 mmol/kg
Phosphorus	2–3 mmol/kg

* Caution with reduced urine output

solutions. Some antibiotics contain potassium and sodium (Table 39).

Table 39. Sodium content of some injectable antibiotics.

Antibiotic	*Sodium* (mmol/100 mg antibiotic)	*Max. daily dose of antibiotic* (mg/kg)	*Daily sodium intake on max. dose* (mmol/kg)
Amoxycillin	0.26	200	0.52
Ampicillin	0.27	200	0.54
Benzylpenicillin	0.28	150	0.42
Cefotaxime	0.21	100	0.21
Ceftazidime	0.23	60	0.14
Cefuroxime	0.22	100	0.22
Cloxacillin	0.21	150	0.31
Flucloxacillin	0.23	150	0.34
Mezlocillin	0.17	150	0.25
Ticarcillin	0.47	150	0.70

ORAL FEEDING

Some groups of infants should be fed early to reduce the likelihood of hypoglycaemia:

1. Small for gestational age infants
2. Well preterm infants
3. Infants of diabetic mothers
4. All large infants (over 3.8 kg)

In general, the well preterm infant should be fed within 2 hours of birth. Expressed breast milk is the best food if available. Donated breast milk is not now used because of the slight risk of transmission of AIDS. For infants over 1500 g one could start with 3 ml/kg/feed every 2 hours and amount of gastric aspirate checked before each successive feed. Feedings can be increased by 1 ml/feed up to a maximum of 20 ml and thereafter the infant may be fed 3 hourly. If gastric residue between feeds is over 2 ml then it should be replaced in the stomach and the next feed reduced by the same amount. Table 40 shows the

Table 40. Constituents of milk.

	Protein * (g/100 ml)	*Energy* kcal/100 ml	kJ/100 ml	*Ca*	*P*	*Na*†	*K*	*Fe*
				mmol/100 ml				
Fresh breast milk	1.2–1.5	65–75	272–313	0.9	0.5	0.8–1.2	1.5	0.001–0.003
Bank breast milk	1.0	50–60	209–251	0.8	0.5	0.6	1.5	0.001
Cow and Gate Premium	1.5	68	284	1.4	1.3	1.0	1.5	0.01
Cow and Gate Plus	1.9	65	272	1.6	1.7	1.3	2.2	0.01
Prematalac	2.4	79	330	1.7	1.7	2.7	2.4	0.01
Prematil	2.0	70	298	2.0	1.2	1.5	2.0	0.001
Aptamil	1.5	67	281	1.4	1.2	0.9	2.3	0.01
SMA LBW	2.0	80	334	1.9	1.3	1.4	1.9	0.01
SMA gold cap	1.5	65	272	1.1	1.1	0.7	1.4	0.01
Osterprem	2.0	80	334	1.8	1.2	2.0	1.6	0.001
Cow's milk	3.3	65	272	3.1	3.1	2.5	3.6	0.002
Nenatal	1.8	76	318	2.5	1.6	0.9	1.5	0.01

* Nitrogen content of milk produced by mothers of 28–30 weeks' gestation is 30% higher than at term

† Preterm breast milk may contain more sodium than that from term mothers

constituents of various forms of milk. Note that banked breast milk has a lower energy value than fresh breast milk because of reduced fat content. Energy value of breast milk is proportional to fat content. To avoid loss of supernatant fat, use fresh breast milk that has been shaken gently before use. If orogastric perfusion is to be used place pump below baby with nozzle pointing up. *Certain drugs are excreted in breast milk* in amounts that may be hazardous to the newborn (see Appendix XVII). If mother is taking any of these drugs she should *not breast feed* or her milk should not be used to feed premature babies.

Collection of Breast Milk

Mothers of all infants of 32 weeks and less should be encouraged to express breast milk manually into sterile containers. This milk may be fed fresh to her newborn, or after culture if risk of contamination is great. If breast milk contains any coliforms, haemolytic streptococci or *Staphylococcus aureus*, then the milk is not used. Cultures of diphtheroids or *Staphylococcus albus* are permissible provided the growth is not heavy ($<10^3$/ml). Manual expression of breast milk is preferred to pump as contamination of milk is less.

Methods of Feeding

Orogastric feeding is better than nasogastric as less obstruction to airway. Continuous feeding may be preferred to intermittent or bolus feeding in the very low birth weight infant, enterohumoral responses are blunted. Start at 1 ml/hour and check gastric aspirates every 2 hours.

If infant becomes active then intermittent orogastric feeding is better as tube less likely to be pulled out by baby causing aspiration. However, it can alter ventilation and lower arterial oxygen tensions.

Orojejunal feeding used when risk of aspiration is high, e.g. for infants on ventilators or those with chronic lung disease. Silastic tube is passed into stomach and through pylorus (infant on right side): check pH of secretions (pH >5.0) and verify position by radiography. We do not routinely take radiographs for tube position but examine the next film taken for other indications (see Nursing Points). It is usually safe to feed after the tube has been passed for 4 hours. Higher volume feeds are possible but necrotizing enterocolitis remains a risk although this has not been our experience. Since adoption of this technique there has been improved outcome for ventilated infants. We now advocate use of transpyloric feeding early in the course of the ventilated very low birth weight infant (about second or third day).

Vitamin Supplements

Routine vitamin supplementation of low birth weight infant probably unnecessary provided one of the newer proprietary milks is used (p. 159). Very low birth weight infant and breast-fed infant may need extra vitamin D provided using a multivitamin preparation. For instance, each 0.6 ml of Abidec (use dropper) contains:

Vitamin A	5000 units
Vitamin C	50 mg
Vitamin D	400 units
Vitamin B_1	1 mg
Vitamin B_2	0.4 mg
Vitamin B_6	0.5 mg
Nicotinamide	5 mg

Children's vitamin drops contain in each 1 ml (35 drops):

Vitamin A	5000 units
Vitamin C	150 units
Vitamin D	2000 units

The very low birth weight infant may need 800–1600 units of vitamin D daily because of poor absorption and this is provided without supplying more than 10 000 units of vitamin A daily (use vitamin D alone).

Rickets in Preterm

Probably not a single entity but comprises frank rickets, osteopenia, phosphate depletion and perhaps vitamin D deficiency. More common now because of increased survival of small babies. Babies at risk:

1. <1200 g birth weight
2. SGA <10th percentile
3. Prolonged jaundice
4. Prolonged parenteral nutrition
5. Associated chronic lung disease
6. Fed expressed breast milk (phosphate depletion)
7. Rapid growth

Check alkaline phosphatase at 2 weeks of age and take radiograph of wrist if alkaline phosphatase > 750 iu or evidence of marked bone demineralization on chest radiographs. Also check serum calcium and phosphate. Start 1α-hydroxyvitamin D supplements (dose 0.05 μg/kg/day) and at same time ensure adequate intake of calcium and phosphate (Table 38). Phosphate supplements do not prevent osteopenia. Vitamin E requirements are discussed on p. 281.

Iron Supplementation

Elemental iron (2 mg/kg/day) is provided to all infants of gestation less than 36 weeks. Ideally, this iron should not be started until the infant is 8 weeks old because serum iron and ferritin levels are high after birth and transferrin may be fully saturated which reduces its bacteriostatic effects (see p. 281). Normal values for haemoglobin and iron status during the first year are shown in Table 106 (see p. 279).

PARENTERAL NUTRITION

Main indications:

1. Severe RDS
2. Most infants <1200 g

3. Necrotizing enterocolitis
4. Surgical conditions

Aim is to provide balanced mixture of carbohydrate, amino acids, fat, electrolytes and vitamins.

In small infants and those with RDS, parenteral nutrition usually begun on day 2.

Carbohydrate

Give as 10% dextrose (100 g/l). Glucose requirements 9–12 g/kg/day. Start with 80 ml/kg/day and increase to 150 ml/kg/day over 7 days, avoiding hyperglycaemia. 150 ml/kg/day of 10% dextrose = 15 g glucose/kg/day = 60 kcal/kg/day (250 kJ/kg/day).

Amino Acids

Given as Vamin or Vamin Newborn, which contains: amino acids, 70 g/l; sodium, 50 mmol/l; potassium, 20 mmol/l. Vamin glucose contains 100 g glucose/l. Start with 14 ml/kg/day (1 g/kg/day) and increase by 7 ml/kg/day to maximum of 33 ml/kg/day by day 4. This will give positive nitrogen balance. Do not increase amino acid infusion if high blood urea or metabolic acidosis. Up to 3.5 g/kg/day may be used if these complications are absent. Amino acid infusions have been associated with transient abnormalities in hepatic function (raised direct bilirubin and transaminases).

33 ml/kg/day of Vamin will provide 2.5 g amino acid/kg/day = 10 kcal/kg/day (4.2 kJ/kg/day).

Fat

Provides high energy food (9 kcal/g; 38 kJ/g) and essential fatty acids, given as 'Intralipid 10%'. Also contains phosphorus supplying about 0.12 mmol/kg/day (3.5 mg).

Contraindications are:

1. High serum bilirubin
2. Liver disease
3. Severe pulmonary disease
4. Coagulation disorder or low platelet count
5. Sepsis

'Intralipid 10%' provides 1.1 kcal/ml (4.6 kJ/ml). Start with 5 ml/kg/day infused over 20 hours.

Check supernatant for turbidity 2 hours after infusion. If supernatant clear, increase to 10 ml/kg/day and so on to a maximum of 20 ml/kg/day.

20 ml/kg/day of Intralipid 10% will provide 22 kcal/kg/day (92 kJ/kg/day).

Vitlipid is given simultaneously to provide fat soluble vitamins (1 ml/kg/day; see below).

INTRALIPID MUST NOT BE MIXED WITH ANY OTHER INFUSATE (p. 101)

Stop Intralipid if supernatant is turbid or if the infant's clinical condition deteriorates.

Electrolytes

Table 38 shows daily requirements of minerals but individual infant should have daily needs calculated after examining serum electrolytes, and serum calcium and magnesium.

Requirements of *magnesium* are not accurately known so supplements are not given unless the serum level is low or seizures present.

Some *phosphate* will be provided in the fat solution. Serum phosphate is usually high for first few days so supplementation should be cautious in the first week.

Electrolytes are conveniently given as 'Ped-El' (4 ml/kg/day). Each 1 ml of 'Ped-El' contains:

Ca^{2+}	0.15 mmol
Mg^{2+}	25 μmol
Fe^{3+}	0.5 μmol
Zn^{2+}	0.15 μmol
Cu^{2+}	0.075 μmol
F^-	0.75 μmol

I^-	0.01 μmol
P	75 μmol
Cl^-	0.35 mmol

Trace elements are also provided in this solution.

Vitamins

Fat soluble. Give 1 ml/kg/day of infant Vitlipid N with the fat emulsion. Each 1 ml of Vitlipid N contains:

Vitamin A	69 μg
Vitamin D	1 μg
Vitamin E	0.64 μg
Vitamin K	20 μg
Fractionated soya bean oil	100 mg
Fractionated egg phospholipids	12 mg
Glycerol	22.5 mg

Water soluble. Give 0.5 ml/kg/day 'Solivito' with the amino acid and glucose solution. Each 0.5 ml of Solivito contains:

Vitamin B_1	1.2 mg
Vitamin B_2	1.8 mg
Nicotinamide	10 mg
Vitamin B_6	2 mg
Pantothenic acid	10 mg
Biotin	0.3 mg
Folic acid	0.2 mg
Vitamin B_{12}	2 μg
Vitamin C	30 mg

Trace Elements

It is unlikely that deficiency will occur if intravenous feeding is required for less than 1 week. However, supplements are given in the form of 'Ped-El' (see above).

Trace elements are also provided in blood or plasma transfusions which most ill infants receive during the first week of life. Normal serum values of copper and zinc during the first year of life are shown in Table 41.

Table 41. Serum copper and zinc levels during the first year: preterm infants.

	Serum copper		*Serum zinc*	
Postnatal age (weeks)	μmol/l	μg/ml	μmol/l	μg/ml
Birth	5.2	0.33	15.8	1.03
3	7.5	0.48	13.0	0.85
6	9.6	0.61	11.5	0.75
9	12.1	0.77	10.9	0.71
12	12.1	0.77	11.9	0.78
15	12.9	0.82	14.1	0.92
24	15.7	1.00	15.6	1.02
36	17.9	1.14	17.9	1.17
52	19.0	1.21	18.2	1.19

Technique (see p. 101)

Monitoring of Parenteral Nutrition

Daily or more frequently:

Glucose strip test: 6 hourly
Urine glucose: 6 hourly
Haematocrit and examine supernatant for lipaemia
Electrolytes and urea

Weekly or more frequently:

Calcium, phosphate, magnesium
Alkaline phosphatase
Protein electrophoresis
Transaminases
Blood culture

Problems with Parenteral Nutrition

These are not uncommon and monitoring above is aimed at early detection of some of them:

1. Bacteraemia, especially *Staphylococcus albus*
2. Systemic candidiasis
3. Local vascular complications, e.g. phlebitis
4. Extravasation and necrosis of skin
5. Cholestatic jaundice
6. Fat embolism
7. Immune suppression
8. In practice difficult to reach full energy needs

Osmolality of Fluids

The osmolality of a solution is a measure of the solute concentration per unit of solvent (the number of dissolved

Table 42. Osmolality of fluids.

Fluid	*Osmolality* (mosmol/kg water)
5% dextrose	280
5% dextrose in N/5 saline	350
10% dextrose	555
10% dextrose/$NaHCO_3$ (1:1 mixture)	1100
25% dextrose	1400
8.4% sodium bicarbonate	1900
Breast milk	280–300
Cow and Gate Premium	290
Cow and Gate Plus	300
Prematalac	342
Prematil	350
Aptamil	305
SMA LBW	268
SMA gold cap	272
Osterprem	300
Cow's milk	300–400
Nenatal	340
Nutramigen	484
Pregestimil	338
Sobee	224

particles). The unit of osmolality is the osmol which is the atomic weight of the solute divided by the number of particles exerting osmotic pressure. The normal osmolality of the serum is 270–280 mosmol/kg and may be calculated as follows:

$$(1.86 \times \text{sodium}) + \text{glucose (mmol/l)} + \text{urea (mmol/l)}$$

Table 42 gives the osmolality of the various intravenous and oral fluids.

Dextrose solutions of 10% and stronger, bicarbonate infusions, cow's milk, Nutramigen and Pregestimil are all hyperosmolar solutions. Infusions of undiluted bicarbonate and dextrose must be avoided as high osmolality of these fluids causes damage to vascular endothelium and necrosis. High osmolality milks have been linked with necrotizing enterocolitis and so should be avoided in the preterm infant.

NURSING POINTS

1. Feeding of preterm babies has been discussed in Chapter 7
2. Encourage mother to express breast milk, instructing her to collect it in sterile containers; manually expressed milk is less likely to be contaminated than using pump
3. Passing a jejunal tube:
    - (a) Measure jejunal tube from lips to stomach and add 8 cm; mark with tape
    - (b) Place baby on right side and pass tube through mouth into stomach; aspirate to obtain acid reaction
    - (c) Leave for 30 min before continuing to pass tube 2 cm every 30 min until mark has been reached
    - (d) Tape firmly in position
    - (e) Aspirate tube to check for alkaline reaction
    - (f) If possible leave for 12 hours before starting feeds; sometimes we would feed earlier than this provided there is no contraindication to giving milk intragastrically. Earlier feeding may help tube to pass through pylorus
    - (g) Radiography may be delayed until next radiograph is indicated for clinical reasons
4. Intravenous fluid volumes should be checked by nurse and

rate in ml/hour calculated. Syringe pumps or drip counters are used to deliver fluids; take care that extravasation does not occur by examining cannula site at least hourly

5. Make sure parenteral nutrition packs are connected up using aseptic technique; gown, gloves and mask
6. If central line is used for parenteral nutrition make sure that it is never broken to administer intravenous drugs; even with peripheral cannula breaking the line for drugs should be avoided unless there is no alternative. Babies on parenteral nutrition need at least one other intravenous line for drug administration

REFERENCES AND FURTHER READING

Baron, D. N., Hamilton-Miller, J. M. T. and Brumfitt, W. (1984). Sodium content of injectable beta-lactam antibiotics. *Lancet* **i**: 1113.

Benda, G. I. M. (1979). Modes of feeding low birth weight infants. *Semin. Perinatol.* **3**: 407.

Bentur, L., Alon, U. and Berant, M. (1987). Bone and mineral homeostasis in the preterm infant: a review. *Pediatr. Rev. Commun.* **1**: 291.

Committee on the Nutrition of the Preterm Infant. European Society of Paediatric Gastroenterology and Nutrition (1987). *Nutrition and Feeding of Preterm Infants*. Oxford: Blackwell Scientific Publications.

Dancis, J., O'Connell, J. and Holt, L. (1948). Grid for recording weight of premature infants. *J. Pediatr.* **33**: 570.

Doyle, L. W. and Sinclair, J. C. (1982). Insensible water loss in newborn infants. *Clin. Perinatol.* **9**: 453.

Gross, S. J. (1983). Growth and biochemical response of preterm infants fed human milk or modified infant formula. *N. Engl. J. Med.* **308**: 237.

Gross, S. J., David, R. J., Bauman, L. and Tomarelli, R. M. (1980). Nutritional composition of milk produced by mothers delivering preterm. *J. Pediatr.* **96**: 641.

Lucas, A. (1984). Hormone, nutrition and the gut. In: *Neonatal Gastroenterology: Contemporary Issues* (eds, Tanner, M. S. and Stocks, R. J.). Newcastle upon Tyne: Intercept.

McMaster, D., Lappin, T. R. J., Halliday, H. L. and Patterson, C. C. (1983). Serum copper and zinc levels in the preterm infant. A longitudinal study of the first year of life. *Biol. Neonate* **44**: 108.

Raiha, N. C. R. (1985). Nutritional proteins in milk and the protein requirement of normal infants. *Pediatrics* **75**: 136.

Rowe, J. C. and Carey, D. E. (1987). Phosphorus deficiency syndrome in very low birth weight infants. *Pediatr. Clin. North Am.* **34**: 997.

Shaw, J. C. L. (1973). Parenteral nutrition in the management of sick low birth weight infants. *Pediatr. Clin. North Am.* **20**: 333.

Shaw, J. C. L. (1988). Growth and nutrition of the very preterm infant. *Br. Med. Bull.* **44**: 984.

Sunshine, P. (1980). Feeding the neonate weighing less than 1500 grams - nutrition and beyond. *Report of 79th Ross Conference on Pediatric Research*. Columbus, Ohio: Ross Laboratories.

12. Glucose, Calcium and Electrolyte Disturbances

Glucose, calcium and electrolyte values for the first few days of life may vary, with low or high levels being found. Low glucose, calcium and sodium levels may cause apnoea and seizures.

GLUCOSE METABOLISM

Glucose is the major energy source of the fetus, crossing the placenta from maternal serum by facilitated diffusion. At birth the maternal source of glucose is lost and the newborn must try to maintain blood sugar from endogenous sources until feeding has been established. The newborn's blood glucose at birth is the same as umbilical venous blood or about 70% of maternal blood levels. After birth, blood glucose level will fall from about 4 mmol/l (70 mg/dl)to between 2 and 3 mmol/l (40 and 50 mg/dl) (see Fig. 1). The reason for this fall is that glucose produced from the breakdown of glycogen in the liver and from gluconeogenesis is insufficient to maintain blood glucose at fetal levels. When feeding is started (2–4 hours of age), blood glucose will slowly rise to 4–5 mmol/l (70–80 mg/dl).

Hypoglycaemia

Hypoglycaemia is defined as a blood glucose level below 1.5 mmol/l (25 mg/dl) in the first 24 hours of life and below 2 mmol/l (40 mg/dl) thereafter. This definition varies from unit to unit and recent evidence suggests that lower levels than those quoted above should not be used because cerebral function is affected. Blood glucose measurements may be made on whole blood in the laboratory, or on capillary blood at the cotside using a variety of glucose strip test methods. Capillary blood samples give lower readings and may be influenced by the method used. If Dextrostix (Ames Co.) is used, a reflectometer gives more accurate measurements; otherwise BM stix (Boehringer) may be more accurate.

Symptomatic hypoglycaemia may cause cerebral damage.

Causes of hypoglycaemia are:

1. Depleted glycogen stores:
   Small for gestational age baby
   Preterm baby
   Delayed feeding
   Chronic asphyxia
   Hypothermia
2. Fetal hyperinsulinaemia:
   Infant of diabetic mother (IDM)
   Severe rhesus isoimmunization
   Beckwith's syndrome
   Nesidioblastosis
3. Others:
   Adrenal insufficiency, exchange transfusion, sepsis, congenital heart disease, galactosaemia

Infants in the first group (e.g. small for gestation) will present with hypoglycaemia at about 2–4 hours of age lasting for 48 hours or longer. Glucose strip test should be checked 3 hourly for 48 hours until feeding has been well-established and glucose levels stable. With fetal hyperinsulinaemia (IDM) increased peripheral utilization of glucose occurs with hypoglycaemia at about 30 min after birth (see Fig. 1). These infants need glucose strip test checked at birth and at 30 min of age (see p. 14). Asymptomatic hypoglycaemia in IDM is relatively common (50%).

Symptoms are lethargy, apnoea, seizures, cyanosis, heart failure.

Treatment

In the newborn, glucose probably forms the main source of energy for brain growth and metabolism. It is possible, however, that ketone bodies and fatty acids may also be utilized by the brain. This may explain asymptomatic hypoglycaemia in the newborn. Blood glucose levels below 1.4 mmol/l (25 mg/dl) should be rapidly corrected, usually by giving intravenous dextrose as 10% solution.

Hepatic output of glucose which is equivalent to glucose

requirement is 6–8 mg/kg/min: 3 ml/kg of 10% dextrose = 300 mg/kg = 40 min requirements.

Once hypoglycaemia has been corrected by infusion of a bolus of glucose, a constant source of glucose must be maintained either by 10% dextrose infusion or by feeding soon afterwards. Failure will lead to rebound hypoglycaemia requiring further dextrose.

In some infants, however, glucose requirements may be greater than 8 mg/kg/min (some small-for-dates infants or some with hyperinsulinaemia or infants with adrenal insufficiency). In these infants, 15–20% dextrose solutions may be given by a central catheter into a large vein.

Very occasionally, it is necessary to use glucagon (300 μg/kg), adrenaline or hydrocortisone to correct intractable hypoglycaemia.

Sequelae of hypoglycaemia

Asymptomatic hypoglycaemia probably does not cause cerebral damage but there is uncertainty. If blood glucose levels stay below 1.1 mmol/l (20 mg/dl) then seizures will occur and at follow up about 30% of these babies will have neurological problems such as cerebral palsy or impaired intellect.

Hyperglycaemia

This is defined as a blood sugar greater than 8 mmol/l (150 mg/dl). It may occur in preterm infant who is having intravenous 10% dextrose or parenteral nutrition. May be an early sign of sepsis. Rarely transient neonatal diabetes.

Reduce dextrose infusion from 10 to 5% and later reduce rate of infusion if blood glucose remains high.

Occasionally, insulin is required to treat this problem, the dose being 0.1 unit/kg of soluble insulin intravenously and repeated as necessary.

CALCIUM AND MAGNESIUM METABOLISM

Calcium, phosphorus and magnesium levels are higher in the fetus than the mother. There is active transport of these minerals against a gradient enabling the fetus to grow. After birth the uptake is interrupted and serum calcium and magnesium levels will fall. In the newborn there is deficient parathyroid response to hypocalcaemia because persistent fetal hypercalcaemia leads to parathyroid suppression. Also, increased serum phosphate as a result of reduced renal excretion exacerbates the hypocalcaemia. Spontaneous increase in parathormone occurs after 3 days.

There is a complex interrelationship between serum magnesium and serum calcium. Hypomagnesaemia is usually accompanied by hypocalcaemia and both may be corrected by the administration of magnesium sulphate.

The normal calcium level in the newborn is 1.8–2.2 mmol/l. Normal magnesium level is 0.6–1.6 mmol/l.

Hypocalcaemia

Early hypocalcaemia occurs within the first 72 hours of life in:

1. Preterm infants
2. RDS
3. Asphyxia
4. Infants of diabetic mothers (IDM)
5. Sepsis

Late hypocalcaemia occurs at about 5–7 days and is usually the result of hyperphosphataemia, caused by feeding of unmodified cow's milk preparations, or of maternal calcium abnormalities (hyperparathyroidism). All calcium levels below 1.8 mmol/l or ionized calcium below 0.7 mmol/l are taken as hypocalcaemia.

Symptoms include irritability, seizures or lethargy and apnoea. Hypocalcaemia of itself would appear to be benign even if seizures are present; underlying cause may determine long-term outcome.

Treatment

If seizures are present then hypocalcaemia should be corrected by slow intravenous infusion of 10% calcium gluconate, 0.2–0.5 ml/kg. Before administration this solution should be diluted 1:4 with 5% dextrose. Bradycardia and arrhythmias can occur during infusion. For asymptomatic hypocalcaemia supplemental calcium may be given orally or intravenously. Normal calcium requirements (see p. 157) may have to be doubled in severe hypocalcaemia. Calcium infusions should be carefully controlled in the presence of renal impairment and any extravasation of the infusate can lead to severe necrosis of the skin. Solutions with more than 8 mmol/100 ml of calcium should not be infused by pump. Avoid mixing with bicarbonate or parenteral nutrition solutions and do not use umbilical vessels for infusion.

Later onset hypocalcaemia is largely prevented by feeding breast milk or modified cow's milk formulas. These have low phosphate content and a calcium:phosphorus ratio of 4:1 or 2:1.

Preterm rickets (see p. 162)

Hypercalcaemia

This may be:

1. Spurious, due to parenteral nutrition or sample taken from catheter
2. Result of renal failure when intake of calcium is not reduced
3. Vitamin D excess
4. Hypophosphataemia

Hypomagnesaemia

Hypomagnesaemia is defined as a serum magnesium level below 0.6 mmol/l and may be corrected by intramuscular administration of 0.2 ml/kg of 50% magnesium sulphate. Only symptomatic infants need be treated and magnesium given deep into the muscle to prevent skin necrosis. Usually associated with hypocalcaemia and both improve when magnesium is given.

ELECTROLYTE DISTURBANCES

Hyponatraemia

The causes of hyponatraemia are given in Table 43. Early hyponatraemia in very low birth weight infants is due to inappropriate ADH secretion and late hyponatraemia due to

Table 43. Causes of neonatal hyponatraemia.

1. Vomiting and diarrhoea
2. Bowel obstruction
3. Inappropriate intravenous fluids:
   - low sodium intake
   - excessive Intralipid
   - hyperglycaemia
   - mannitol infusions
4. Inappropriate ADH secretion:
   - asphyxia
   - meningitis
   - brain injury
   - pneumonia
   - mechanical ventilation
5. Congestive heart failure, e.g. PDA
6. Diuretic or indomethacin treatment
7. Renal failure
8. Sepsis, sick cell syndrome
9. Cystic fibrosis
10. Maternal hyponatraemia:
    - 5% dextrose in labour
    - oxytocin in labour
11. Adrenal insufficiency:
    - acute
    - congenital adrenal hyperplasia
12. Severe hypoproteinaemia

inadequate sodium intake. Severe hyponatraemia (serum sodium below 120 mmol/l) is associated with apnoea or seizures and should be treated promptly. Other symptoms include apathy, hypotonia, hypotension and paralytic ileus. Treat first by fluid restriction and later sodium supplementation with hypertonic saline. Hypertonic saline is available as 2.7 or 3% solutions which are infused at 4 ml/kg slowly over 1 hour. Hypertonic saline should be reserved for treatment of serious symptoms. It is better to use 0.9% saline. Insulin and glucose treatment (p. 178) may have a role in treatment of sick cell syndrome.

Table 44. Causes of neonatal hypernatraemia.

1. Mismanaged intravenous fluids
2. Dehydration: radiant warmers, very immature infants
3. Vomiting and diarrhoea
4. Bowel obstruction: NEC
5. Osmotic diuresis: hyperglycaemia
6. Excessive use of sodium bicarbonate
7. Congenital hyperaldosteronism: Conn's syndrome, congenital adrenal hyperplasia

Hypernatraemia

Causes are listed in Table 44.

Preterm infants become rapidly dehydrated if fluid is withheld or abnormal losses occur. The preterm infant has a very high insensible water loss which is increased with radiant warmers or phototherapy. Hypernatraemia also caused by loss of extracellular fluid from vomiting, diarrhoea, or 'third-spacing' of fluid in intestinal obstruction.

With normal blood glucose, serum osmolality correlates well with serum sodium (osmolality = approximately 2 × serum sodium) (see also p. 168).

When hypernatraemia is present osmolality will be high and there is association with intraventricular haemorrhage in premature infant. Reduction of serum sodium should be gradual to prevent seizures. Use slow infusion of dextrose or one-fifth N saline and dextrose solutions.

Hyperkalaemia

The causes of hyperkalaemia are shown in Table 45. Apart from spurious hyperkalaemia caused by haemolysis during blood sampling, renal failure is the next commonest cause. Serum potassium levels above 7 mmol/l are associated with ECG changes of tall T waves and widening of QRS complex.

Treatment should be prompt; metabolic acidosis should be

Table 45. Causes of neonatal hyperkalaemia.

1. Haemolysis: heel stab blood
2. Acidosis, shock, hypoxia
3. Increased intake: intravenous fluids, blood transfusion, penicillin
4. Renal failure
5. Drugs, e.g. indomethacin
6. Adrenal insufficiency

Table 46. Causes of neonatal hypokalaemia.

1. Inadequate intake
2. Alkalosis
3. Diuretic treatment
4. Vomiting and diarrhoea
5. Hyperadrenalism

corrected with sodium bicarbonate and 10% calcium gluconate 1–2 ml/kg diluted solution infused over 3 min. If ECG changes remain, glucose and insulin should be given: 1 g/kg of glucose (10 ml/kg of 10% dextrose) mixed with 0.25–0.5 units of insulin/kg is given intravenously. Other effective therapies are ion exchange resin (sodium polystyrene sulphonate (Resonium A) 1g/kg/day orally or rectally) or peritoneal dialysis (see also p. 261). Ion exchange resins exchange K^+ for either Na^+ or Ca^{2+}; the choice should depend upon serum levels of Na^+ and Ca^{2+}.

Hypokalaemia

The causes of hypokalaemia are listed in Table 46. Hypokalaemia should be corrected with potassium replacement therapy provided renal function is normal (see p. 157). Avoid infusing solutions with more than 5 mmol/100 ml of potassium.

Hypo- and Hyperchloraemia

Tables 47 and 48 list the causes of hypochloraemia and hyperchloraemia. In hypochloraemia, increasing intake is effective and in hyperchloraemia correction of the underlying cause is essential.

Table 47. Causes of neonatal hypochloraemia.

1. Metabolic alkalosis: bicarbonate therapy, hypokalaemia
2. Respiratory alkalosis: mechanical hyperventilation
3. Inadequate intake
4. Vomiting and diarrhoea
5. Diuretic therapy
6. Chloridorrhoea

Table 48. Causes of neonatal hyperchloraemia.

1. Excessive intake
2. Metabolic acidosis: shock, hypoxia, diarrhoea, renal failure
3. Respiratory acidosis: RDS, pneumonia

NURSING POINTS

1. Glucose strip test measurements: very important to use correct technique: we prefer BM test strips and capillary blood obtained from heel prick. A large drop of blood completely covering the test area must be used. For Dextrostix measurements a glucometer (reflectometer) should be used
2. Blood glucose measured on all babies admitted to NICU: if level < 2 mmol/l medical staff are informed and if baby is well a milk feed is given and BM stix repeated in 1 hour. For frequency of repeat glucose estimations see beginning of chapter
3. Babies having parenteral nutrition have glucose measured every 4–6 hours and readings above 9 mmol/l warrant

medical staff attention and urine sample for glycosuria. Hyperglycaemia may be an early sign of sepsis. For management see text

4. Calcium containing solutions should be very carefully observed with half-hourly inspection of infusion site as extravasation can cause quite severe skin necrosis. Any redness or swelling warrants stopping infusion and reporting to medical staff

REFERENCES AND FURTHER READING

Cornblath, M. and Schwartz, R. (1976). *Disorders of Carbohydrate Metabolism in Infancy*, 2nd edn. Philadelphia: W. B. Saunders.

Cornblath, M., Ganzon, A. F., Nicolopoulos, D. *et al.* (1961). Study of carbohydrate metabolism in the newborn infant III. Some factors affecting capillary blood sugar and the response to glucagon during the first hours of life. *Pediatrics* **27**: 378.

Hirata, T. and Brady, J. P. (1977). *Newborn Intensive Care: Chemical Aspects*. Springfield, IL: Charles C. Thomas.

Louik, C., Mitchell, A. A., Epstein, M. F. and Shapiro, S. (1985). Risk factors for neonatal hyperglycaemia associated with 10% dextrose infusion. *Am. J. Dis. Child* **139**: 783.

Lyon, A. J., McIntosh, N., Wheeler, K. and Brooke, O. G. (1984). Hypercalcaemia in extremely low birthweight infants. *Arch. Dis. Child* **59**: 1141.

Reid, M. Mc. C., Reilly, B. J., Murdock, A. I. and Swyer, P. R. (1971). Cardiomegaly in association with neonatal hypoglycaemia. *Acta Paediatr. Scand.* **60**: 295.

Tsang, R. C., Donovan, E. F. and Steichen, J. J. (1976). Calcium physiology and pathology in the neonate. *Pediatr. Clin. North Am.* **23**: 611.

13. Jaundice

BILIRUBIN METABOLISM

Red cell destruction releases globin, iron and unconjugated bilirubin (indirect reacting). This bilirubin exists in two forms: albumin-bound and free. Free bilirubin causes kernicterus (see p. 189). In liver cells, bilirubin is conjugated by glucuronyl transferase, becomes water-soluble and direct reacting. Bilirubin is excreted in bile into duodenum where stercobilinogen is

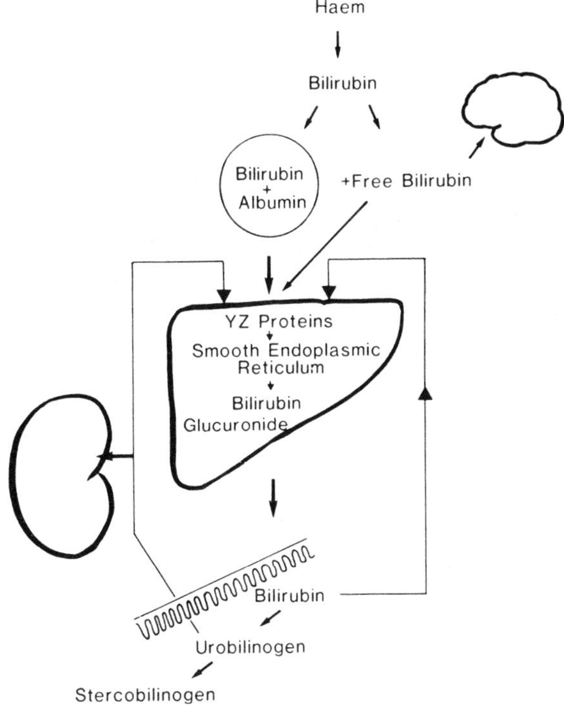

Fig. 47. Bilirubin metabolism.

formed which may be reabsorbed and excreted in urine as urobilinogen (Fig. 47).

In newborns, conjugated bilirubin may become unconjugated by action of β-glucuronidase in gut and be reabsorbed to undergo reconjugation in the liver - the *enterohepatic circulation of bilirubin*. Factors involved in physiological jaundice are shown in Fig. 47 and Table 49.

Table 49. Aetiology of physiological jaundice.

1. Decreased red cell survival (40–60 days)
2. Polycythaemia, bruising, cephalhaematoma
3. Decreased Y and Z proteins (ligandins)
4. Inadequate calories, dehydration
5. Decreased glucuronyl transferase
6. Enterohepatic circulation
7. Shunt bilirubin (20%) from haem pigments

Jaundice of the newborn is frequently benign and may settle with no treatment, but may indicate serious underlying disease and may cause brain damage. Commoner causes are listed in Table 50.

Those babies at greatest risk and who require close observation and bilirubin monitoring are:

1. Preterm infants
2. Ill infants
3. Infants whose jaundice begins within 24 hours of birth
4. Infants with blood group incompatibility
5. Infants with prolonged jaundice.

PRETERM INFANTS

Jaundice commoner because of hepatic immaturity and increased red cell breakdown. Preterm infants at greater risk of kernicterus because of reduced bilirubin binding. Drugs that displace bilirubin from its albumin-binding sites (Table 51) should be used with caution in the preterm infant. Free fatty

Table 50. Causes of neonatal jaundice.

1. Physiological jaundice	Aetiology: Table 49. Onset after 24 hours and reaches peak at 4–5 days but lasts longer in preterms. Peak levels usually 200 μmol/l but exaggerated in dehydration, poor energy intake and breast fed infants
2. Isoimmune haemolytic disease	Rhesus, ABO or rarer ones: c. E, Duffy, Kell, Jaundice onset within 24 hours of birth, and Coombs' test positive. Maternal O and infant A causes most trouble of ABO compatibility
3. Other haemolytic disease	Glucose-6-phosphate dehydrogenase deficiency, (aspirin, sulplas) pyruvate kinase deficiency, congenital spherocytosis or elliptocytosis, thalassaemia. May occur in infants of Mediterranean, African or Chinese origin
4. Infection	Septicaemia, urinary infection, TORCH infections, viral hepatitis, syphilis
5. Haemolysis from	Haematoma, excessive bruising, polycythaemia
6. Galactosaemia	Urine Clinitest positive but Clinistix negative
7. Hypothyroidism	Prolonged jaundice and absent femoral epiphyses (see Table 56)
8. Drugs	Phenothiazines, novobiocin, vitamin K
9. Cystic fibrosis	
10. Biliary atresia or hepatitis	Prolonged jaundice with raised direct bilirubin
11. Breast milk	Low fluid intake may accentuate 'physiological jaundice'. Also prolonged jaundice from abnormal progesterone metabolite in breast milk which competes with bilirubin for conjugation with glucuronyl transferase. Kernicterus has not been reported even though bilirubin levels as high as 350 μmol/l may occur
12. Rare inherited enzyme deficiencies	Inborn errors of metabolism: send urine for amino acid and sugar chromatograms
13. Pyloric stenosis	

Table 51. Drugs that displace bilirubin from albumin.

Sulphonamides	Indomethacin
Salicylates	Oxacillin
Sodium benzoate (parenteral diazepam)	Gentamicin
Frusemide	Digoxin

Table 52. Maximum safe bilirubin levels.

Under 1000 g	140–170 μmol/l
Under 1500 g	170–270 μmol/l
Under 2000 g	220–270 μmol/l
Under 2500 g	270–310 μmol/l

acids and haematin also displace bilirubin from albumin. Lower albumin levels and increased risk of acidosis, hypoxia and hypoglycaemia mean that exchange transfusion must be performed at lower total bilirubin levels (Table 52, Fig. 48). Preterm infants tolerate exchange transfusion less well than term infants. Hypoxia and hypoglycaemia cause increased free fatty acid levels which may displace bilirubin from albumin. Acidosis decreases bilirubin binding and facilitates entry of free bilirubin into cerebral cells. Preterm babies are at greater risk of kernicterus as a result (p. 189).

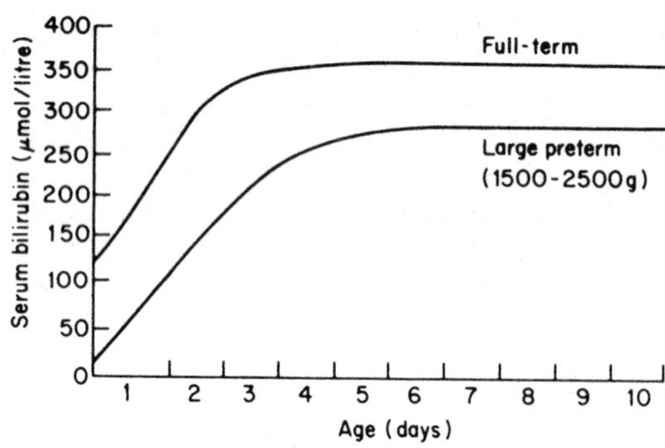

Fig. 48. Maximum safe bilirubin levels for well-term and preterm infants.

ILL INFANTS

Infants who are clinically unwell and who are jaundiced must have full investigation. Infection may be underlying cause and full sepsis work-up should be done (see Table 62). Acidosis reduces albumin binding and increases uptake of free bilirubin by cerebral cells.

Blood film, blood groups of mother and infant and Coombs' test should be done.

In sick infant, if these initial investigations are negative then seek further advice.

INFANTS JAUNDICED DURING FIRST 24 HOURS OF LIFE

Probably due to blood group incompatibility but intrauterine infection may also be cause. All require investigation but no cause may be found. Initial investigations include:

1. Haemoglobin
2. Blood groups, mother and father
3. Coombs' test

If these tests are unhelpful or infant ill, look for intrauterine infection (bacterial or viral, p. 193).

BLOOD GROUP INCOMPATIBILITY

Rhesus Isoimmunization

Fifteen per cent of women are rhesus negative (D antigen). Other rhesus antigens can cause haemolysis (c, E). Before anti-D prophylaxis, about 1% of primigravidae developed antibodies after the first pregnancy, 7% during second, 17% in third and 35% in sixth pregnancy. With the introduction of anti-D in 1969, the number of affected babies has fallen dramatically (the number of exchange transfusions has dropped to one-tenth of peak in 1970).

ABO Incompatibility

About 10% of group O women have IgG anti-A and anti-B haemolysins which cross the placenta (normally anti-A and anti-B are IgM antibodies and do not cross the placenta). First babies may be affected (unlike rhesus) and the severity does not usually increase in subsequent pregnancies (again unlike rhesus). ABO incompatibility is three to four times more common than rhesus isoimmunization but rarely causes problems. Presentation is usually within the first 24 hours with highest bilirubin levels on third and fourth days. Coombs' test is usually weakly positive and anaemia, while not present at birth, may develop later at 4 to 6 weeks as a result of continuing chronic haemolysis.

MANAGEMENT OF EARLY JAUNDICE

The primary aim of management is to keep bilirubin below neurotoxic levels. Maximum safe levels of bilirubin are not known but suggested levels for different birth weights are given in Table 52 and Fig. 48. There are three methods of reducing high bilirubin:

1. Exchange transfusion
2. Phototherapy
3. Phenobarbitone

Exchange Transfusion

This technique is described in Chapter 9, p. 108. Indications are shown in Table 53.

Table 53. Suggested indications for early exchange transfusion.

1. Obviously ill infant at birth	Anaemia, hydrops, etc. Intrauterine fetal transfusion. Exchange started soon after resuscitation and before cord blood results available
2. Cord blood findings	Haemoglobin less than 11 g/dl. Bilirubin over 80 μmol/l, Coombs' test positive

When hydrops is due to rhesus isoimmunization, the causes are interrelated: anaemia, heart failure and hypoproteinaemia as a result of liver damage. Obstetric management involves a balance of early delivery against intrauterine fetal transfusion

(IUFT). IUFT may now be performed by direct cannulation of umbilical vessels at fetoscopy. Prevention of anaemia is beneficial to the fetus and major risk of early delivery is respiratory distress syndrome. Direct fetal transfusion has definite benefits for severely affected infants early in the second trimester.

Emergency management of the baby with severe erythroblastosis (hydrops fetalis)

1. Most delivered by caesarean section. Experienced personnel should be present
2. Resuscitate as Chapter 4. May need intubation to stabilize. May need aspiration of pleural and peritoneal effusions. If IUFT has been performed within the last 7 days, unabsorbed blood may splint the diaphragm and should be removed by paracentesis (p. 120). Babies born after IUFT have other problems: abnormal cord blood result with negative Coombs' test, increased risk of obstructive jaundice (p. 190), high incidence of inguinal hernias and possibly increased risk of graft versus host reaction
3. Catheterize umbilical vein. Check haemoglobin, bilirubin, Coombs' test. If central venous pressure over 10 cmH_2O, remove 10 ml/kg; if normal or low, stabilize and transfer to nursery
4. Mechanical ventilation if any evidence of RDS, severe heart failure or pulmonary hypoplasia, all of which are associated with hydrops
5. Early exchange transfusion with semi-packed cells to raise haemoglobin; no deficit unless CVP high. Blood should be donor fresh if possible but certainly < 48 hours old, X-matched and CMV negative
6. May also need digoxin and diuretics (p. 237) or peritoneal dialysis (p. 261)

Later exchange transfusion when bilirubin approaches neurotoxic levels and other methods have failed.

Exchange transfusion should lower bilirubin levels by over 60%. About 2 hours after the procedure there will be a rebound rise in bilirubin level as tissue bilirubin equilibrates with plasma level. Hypoglycaemia may occur after exchange transfusion because rhesus babies have hyperinsulinaemia (hypertrophy of islet cells perhaps due to glutathione released from haemolysed red cells) and acid citrate dextrose (ACD) blood provides a glucose load which stimulates insulin release.

Phototherapy

Reduces bilirubin levels, but may also be used prophylactically in very immature infants with marked bruising. Probably works by converting bilirubin into water-soluble compounds but may also allow unconjugated bilirubin to bypass hepatic glucuronidation.

This treatment has some risks, including:

1. Retinal damage
2. Increased insensible water loss
3. Thermal instability
4. Masking of sepsis
5. Loose stools
6. Rashes
7. Bronzing if direct bilirubin raised
8. Possible long-term effects

Tables 54 and 55 give indications and precautions to be used in phototherapy.

Table 54. Indications for phototherapy.

	Bilirubin levels (μmol/l)	
	Phototherapy at	*Exchange at*
Normal term infant (no incompatibility)	250–270	340–360
Normal term infant but incompatibility	180–200	340
Well preterm infant over 1500 g	140–170	220–270
Well preterm infant under 1500 g	100–130	170–220
Sick preterm infant over 1500 g	80–110	170–220
Sick preterm infant under 1500 g	Birth–100	140–200

Table 55. Precautions with phototherapy.

1. Do not use if direct bilirubin is high (bronzing)
2. Cover the eyes without pressure (pad and bandage)
3. Watch fluid balance carefully (increase fluid intake)
4. Watch for temperature instability (check temperature 4-hourly)
5. Watch for 'masked' sepsis (examine infant every 6 hours)

Phenobarbitone

Ineffective unless used prenatally. Works by inducing glucuronyl transferase.

KERNICTERUS

No specific clinical picture is pathognomonic of kernicterus but it should be considered in any unwell and jaundiced infant. There may be hypotonia or hypertonia with opisthotonus and convulsions. Downward rolling of the eyes or setting-sun sign may occur. The Moro reflex may be abnormal with brisk extension of the arms but not flexion. Apnoea may occur in the immature infant but the finding of unsuspected kernicterus at postmortem is probably commoner than clinical presentation. If kernicterus is suspected immediate exchange transfusion should be done after infusion of albumin 1 g/kg. The presence of signs of kernicterus is not an indication to abandon treatment as permanent neurological damage may be lessened or even prevented by prompt action. Failure to treat may result in the full-blown syndrome of choreoathetosis, spastic dysplegia, deafness, mental retardation, failure of upward gaze and green teeth.

Predisposition to Kernicterus

Low serum albumin, acidosis, hypoxia, hypoglycaemia, co-existent sepsis or haemolytic disease, certain drugs (see Table 51). Test of bilirubin binding may be helpful, e.g. HBABA (hydroxybenzeneazobenzoic acid) or Sephadex gel, but these are not in common routine use.

INFANTS WITH PROLONGED JAUNDICE

Defined as clinically apparent jaundice present 10 days after birth in a term infant and 14 days after birth in a preterm infant. The causes are listed in Table 56. Breast feeding is the commonest cause in the term infant and non-specific 'hepatitis' in the very low birth weight infant. If due to breast feeding there is an association with haemorrhagic disease of the newborn and infant should be given 1 mg of vitamin K (Konakion). Rarely is there a need to stop breast feeding and kernicterus has not been reported in the absence of coexistent haemolytic disease. Ensure adequate fluid intake and reassure mother. Occasionally phototherapy is needed.

Table 56. Causes of prolonged jaundice.

1. Sepsis	Especially in ill infant, urinary infection or septicaemia
2. Breast milk	Breast milk jaundice
3. Hypothyroidism	Screen T_4 and TSH. Other clinical signs often absent*
4. Galactosaemia	Usually vomiting and sepsis picture. Test urine and send urinary chromatogram
5. Inspissated bile syndrome	Follows severe haemolytic disease especially if exchange transfusion needed. Raised direct bilirubin; usually responds to conservative management. Liver biopsy may show giant cell hepatitis
6. Cystic fibrosis	Uncommon presentation of this disorder
7. Very immature infant	Especially if bruised and fed with intravenous amino acids
8. Obstructive jaundice	Biliary atresia. Hepatitis: infections, errors of metabolism, galactosaemia, drugs, cholestasis, inspissated bile syndrome, parenteral nutrition, α_1-antitrypsin deficiency. Choledochal cyst
9. Delayed passage of stool	Increased enterohepatic circulation. Intestinal obstruction or extreme immaturity
10. Pyloric stenosis	Occasional early presentation

* Neonatal signs of hypothyroidism: prolonged pregnancy, high birth weight, large fontanelle, hypothermia, peripheral cyanosis, lethargy, poor feeding, delayed passage of meconium, prolonged jaundice, oedema, respiratory distress. Treatment with thyroxine (see p. 352)

Raised direct bilirubin in the very low birth weight infant recovering from intensive care is very common. Probably due to a combination of problems: intravenous feeding, chronic infection and possibly ascending cholangitis. Often coexists with rickets of prematurity (p. 162) and bronchopulmonary dysplasia (p. 148). Conservative management usually leads to resolution: treat any underlying infection, ensure adequate oral nutrition, especially fat-soluble vitamins A, D, E and K, consider treatment with metronidazole. For infants with prolonged jaundice do the following investigations:

1. Urine culture
2. Thyroid function tests
3. Clinitest/Clinistix on urine and chromatogram
4. Full blood count and film
5. Total and direct bilirubin

If direct bilirubin raised and biliary atresia suspected, there is some urgency in differentiating this from hepatitis. Laparotomy and corrective surgery are more successful if done before 6–8 weeks.

1. Rose bengal test (now obsolete)
2. Liver enzymes
3. Ultrasonic scan
4. Liver biopsy

NURSING POINTS

1. Phototherapy: keep baby warm in incubator (check temperature 3 hourly); ensure extra fluid intake by 10% either orally or intravenously; keep eyes covered except when mother visiting and lights can be turned off (watch for damage to eyes and nasal obstruction); reassure parents and carefully explain precautions being taken
2. Exchange transfusion: incubator or radiant warmer (easier access); attach cardiorespiratory monitor; empty stomach; check temperature and blood pressure half hourly; have emergency drugs checked and readily available (calcium gluconate, sodium bicarbonate, adrenaline, atropine, frusemide and dopamine); resuscitation trolley including defibrillator should be at hand; accurately record input/output during procedure and keep doctor informed of

baby's condition (act as the anaesthetist); after procedure send catheter tip for culture and withhold feeds for about 4 hours, especially if abdominal distension present

REFERENCES AND FURTHER READING

Auerbach, K. G. and Gartner, L. M. (1987). Breast feeding and human milk; the association with jaundice in the neonate. *Clin. Perinatol.* **14**: 89.

Cashore, W. J. and Stern, L. (1982). Neonatal hyperbilirubinemia. *Pediatr. Clin. North Am.* **29**: 1191.

Cockington, R. A. (1979). A guide to the use of phototherapy in the management of neonatal hyperbilirubinemia. *J. Pediatr.* **95**: 281.

Diamond, L. K., Allen, F. H. and Thomas, W. O. (1951). Erythroblastosis fetalis VII: treatment with exchange transfusion. *N. Engl. J. Med.* **244**: 39.

Gartner, L. M. (1983). Cholestasis of the newborn (obstructive jaundice). *Pediatr. Rev.* **5**: 163.

Kramer, L. I. (1969). Advancement of dermal icterus in the jaundiced newborn. *Am. J. Dis. Child* **118**: 454.

Levine, R. L. (1979). Bilirubin: worked out years ago? *Pediatrics* **64**: 380.

Levine, R. L. (1988). Neonatal jaundice. *Acta Paediatr. Scand.* **77**: 177.

Lucey, J. F. (1982). Bilirubin and brain damage: a real mess. *Pediatrics* **69**: 381.

Murphy, J. F., Hughes, I. A., Verrier-Jones, E. R. *et al.* (1981). Pregnanediols and breast milk jaundice. *Arch. Dis. Child* **56**: 474.

Odell, G. B. (1980). *Neonatal Hyperbilirubinemia.* New York: Grune and Stratton.

Tsao, Y. C. and Yu, V. Y. H. (1972). Albumin in management of neonatal hyperbilirubinaemia. *Arch. Dis. Child* **47**: 250.

Watchko, J. F. and Oski, F. A. (1983). Bilirubin 20 mg/dl = vigintiphobia. *Pediatrics* **71**: 660.

14. Fetal and Neonatal Infection

For discussion of cross-infection measures see p. 61. Infection with HIV (AIDS) and maternal bacterial sepsis are discussed in Chapter 3. Early fetal infections are often viral and remembered by the mnemonic (TORCH) (see below). These are uncommon by comparison to perinatal bacterial infection (Table 57).

Table 57. Incidence of perinatal infection.

Organism	*Mother/1000 pregnancies*	*Fetus/1000 pregnancies*	*Newborn/1000 live births*
Toxoplasma	1.5–6.4	1.3–7.0	0.05–1.0
Rubella virus			
epidemic year	20–40	4–30	2–6
interepidemic	0.1–1.0	0.2–0.5	0.25
Cytomegalovirus	30–140	5–15	1–5
Herpes simplex virus	1–10	rare	0.1–0.5
Treponema pallidum	0.2	0.1	0.2
All bacterial infections	—	—	3–5

TORCH INFECTIONS

TORCH stands for *to*xoplasmosis, *r*ubella, *c*ytomegalovirus and *h*erpes simplex infections.

Infants with TORCH infection are usually small-for-dates and have rashes, hepatitis, CNS findings, chorioretinitis and failure to thrive (Table 58).

Screen by cord blood IgM (normal < 0.2 g/l). If TORCH infection, cord IgM > 0.25 g/l in about 60%.

Table 58. Clinical features of TORCH infections.

	TO	*R*	*C*	*H*
Central nervous system				
Encephalitis	+	+	+	+
Microcephaly	+	+	+	+
Hydrocephaly	+	+	+	+
Intracranial calcification	+	+	+	+
Psychomotor retardation	+	+	+	+
Hearing loss	+	+	+	?
Eye				
Chorioretinitis	+	0	+	+
Pigmented retina	0	+	0	0
Keratoconjunctivitis	0	0	0	+
Cataracts	0	+	0	+
Glaucoma	+	+	0	0
Visual impairment	+	+	+	+
Reticuloendothelial system				
Hepatosplenomegaly	+	+	+	+
Liver calcification	+	?	+	+
Jaundice	+	+	+	+
Haemolytic anaemia	+	+	+	+
Petechiae	+	+	+	+
Heart				
Myocarditis	+	+	+	+
Congenital heart disease	+	+	+	+
Bone lesions	+	+	+	?
Skin				
Vesicular lesions	0	0	0	+
Pregnancy complications				
Abortions, stillbirths prematurity, IUGR	+	+	+	+

+ = occurs; 0 = does not occur; ? = uncertain
After Kadar (1979)

Toxoplasmosis

Uncommon in UK, but more common in France and Spain where undercooked meat may be the source. May also be contracted from young cats and their faeces.

Acquired toxoplasmosis is treated with sulphadiazine, pyrimethamine and folic acid (see p. 352). Spiramycin has been used in pregnancy to reduce effects of infection on the fetus.

Rubella

Comes in epidemics about every 7 years. First trimester infections are most serious causing CNS and cardiovascular defects. After 14 weeks of pregnancy, only adverse effect on fetus is deafness. Prevention by rubella vaccination of seronegative women and girls. Rubella vaccination of children has recently been introduced in the UK and this should reduce the prevalence of congenital rubella syndrome.

Cytomegalovirus (CMV)

Probably the commonest fetal infection although most are subclinical at birth. Severe infections can cause hydrops and gross CNS defects. Less severe infections lead to neurological deficits in later childhood. Postnatal infection (pneumonitis and jaundice) may be acquired from blood transfusions: about 7% of donor packs are infected. Use CMV negative blood for all neonatal transfusions. There is no effective treatment for established disease.

Herpes Simplex Virus (HSV)

Risk after vaginal delivery when mother has genital and especially cervical herpes infection (usually Type II virus). Risk may be great enough to consider caesarean section before labour or within 6 hours of membrane rupture. Mildest infection is vesicular rash on the presenting part. With disseminated infection the signs mimic bacterial sepsis (see Table 61), with jaundice, bleeding, collapse and cerebral signs. Diagnosis by electron microscopy of vesicle scraping and culture of virus. Intravenous adenosine arabinoside may help, but mortality and morbidity are high.

HEPATITIS B VIRUS (HBV)

High carrier rate in mothers from Far East, especially Chinese. Screening is routine during pregnancy and e antigen positive means high risk of vertical transmission to baby at birth.

Prevention by vaccinating infants at risk: Give 1 ml (2 μg) anti-HBV vaccine intramuscularly into anterolateral thigh at birth and repeat at 1 and 6 months. To give protection until vaccine effective give 2 ml (100 iu) of anti-HBV globulin intramuscularly in a different muscle at birth.

Breast feeding should be discouraged in UK but may be important for other reasons in less-developed countries. Precautions to avoid self-innoculation include care with contaminated needles, wearing gloves and visor at delivery and careful handling of infected secretions.

HIV (AIDS)

See Chapter 3.

SEVERE BACTERIAL INFECTIONS

Severe bacterial infections in newborn in 3–5/1000 births, though less in full term (about 1/1000). The incidence in preterm babies varies from 2 to 4%. In babies having intensive care, incidence is up to 30%.

The newborn has reduced defence against infection (Table 59).

Risks of congenital bacterial infection are increased in presence of factors listed in Table 60. Consider sepsis work-up and antibiotic cover if any of these are present.

Table 59. Neonatal defence against infection.

1. Decreased humoral immunity: only IgG crosses the placenta (IgM contains specific bactericidal antibodies to Gram-negative organisms)
2. Decreased cellular immunity: still debated but the preterm infant probably has impaired cell-mediated immunity
3. Decreased white cell activity: phagocytosis reduced due to deficient opsonizing antibody and impaired chemotaxis. Newborn white cells function in adult serum
4. Deficient complement system
5. Secretory IgA from colostrum and breast milk will not be provided for bottle-fed baby

Table 60. Risk factors for congenital bacterial infection.

1. Prolonged rupture of membranes >24 hours (see p. 24)
2. Maternal infection — fever, leucocytosis, tender uterus, foul discharge suggesting chorioamnionitis:
   - recent urinary tract infection
   - colonization with group B streptococcus
   - Shirodkar suture
   - poor socioeconomic status
3. Antepartum haemorrhage especially abruption
4. Preterm infant, especially male sex
5. Early respiratory distress (p. 145)

The commonest pathogens are coliforms, staphylococci, group β-haemolytic streptococci, *Pseudomonas*, *Listeria* and others, e.g. *Klebsiella*, *Haemophilus*, *Serratia*, pneumococci, enterococci and anaerobes.

Route of infection may be:

1. Ascending ± rupture membranes 2. Transplacental 3. Aspiration during birth	Congenital infection
4. Direct invasion after birth: either via umbilical cord, skin lesions or aspiration or from apparatus	Nosocomial infection

Signs of sepsis in the newborn are listed in Table 61. The predominant sign of congenital infection is respiratory distress or apnoea. These infections present as bacteraemia, pneumonia or meningitis or any combination of these.

Nosocomial infections (acquired from the environment, late onset, therefore not congenital) may present as septicaemia, pneumonia or meningitis also, but in addition may be osteomyelitis, urinary tract infection, skin infections and conjunctivitis. Laboratory investigations of suspected sepsis given in Table 62. Table 63 shows abnormalities that may occur on blood film in neonatal sepsis.

Table 61. Signs of sepsis.

1. Pallor or mottling, shock	10. Abdominal distension
2. Hypotonia or poor Moro	11. Splenomegaly, hepatomegaly
3. Lethargy	12. Enlarged kidneys
4. Poor feeding	13. Bradycardia
5. Vomiting	14. Bloody stools or diarrhoea
6. Hypothermia or fever	15. Seizures
7. Jaundice	16. Omphalitis
8. Apnoea or tachypnoea	17. Sclerema
9. Tachycardia	18. Abnormal bleeding, petechiae

Table 62. Laboratory investigation of suspected infection.

1. Cultures: blood, CSF, urine, skin, external ear, throat, rectum, cord, amniotic fluid, gastric aspirate, catheter tips
2. Microscopy: CSF, urine and gastric aspirate (Gram stain)
3. Full blood picture (see Table 63)
4. Acute phase reactants:
   C-reactive protein
   erythrocyte sedimentation rate (ESR)
5. Radiographs:
   chest if respiratory signs
   abdomen if NEC suspected
6. Others (if indicated): immunoglobulins, blood gases, calcium, electrolytes, coagulation studies
7. Histopathology of placenta and cord

NEC: Necrotizing enterocolitis

Treatment of Infection (see also p. 206)

Antibiotic treatment is the mainstay. Any baby with suspected infection (Tables 60, 61) should have sepsis work-up (Table 62) and be given antibiotics. If all cultures subsequently prove negative, antibiotics can be stopped in 2–3 days if the baby is well. Proven infections (positive cultures) should be treated for 7–10 days with appropriate antibiotics by intravenous route. A combination of antibiotics should be given, usually a penicillin

Table 63. Blood film in neonatal sepsis.

1. Extreme shift to the left: band: segmented neutrophil ratio >0.2*
2. Leucocytosis over 20 000/mm^3 and over 60% neutrophils
3. Leucopenia under 5000/mm^3
4. Toxic granulation of neutrophils
5. Fragmentation of red cells
6. Reticulocytosis
7. Thrombocytopenia under 100 000/mm^3

* See Table 104, p. 277

and an aminoglycoside (see Appendix V, p. 353). The choice of penicillin is determined by the likely organism, e.g. group B streptococcus - penicillin G; *Staphylococcus* - flucloxacillin; *Pseudomonas* - ticarcillin; listeriosis and enterococcus - ampicillin. The newer, third-generation cephalosporins are now finding a place in the treatment of neonatal infection (p. 208). For late onset infections *Staphylococcus albus* and *aureus* (sometimes methicillin resistant, MRSA) are most common and a combination of flucloxacillin and netilmicin or vancomycin may be needed (see later).

In addition to antibiotics, infants with infections need supportive care with intravenous fluids and nutrition, electrolyte correction and acid–base balance. Hypotension should be corrected by volume expansion or infusion of dopamine if due to myocardial depression. Bleeding disorder may be improved by giving fresh plasma and vitamin K (Konakion). Exchange transfusion with fresh blood provides opsonins and is useful in septicaemia and sclerema (p. 204). A single volume exchange transfusion (80 ml/kg) should be performed as described on p. 108. Recently, granulocyte transfusions or buffy coat have been shown to be of benefit. Prophylaxis with immunoglobulin infusions is promising but further studies are needed and this treatment is costly.

COLIFORM INFECTIONS

Preterm infant susceptible because of reduced specific IgM antibody, increased use of broad spectrum antibiotics and equipment with high humidity. Infection may be congenital or nosocomial. Umbilicus often the portal of entry leading to septicaemia with meningitis in 30% of babies with positive blood cultures.

Congenital Pneumonia

Congenital infection may mimic RDS (p. 145).

Septicaemia

Later symptoms are often non-specific (Table 61) or may present as sudden deterioration. Jaundice may increase or reappear.

Investigate with cultures (Table 62) and start antibiotics: gentamicin or netilmicin and ampicillin in combination are preferred. Cephalosporin such as cefotaxime or ceftazidime may also be used but these are better reserved as second-line treatment unless meningitis or *Pseudomonas* infection are strongly suspected. Duration of treatment if proven septicaemia is 10–14 days. Doses of antibiotics are given in Appendix V. Aim to keep trough (after 12 hours) serum gentamicin level in therapeutic range 0.5–1.0 μg/ml. Peak levels should be 4–5 μg/ml (Table 64). About 30% of babies with septicaemia will also have meningitis.

Table 64. Toxic levels of aminoglycosides.

	Gentamicin (μg/ml)	*Netilmicin* (μg/ml)	*Amikacin* (μg/ml)
Peak	>10	>16	>32
Trough	> 3	> 4	>10

Peak taken 60 min after im injection or 15 minutes after iv injection. Trough taken just before injection

Meningitis

Symptoms usually non-specific, e.g. vomiting and lethargy. Seizures, high-pitched cry and tense anterior fontanelle occur late. If in doubt do a lumbar puncture (p. 114).

Dosage of antibiotics (usually a penicillin and an aminoglycoside, but newer cephalosporins such as cefotaxime penetrate well into CSF) should be increased but intrathecal and intraventricular therapy with gentamicin is not usually helpful (see Appendix V). If deterioration, persistent fever, increasing head size or ultrasound scan suggests ventriculitis, then intraventricular antibiotics may be given, if ventriculitis present, Rickham reservoir may be inserted by paediatric surgeon. Duration of parenteral therapy is usually 3 weeks. Lumbar puncture should be repeated after 3 days and possibly again after 2 weeks to help determine duration. For poor responders chloramphenicol may be helpful as it penetrates well into CSF. If chloramphenicol is used, serum should be assayed (therapeutic range 10–25 μg/ml; toxic levels > 50 μg/ml.

Despite intensive care and newer antibiotics, outcome remains disappointing with 30–50% mortality and a significant proportion of survivors (perhaps 30–50%) have handicaps.

Urinary Tract Infection (UTI)

Incidence 1–2% of newborns; commoner in boys. Often presents with poor feeding, vomiting and jaundice.

Urine for culture obtained by:

1. Suprapubic aspiration (see Chapter 9; Fig. 40)
2. Clean catch
3. Uribag

Urine obtained by suprapubic aspiration is least likely to be contaminated. Culture of urine collected by clean catch or Uribag method may be contaminated, so take several specimens for culture and transport rapidly to the laboratory. All cultures should reveal same organism > 10^5 ml, with pus cells. Treat with parenteral antibiotics for 7–10 days. Renal ultrasound scan and contrast radiography (intravenous pyelogram (IVP) and micturating cystogram (MCU)) to look for renal anomalies (10–20%) and reflux. Babies need follow up for recurrence of UTI (25–50%).

PSEUDOMONAS INFECTIONS

Pseudomonas may cause infections like *E. coli* but mortality is higher. May present with a pink macular rash associated with a marked vasculitis and necrotic lesions. *Pseudomonas* may cause pneumonia. Gentamicin usually effective; but sometimes need netilmicin or ceftazidime (Appendix V). Infections with *Serratia* often resemble *Pseudomonas* and occur in very immature infants who have been treated with broad-spectrum antibiotics.

STAPHYLOCOCCAL INFECTIONS

Infections range from severe systemic illness with MRSA to superficial skin sepsis.

Pneumonia

Infant is often very ill. Sclerema may be present. Chest radiograph initially may show non-specific changes and later lobar consolidation with pneumatoceles. Complications are pneumothorax and empyema.

Treatment with flucloxacillin; if sclerema present, exchange transfusion may help. The pneumatoceles may take weeks to disappear. Assisted ventilation is often needed.

Recently, multi-resistant staphylococci (MRSA) have re-emerged in neonatal intensive care units and these are cloxacillin and methicillin resistant. Vancomycin is the drug of choice under these circumstances but the dose must be carefully adjusted (Appendix V and p. 208). Start with 20 mg/kg/day in two divided doses and check serum levels after 48 hours. These organisms are occasionally sensitive to fusidic acid and rifampicin. Local treatment with mupirocin helps to reduce skin colonization (see below).

Osteomyelitis

May present up to 6 weeks after a staphylococcal septicaemia or bacteraemia. Bones most commonly affected are tibiae, the other long bones, vertebrae and maxilla. Others are skull bones (scalp electrodes) and os calcis (heel stab). Signs are usually non-specific but later localized redness, tenderness, local oedema and loss of movement. Aspiration of infected area for culture.

Treatment with flucloxacillin or fusidic acid in high doses and orthopaedic opinion. May lead to deranged bone growth if metaphyseal plate damaged. The duration of antibiotic therapy is 6 weeks.

Skeletal survey should be performed on all infants about 4–6 weeks after a proven staphylococcal septicaemia.

Pemphigus

Also called scalded skin syndrome. Generalized bullous eruption which is often rapidly fatal. Prompt treatment with intravenous fluids and antibiotics imperative.

Superficial Infection

Septic spots should be differentiated from erythema toxicum by smear for Gram stain examination. Septic spots contain polymorphs and staphylococci, and erythema toxicum lesions contain eosinophils with no organisms.

Paronychia is infection along the side of the nail beds.

Omphalitis presents as an erythematous and indurated area around the cord stump which may have a serous or purulent exudate. Danger from local and systemic spread.

Breast abscess may present as a red, tender swelling and need drainage and antibiotic therapy.

Superficial staphylococcal infections are potentially dangerous and isolation with strict handwashing is essential. Local therapy with alcohol swabs and antiseptics like hexachlorophane is helpful but ill infant should also have systemic antibiotics. Mupirocin (pseudomonic acid) is a local antibacterial agent with powerful activity against MRSA. To reduce colonization it should be applied liberally to carrier sites (nares, umbilicus, groins and perianal area).

GROUP B β-HAEMOLYTIC STREPTOCOCCAL INFECTIONS

Early onset infection: septicaemia or pneumonia – has been previously discussed (see p. 145). The illness is rapidly fatal in untreated cases.

Late onset infection: meningitis with septicaemia – prognosis somewhat better. CSF examinations will show increase in polymorphs and Gram-positive cocci. Treatment is high-dose intravenous penicillin or ampicillin/gentamicin in combination for 3 weeks (see Appendix V and p. 206).

Osteomyelitis may be a complication and become the source for re-infection.

LISTERIOSIS

Discussed on p. 146. Also a late onset form presenting with septicaemia and meningitis.

SCLEREMA

Woody hardening of the subcutaneous tissues that is now seen much less commonly. The changes first appear in the buttocks and legs but spread to back and chest. Associated with a poor prognosis but exact cause of changes in subcutaneous fatty tissues is unknown. Both hypothermia and reduced peripheral circulation may be underlying factors. Staphylococcal or streptococcal infections are often found.

Therapy to correct metabolic and other abnormalities (hypoxia, hypothermia, acidosis, hypoglycaemia and coagulation upsets). Antibiotics should always be started if not already being administered. Exchange transfusion with fresh blood may help perhaps by providing opsonins and other serum factors enhancing ability to fight underlying infection. Steroids are unhelpful and should not be given.

CONJUNCTIVITIS

Caused by chemical, bacterial or viral agents. Chlorhexidine to swab the maternal perineum or silver nitrate to prevent ophthalmia neonatorum may cause a purulent-looking neonatal conjunctivitis. This will be present on first day and cultures will be negative.

Ophthalmia neonatorum caused by *Neisseria gonorrhoeae* (gonococcus) is increasing in the UK. Severe conjunctivitis presenting within 48 hours, especially if bilateral and with oedema of the eyelids, may be gonococcal infection. Swabs from both infant and mother should be taken (Gram stain shows Gram-negative, intracellular diplococci) and penicillin eye drops should be started. These are given half hourly for the first 8 hours and then 4 hourly for 7 days. Systemic penicillin should also be given until results of culture are available (50 000 units/mg/kg/day). Prompt and aggressive therapy is necessary to prevent blindness. The mother and her contacts will also need treatment.

Conjunctivitis is also caused by staphylococci, chlamydiae and coliforms. Chloramphenicol eye ointment treats staphylococcal conjunctivitis and tetracycline ointment is best for chlamydiae (sulphonamide eye drops may also be used).

Chlamydia has also been implicated as a cause of neonatal pneumonia. The illness seems mild and radiological findings much worse than the clinical picture. Treated with erythromycin (40 mg/kg/day).

ANAEROBIC INFECTIONS

Anaerobic infections (see p. 147), e.g. *Bacteroides*, suspected when maternal illness, prolonged rupture of membranes, foul-smelling baby and scalp abscesses. Penicillin, chloramphenicol, clindamycin and metronidazole may be used.

CANDIDA INFECTIONS

Infection encouraged by broad spectrum antibiotics and parenteral nutrition. Superficial infection of mouth with thrush may make infant reluctant to feed and candidiasis of the perineum may cause a fiery-red scaly rash affecting the intertriginous areas. Nystatin suspension 100 000 units/ml given after feeds for 7 days and nystatin ointment applied to perineal infection.

Systemic candidiasis in the preterm infant may be associated with parenteral nutrition, broad spectrum antibiotics and chronic illness. The signs are non-specific (lethargy, apnoea, poor colour, abdominal distension) but in severe cases joint effusions or renal failure may occur.

Candida is cultured from the blood, urine, faeces and CSF. Organism is difficult to grow so several samples for culture should be sent and high suspicion in very immature baby who deteriorates but has negative bacterial cultures. Urine and arterial blood are best for culture. Budding yeasts may be seen on direct microscopy of urine. Treatment is with anti-fungal agents amphotericin B and flucytosine: amphotericin B gradually increased to 0.5 mg/kg/day and flucytosine to 150 mg/kg/day in four divided doses. Occasional side-effects of thrombocytopenia and hepatic and renal dysfunction. Mortality is now less than 15%. Amphotericin B has been given intraventricularly in a dose of 5 μg into each ventricle on alternative days when *Candida* meningitis has been diagnosed.

ANTIBIOTICS IN THE NEWBORN

Absorption, distribution, metabolism and excretion of drugs are different in neonatal period. Many physiological factors influence the pharmacokinetics of antibiotics in the newborn: biotransformation, extracellular fluid volume, protein binding and renal function. Also, enzyme systems may be deficient, e.g. glucuronyl transferase. Antibiotic dosage depends upon gestational and postnatal age as well as weight and renal maturity. Appendix V gives dosage recommendations for newborns based on birth weight and postnatal age. The duration of antibiotic therapy depends on diagnosis and result of cultures.

Penicillins

In general, safe and effective for treatment of streptococcal, pneumococcal and staphylococcal infections. Ampicillin has broad spectrum and used against pathogens such as enterococci, coliforms, *Proteus* and *Listeria monocytogenes*. Carbenicillin and ticarcillin have been replaced by netilmicin and ceftazidime for treatment of *pseudomonas* infections. Adverse reactions to the penicillins rare in the newborn, though bolus injections have caused seizures from CNS toxicity. Benzylpenicillin (Penicillin G) does not penetrate well into CSF and the dose should be doubled for treatment of meningitis (150 000–250 000 units/kg/day). Procaine penicillin G used to treat congenital syphilis (50 000 units/kg/day). Cloxacillin is an anti-staphylococcal penicillin, resistant to β-lactamase produced by hospital staphylococci. Cloxacillin greater activity *in vitro* than methicillin but this is offset by greater protein-binding *in vivo* of former. Nephrotoxicity reported in older infants treated with methicillin but very uncommon in newborn. Flucloxacillin is antibiotic of choice for staphylococcal infections unless methicillin-resistant *Staphylococcus aureus* (MRSA) which should be treated with vancomycin (p. 208).

A penicillin and aminoglycoside combination is commonly used as initial treatment for suspected or confirmed bacterial infections in newborn.

Aminoglycosides

These antibiotics act on microbial ribosomes to inhibit protein synthesis. There is risk of renal or ototoxicity unless correct doses used (see Appendix V). Risk of ototoxicity is related to both peak and trough serum levels of antibiotic and to cumulative effects. Aminoglycosides given intramuscularly if infant has large enough muscle mass and not shocked. If drug is given intravenously, a 20 min infusion results in serum concentrations comparable to those after intramuscular injection. Netilmicin closely resembles gentamicin in antimicrobial activity, pharmacology, clinical efficacy and toxicity. However, it is more effective *in vitro* against *Pseudomonas* than gentamicin or amikacin and may be less likely to cause ototoxicity. It is more expensive than gentamicin but may be preferred for late onset infections as activity against *Staphylococcus albus* is greater (total daily dose 6 mg/kg/day).

When using aminoglycosides, serum levels should be measured in very preterm infants or those with renal impairment. Toxic levels of various aminoglycosides are shown in Table 64.

Cephalosporins

New third-generation cephalosporins achieve significant concentration in CSF. Effective *in vitro* against most Gram-positive and Gram-negative bacteria, but antimicrobial activity approximately one-tenth that of benzylpenicillin. Possible indication for use is treatment of ampicillin-resistant *Klebsiella–Enterobacter* infections in combination with aminoglycoside. Now used as second-line antibiotics in treatment of neonatal infections in combination with broad-spectrum penicillin antibiotic or aminoglycoside. Cefotaxime or cefuroxime are effective and ceftazidime has activity against *Pseudomonas*. Penetration of CSF by cefotaxime is good.

Chloramphenicol

Few indications for use of chloramphenicol in newborn. May be given for infection caused by organisms resistant to aminoglycosides or to infants not responding to conventional antibiotics after trial period. Adequate antibiotic levels in CSF achieved after oral administration in appropriate doses and chloramphenicol may be used to treat neonatal meningitis. 'Grey baby syndrome' was complication of chloramphenicol therapy due to increased serum concentration of free and conjugated drug leading to collapse. Excessive doses, immaturity of glucuronyl transferase and reduced renal function combined to cause this complication. Early signs of 'grey baby syndrome' were vomiting, poor sucking, respiratory distress, abdominal distension and diarrhoea. In appropriate doses, 'grey baby syndrome' is *not* seen (see Appendix V). Because of long half-life, chloramphenicol is given at 24-hour intervals for the first week and 12 hourly in the second. Blood dyscrasias have not been reported in newborn. Serum levels should be measured (see p. 201).

Vancomycin

Effective against methicillin-resistant *Staphylococcus* (MRSA) and *Clostridium difficile*. Total daily dose 20–30 mg/kg/day in divided doses. Check serum levels after 48 hours. Aim to keep peak levels in the range of 20–30 μg/ml and trough < 12 μg/ml.

Other Antibiotics

Metronidazole is effective against anaerobes and is sometimes used to treat necrotizing enterocolitis, and congenital pneumonia in 'smelly' babies.

Trimethoprim is now available for intravenous use and is occasionally used to treat septicaemia in susceptible cases.

Ciprofloxacin is a new synthetic quinolone antibiotic which is bactericidal and works by inhibiting bacterial DNA-gyrase. Ciprofloxacin has a wide spectrum of activity including *Pseudomonas* and *Serratia* but its use in the newborn may be limited because it inhibits the metabolism of theophylline in the liver and may also damage joint cartilage in growing animals.

MATERNAL INFECTIOUS DISEASES

Appendix XI lists the infectious diseases that are notifiable.

Only for varicella infection should baby be isolated from mother. Treat baby with 0.05 ml/kg of zoster immune globulin (ZIG) and acyclovir (10–15 mg/kg/day) 8 hourly in divided doses by slow intravenous infusion over 1 hour.

For maternal hepatitis A and B, immune globulin should be given to the baby to prevent transmission (see above). Precautions to prevent spread of HBV and HIV are similar (see p. 24 and above).

For active tuberculosis, give isoniazid to baby and check for Mantoux conversion at 6 months. If no conversion then give BCG. If mother's TB is inactive or adequately treated then give baby BCG at birth.

If mother has malaria and baby's blood contains parasites treat with chloroquine.

For rubella infections isolate mother and baby from others.

NURSING POINTS

1. Early diagnosis of infection, particularly late onset relies on high level of suspicion and observation of subtle and indefinable signs such as 'handles poorly'
2. Temperature instability is a useful sign that may be masked by use of servo-control
3. High blood glucose (glucose stix readings) may be an early sign of sepsis
4. Abdominal distension and increased gastric aspirates may indicate sepsis or NEC
5. Prolonged bleeding from puncture sites may be first noted by nursing staff

REFERENCES AND FURTHER READING

Anonymous (1988). HIV infection, breastfeeding, and human milk banking. *Lancet* ii: 143.

Chirico, G., Rondini, G., Plebani, A. *et al.* (1987). Intravenous gammaglobulin therapy for prophylaxis of infection in high-risk neonates. *J. Pediatr.* **110**: 437.

Halliday, H. L. (1989). When to do a lumbar puncture in a neonate. *Arch. Dis. Child* **64**: 313.

Kadar, N. (1979). TORCH infections: a significant health hazard to pregnant women. *J. Mat. Child. Health* **4**: 430.

Kite, P., Millar, M. R., Gorham, P. and Congdon, P. (1988). Comparison of five tests used in diagnosis of neonatal bacteraemia. *Arch. Dis. Child.* **63**: 639.

McCracken, G. H. and Nelson, J. D. (1989). *Antimicrobial Therapy for Newborns*, 3rd edn. New York: Grune and Stratton.

Preece, P. M., Pearl, K. N. and Peckham, C. S. (1984). Congenital cytomegalovirus infection. *Arch. Dis. Child.* **59**: 1120.

Remington, J. S. and Klein, J. O. (1983). *Infectious Disease of the Fetus and Newborn Infant*. Philadelphia: W. B. Saunders.

15. Apnoeic Attacks

Apnoea in newborn is cessation of breathing for more than 15 sec. May be associated bradycardia (heart rate less than 100 beats/min) and cyanosis. The commonest cause is apnoea of prematurity but this diagnosis made only after exclusion of other causes (Table 65). Apnoeic attacks occur in at least 30%

Table 65. Causes of apnoea (and bradycardia).

1. Hypoxia, especially severe RDS
2. Sepsis, especially group B streptococcal septicaemia and meningitis
3. Airway obstruction: aspiration, blocked nares, neck flexion or extension, face mask
4. Hypoglycaemia
5. Hypocalcaemia
6. Hypovolaemia
7. Hypothermia and hyperthermia
8. Excessive pharyngeal suctioning
9. Excessive handling and/or accidental alteration of environment, e.g. during radiography, opening incubator door
10. Maternal narcotic and analgesic drugs
11. Cerebral birth trauma
12. Intraventricular haemorrhage
13. Anaemia
14. Polycythaemia
15. Hyponatraemia
16. Overdose of anticonvulsant drugs, especially diazepam and phenobarbitone mixtures
17. Seizures (see Table 72)
18. Patent ductus arteriosus
19. Kernicterus
20. Apnoea of prematurity

of newborn infants of < 34 weeks gestation, so all should be monitored until no longer having them. Onset of apnoea of prematurity may be delayed until the third day of life or later. Apnoea within the first 24 hours should suggest infection or severe RDS as an underlying cause.

Periodic breathing is a regular sequence of respiratory pauses of 10–20 sec interspersed with periods of hyperventilation of 4–15 sec, and occurring at least 3 times/min. It is not associated with cyanosis or bradycardia.

INVESTIGATION OF APNOEA (AND BRADYCARDIA)

1. Examine infant closely, looking for signs of infection, airway obstruction, seizures or patent ductus arteriosus. Note incubator temperature and oxygen concentration
2. Laboratory investigations: full blood picture and platelets; blood culture; glucose stix; electrolytes and calcium. Chest radiography, blood gas analysis and pH and examination of CSF may also be indicated if meningitis is suspected. In previously well infant who suddenly deteriorates with apnoea ultrasound scan of brain and/or a lumbar puncture should be performed to exclude meningitis or intraventricular haemorrhage

Only after exclusion of infection, biochemical or drug causes of apnoea can infant confidently be labelled as having apnoea of prematurity.

APNOEA OF PREMATURITY

Apnoea and periodic breathing are very common in the preterm infant. The aetiology is not completely understood but immaturity of medullary respiratory centres or chemoreceptors may cause irregular stimulation of breathing. Inspiratory and expiratory centres in the brainstem control ventilation (Fig. 49). They are influenced by sensors (central and peripheral chemoreceptors) which monitor arterial blood to maintain normal arterial oxygen tensions and pH despite wide variations in oxygen demand and carbon dioxide production. Central chemoreceptors respond to hypercapnia and acidosis, and

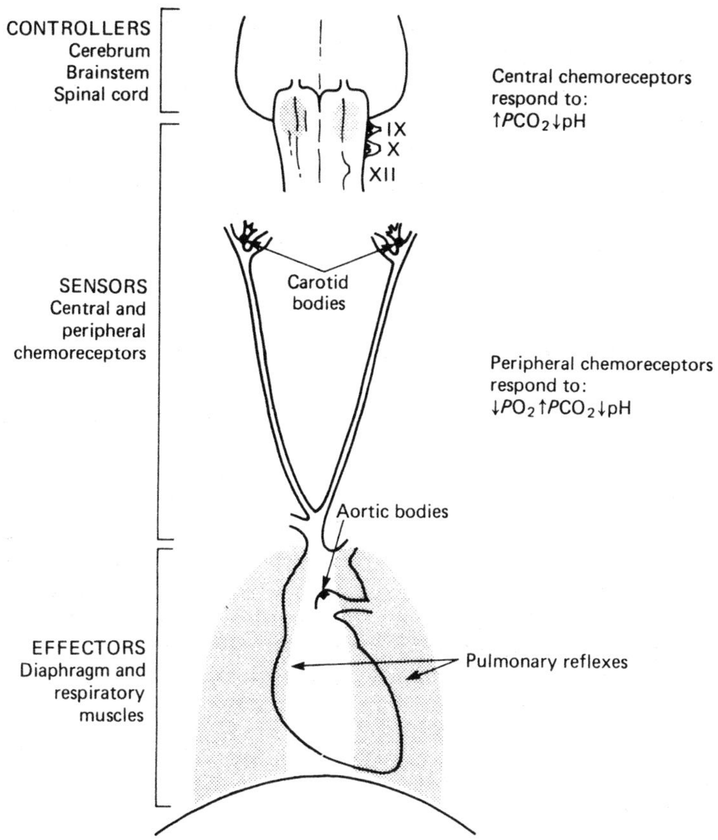

Fig. 49. Control of breathing: brain centres, peripheral chemoreceptors and effectors in man. Adapted from Brady and Gould (1984).

peripheral chemoreceptors (carotid and aortic bodies) to hypoxaemia, by stimulation of effectors to increase respiratory effort (Fig. 49). These responses are modified by maturity, sleep state, environmental temperature, level of oxygenation and drugs. During REM (rapid eye movement) sleep there is a lot of intrinsic drive but little chemical control. During non-REM sleep, respiration depends upon chemical control. Periodic breathing disappears after a few weeks as infant approaches term (40 weeks) and this may coincide with maturation of the respiratory centres. Response of the preterm respiratory centre to hypercapnia and hypoxia is different from that of the mature infant or older child. Normally these chemical changes cause stimulation of respiration with increase in rate and depth of breathing (increased minute ventilation) but in the preterm infant the opposite often occurs: hypercapnia causing no response and hypoxia depressing respiration in preterm infant. Hypoxia has a dual effect on breathing: stimulation via peripheral chemoreceptors and central depression. Normal response to hypoxia is immediate increase in ventilation by 25% followed by decrease due to overriding influence of central depressant effect during the first month of life. Apnoea of prematurity often has its onset on the third day of life, coinciding with lowest thoracic gas volume of the preterm baby. Patchy atelectasis caused by pliable chest wall may cause hypoxaemia and subsequent apnoea.

TREATMENT OF APNOEA

Any underlying cause should first be corrected (see Table 65). Infant who is having apnoea should be monitored with continuous recording of heart and respiratory rate. Continuous measurement of oxygen saturation or transcutaneous oxygen tension is also desirable. Apnoea of 15 sec or more, especially with bradycardia, is serious and needs action. Heat shield to reduce temperature swings may reduce number of attacks. Table 66 outlines a plan of management.

Table 66. Plan for management of apnoea.

1. Search for underlying cause(s) and correct. Raise ambient O_2 2% if P_aO_2 <8 kPa (60 mmHg)
2. Careful monitoring of heart and respiratory rate
3. Intermittent stimulation: stroking, rocking
4. Intermittent bag and mask ventilation
5. Continuous stimulation: inflatable rubber glove, water bed
6. Continuous positive airways pressure (CPAP)
7. Drugs: theophylline/aminophylline, caffeine, doxapram
8. Mechanical ventilation

Repeated Stimulation

Repeated stimulation of infant by stroking, gentle rubbing or rocking will often prevent or shorten apnoeic attacks. Rocking water beds reduce frequency of short apnoeic attacks but require adequate and safe method of heating them. All forms of stimulation work by increasing input to immature respiratory centre via cutaneous, vestibular or proprioceptive pathways. Should intermittent stimulation fail then continuous methods may be tried, e.g. regular inflation of a rubber glove placed under the infant.

Intermittent Bag and Mask Ventilation

This may be used for infrequent apnoeic episodes when continuous stimulation has failed. The technique is described on p. 73 but always ventilate infant with same concentration of oxygen as the ambient oxygen concentration in order to reduce possibility of retinopathy of prematurity. Use Cardiff or Ohio self-inflating bags.

Continuous Positive Airways Pressure (CPAP)

Use either nasopharyngeal tube, nasal prongs or Bennett mask (see Chapter 9). CPAP reduces frequency of apnoeic attacks by improving oxygenation and correcting alveolar collapse. CPAP may also stabilize the chest wall and stimulate receptors in nose, mouth and pharynx.

Respiratory Centre Stimulants

Aminophylline, theophylline, caffeine and doxapram have been used. Theophylline compounds, which are phosphodiesterase inhibitors, probably work by increasing the sensitivity of the respiratory centre to raised carbon dioxide tensions. Other effects are stimulation of the diaphragm, positive inotropic and chronotropic actions on the heart, mild diuresis (improved cardiac output) and increased heat production through utilization of brown fat. Unwelcome effects include decreased cerebral blood flow and uncertainty of long-term use.

Recommended doses of theophylline are 5 mg/kg by slow intravenous infusion as a loading dose and 1 mg/kg 6 hourly as maintenance. A 4 mg dose of theophylline is equivalent to 5 mg of aminophylline. After 24–48 hours of theophylline therapy, serum levels should be measured to keep them in therapeutic range (10–18 μg/ml). Theophylline levels over 20 μg/ml or signs of toxicity (heart rate over 180 beats/min, vomiting or seizures) are indications to reduce dose. Alternative routes of administration are oral or rectal (5 mg suppositories are available). Dose of rectal aminophylline varies in each infant and serum levels should be measured. Half a suppository (2.5 mg) is the starting dose for infants less than 1800 g, usually given 6 hourly. Rectal treatment is now only occasionally used. Side-effects are proctitis and variable absorption giving erratic effects. Once apnoeic attacks have been controlled, aim to gradually reduce frequency and dose of theophylline or aminophylline.

In the neonate theophylline is methylated to caffeine which also reduces apnoea frequency. Caffeine has a wider margin of safety than theophylline but is probably less effective. Loading dose is 10 mg/kg orally, followed by 2.5 mg/kg once daily.

Doxapram is a direct respiratory stimulant which has undergone limited study in treatment of neonatal apnoea. Dose is 2.5 mg/kg/hour by infusion and side-effect is jitteriness.

Mechanical Ventilation

Used for babies with apnoea resistant to treatment with xanthines and repeated stimulation. Often needed for very immature babies, those with septicaemia and respiratory failure with acidosis.

REFERENCES AND FURTHER READING

Aranda, J. V., Grondin, D. and Sasyniuk, B. I. (1981). Pharmacologic considerations in the therapy of neonatal apnea. *Pediatr. Clin. North Am.* 28: 113.

Brady, J. P. and Gould, J. B. (1984). Sudden infant death syndrome. In: (ed., Barness, L. A.) *Advances in Pediatrics*, Vol. 31. Chicago: Year Book Medical.

Bucher, H. U. and Duc, G. (1988). Does caffeine prevent hypoxaemic episodes in premature infants? A randomized controlled trial. *Eur. J. Pediatr.* **147**: 288.

Eyal, F., Alpan, G., Sagi, E. *et al.* (1985). Aminophylline versus doxapram in idiopathic apnea of prematurity: a double blind controlled study. *Pediatrics* **75**: 709.

Jones, R. A. K. (1981). A controlled trial of a regularly cycled oscillating waterbed and a non-oscillating waterbed in the prevention of apnoea in the preterm infant. *Arch. Dis. Child.* **55**: 889.

Jones, R. A. K. (1982). Apnoea of immaturity. I. A. controlled trial of theophylline and face mask with aminophylline. *Arch. Dis. Child* **57**: 761.

Kattwinkel, J. (1980). Apnea in the neonatal period. *Pediatr. Rev.* **2**: 115.

Kuzemko, J. A. and Poala, J. (1973). Apnoeic attacks in the newborn treated with amonophylline. *Arch. Dis. Child* **48**: 404.

Levitt, G. A., Mushin, A., Bellman, S. and Harvey, D. R. (1988). Outcome of preterm infants who suffered neonatal apnoeic attacks. *Early Hum. Develop.* **16**: 235.

Miller, M. J., Carlo, W. A. and Martin, R. J. (1985). Continuous positive airways pressure selectively treduces obstructive apnea in preterm infants. *J. Pediatr.* **1066**: 91.

Rigatto, H. (1982). Apnea. *Pediatr. Clin. North Am.* **29**: 1105.

16. Neurological Problems

Neurological disorders in the newborn may be primary or secondary in origin (Table 67). Secondary disorders are of greater importance in that it may be possible to prevent extension of cerebral damage and thus minimize handicap. Cerebral hypoxia and bacterial infection are of prime importance. Of these, cerebral hypoxia is commoner and more difficult to diagnose.

Table 67. Types of neurological disorder.

Primary causes (prenatal and birth):

1. *Congenital anomalies*: microcephaly, hydrocephaly, hydranencephaly, encephalocele, porencephalic cysts, chromosomal anomalies, or myopathies
2. *Infections*: CMV, rubella, toxoplasmosis, syphilis
3. *Neurocutaneous syndromes*: tuberous sclerosis, neurofibromatosis, Sturge–Weber syndrome
4. *Trauma*: torn falx cerebri, subdural, subarachnoid haemorrhages, skull fractures, spinal cord and brachial plexus injuries

Secondary causes (postnatal):

1. *Infections*: meningitis, herpes simplex encephalitis
2. *Drugs*: narcotics, barbiturates, general anaesthesia, local anaesthesia (direct)
3. *Hypoxia*: asphyxia, RDS, recurrent apnoea, intraventricular haemorrhage
4. *Metabolic*: hypoglycaemia, acidosis, hypocalcaemia, hyponatraemia, hypernatraemia, hypomagnesaemia, aminoacidurias, galactosaemia, hypothyroidism, hypothermia, malnutrition and vitamin deficiency
5. *Secondary bleeding*: intracranial haemorrhages from thrombocytopenia or disseminated intravascular coagulation

CEREBRAL HYPOXIA AND ISCHAEMIA (see also p. 34)

May occur in antepartum, intrapartum or neonatal period. Major problem is to determine the nature and extent of cerebral damage. The most satisfactory neurological assessment seems

Table 68. Sarnat staging of hypoxic/ischaemic encephalopathy (HIE).

	Stage 1	*Stage 2*	*Stage 3*
1. *Level of consciousness*	Hyperalert	Lethargic or obtunded	Stupor or coma
2. *Neuromuscular control*:			
Muscle tone	Normal	Mild hypotonia	Flaccid
Posture	Mild distal flexion	Strong distal flexion	Intermittent decerebration
Tendon reflexes	Over-active	Over-active	Decreased or absent
Segmental myoclonus	Present	Present	Absent
3. *Complex reflexes*:			
Suck	Weak	Weak or absent	Absent
Moro	Strong	Weak	Absent
Oculovestibular	Normal	Over-active	Weak or absent
Tonic neck	Slight	Strong	Absent
4. *Autonomic function*:	General sympathetic	General parasympathetic	Both depressed
Pupils	Dilated	Constricted	Variable, poor light reflex
Heart rate	Tachycardia	Bradycardia	Variable
Bronchial and salivary secretions	Sparse	Profuse	Variable
GI motility	Normal or reduced	Increased, diarrhoea	Variable
5. *Seizures*	None	Common	Uncommon, decerebrate

Adapted from Sarnat and Sarnat (1976)

to be that described by Sarnat and Sarnat in 1976 (see Table 68). This assessment places the infant in one of three stages of hypoxic–ischaemic encephalopathy (HIE). The examination is based upon five clinical areas:

1. Level of consciousness
2. Neuromuscular control: tone and posture
3. Complex reflexes: primitive reflexes
4. Autonomic function
5. Presence of seizures

EEG examination may be used in doubtful cases but clinical staging alone has been shown to correlate well with outcome. (Table 69). Sarnat scoring should be done within 12 hours of birth and repeated daily until normal. We have found that 0.6% of term babies have an Apgar score at 5 min < 5 but only one-third of these babies develop encephalopathy (two-thirds, Stage 1; one-quarter, Stage 2; 10%, Stage 3).

Table 69. Outcome of hypoxic/ischaemic encephalopathy (HIE) by Sarnat Stage.

Sarnat Stage		*Mortality* (%)	*Normal development* (%)
1		0	90
2		10	50
3		90	0
Stage 2	< 5 days	0	90
	≥ 5 days	20	10

Sarnat staging predicts outcome well (Table 69). Stage 1 or 2 for less than 5 days: low mortality and 90% normal development. There is a poor outcome for babies in Stage 3: 90% mortality and no normal survivors. For Stage 2 > 5 days: only 10% with normal development. Sarnat staging also predicts the severity of the handicap: Stage 1, mild handicap if any, and Stage 3, moderate or severe handicap.

Investigation for confirmation of diagnosis and detection of secondary upsets may include:

1. Lumbar puncture
    Subarachnoid haemorrhage
    Meningitis (normal CSF findings are shown in Table 70)

Table 70. Normal CSF findings.

	Term		Preterm	
	Range	*Mean*	*Range*	*Mean*
Red cells (per HPF)	0–600	9	0–800	15
White cells (per HPF)	0–32	8	0–29	9
Protein (g/l)	0.20–1.70	0.90	0.65–1.50	1.15
Sugar (mmol/l)	1.8–4.3	2.8	1.5–4.1	2.4

After Sarff *et al.* (1976)

2. Ultrasonic and CT scan:
   Ventricular size
   Intracerebral bleeding
   Increased echodensity (see Chapter 24)
3. Skull transillumination
   Subdural haematoma
   Hydrocephalus and hydranencephaly
4. Auditory brainstem evoked responses (ABER)
5. EEG
6. Skull radiography usually of little help

Investigation of secondary upsets (Table 67) includes blood glucose, calcium, electrolyte and coagulation measurements.

Treatment of Hypoxic–Ischaemic Encephalopathy

1. Maintain neutral thermal environment, normoxaemia, and normoglycaemia (both hypo- and hyperglycaemia are harmful)
2. Fluid, electrolye and acid–base balance very important: maintain urine specific gravity at 1010
3. Adequate blood pressure and cerebral perfusion pressure should be maintained using dopamine if necessary (5–15 μg/kg/min)
4. Attempt to minimize damage:
   Treatment of cerebral oedema (Table 72)
   Treatment of seizures (Table 75)
   Treatment for other organ systems (p. 34)

5. Gentle infrequent handling by staff
6. Good support of mother, father and baby with frequent visits and communication

PREDICTION OF OUTCOME OF HYPOXIC–ISCHAEMIC ENCEPHALOPATHY

Several methods currently available (Table 71). Clinical examination is of value (see Sarnat Staging, Table 69). Imaging with ultrasound and CT scans has limitations with the latter being more valuable in term babies. Persistent generalized hypodensities and focal infarcts on CT scan carry a poor prognosis.

Table 71. Prediction of outcome of HIE.

1. Clinical methods: Apgar score at 10 or 20 min, neurological examination (e.g. Sarnat)
2. Imaging techniques: ultrasound and CT scanning, MRI
3. Biochemical methods: hypoxanthine, ammonia, lactate dehydrogenase, brain-specific creatine kinase (CKBB)
4. Electrophysiological techniques: EEG, auditory and visual evoked potentials, somatosensory evoked responses

The best biochemical test is brain-specific creatine kinase (CKBB) which can be measured in blood and CSF. Blood CKBB level is a sensitive indicator of cerebral damage but is unable to predict outcome.

Electrophysiological techniques (EEG and evoked responses) help in diagnosis but only EEG and auditory evoked brainstem potentials have been used to predict outcome following asphyxia. Persistent abnormalities are associated with poor prognosis.

Treatment of Cerebral Oedema (Table 72)

Cerebral oedema is difficult to diagnose in the newborn but signs are tense anterior fontanelle, low heart rate

Table 72. Treatment of cerebral oedema.

1. Correct hypoxia and acidosis
2. Control seizures (Table 75)
3. Fluid restriction 60 ml/kg/day
4. Mannitol infusion 7 ml/kg 20% solution over 20 min
5. Dexamethasone 1 mg/kg loading dose then 0.3 mg/kg 8 hourly for 3 days
6. Hyperventilation: lower $P\text{CO}_2$ 4 kPa (25–30 mmHg)
7. High dose barbiturate or thiopentone

(<110/min), raised blood pressure (>80 mmHg) systolic), seizures. Ultrasound scan shows small ventricles, decreased vascular pulsation and generalized increase in echodensity (Chapter 24).

The benefits of treatment of cerebral oedema as outlined above are unproven but nevertheless often used. May be treated acutely with mannitol infusions (7 ml/kg of 20% mannitol over 20 min) which may be repeated 4 hourly if necessary. For mannitol to be effective serum osmolality must be less than 300 mosm/l. Mechanical hyperventilation may be used to reduce cerebral blood flow by lowering $P\text{CO}_2$ to 4–5 kPa (25–30 mmHg). Alternatively, dexamethasone as a 1 mg/kg loading dose followed by 0.3 mg/kg 8 hourly may be used. Takes time to work and may not be effective. Should be gradually tailed off after 3 days. Other potential therapies include high-dose barbiturates (lower cerebral metabolic needs but cause hypotension), calcium channel blockers and oxygen free radical scavengers.

Periventricular Leucomalacia

Cerebral hypoxia and/or ischaemia may result in periventricular leucomalacia (PVL) which is seen on ultrasound scan in 2–15% of infants < 1500 g. Rarely occurs in term infants. Has a predilection for watershed areas in deep white matter and occipital radiation at trigone of lateral ventricles. Initial lesion is an area of coagulation necrosis perhaps due to venous infarction or cerebral ischaemia and which may progress to cavitation. In 25% of cases haemorrhage into an area of ischaemic necrosis may be involved. Predisposing factors: IRDS, birth asphyxia, APH, septic shock, hypotension and PDA.

Diagnosis is by US scan (see Chapter 24). Prognosis is poor with a high incidence of major handicap in infants with cystic PVL. Those with transient echodensities (< 2 weeks) have a good outcome but outcome is not clear for infants with persistent echodensities without cyst formation.

NEONATAL SEIZURES

Seizures in the newborn relatively common (0.6–1/1000 births) but difficult to diagnose as can present in unusual ways ('subtle seizures'). Classical repetitive jerky movements of limbs may be seen but more subtle presentation with apnoea, hypotonia, bradycardia, rigidity and rolling of the eyes. The causes of neonatal seizures are listed in Table 73 and underlying cause

Table 73. Causes of neonatal seizures.

1. Hypoxia/ischaemia: antepartum, intrapartum, neonatal (RDS, apnoeic attacks) (40%)
2. Intracranial bleeding: subdural, extradural, subarachnoid, intraventricular (30%)
3. Metabolic: hypoglycaemia, hypocalcaemia, hypomagnesaemia, hyponatraemia, hypernatraemia (12%)
4. Meningitis (8%)
5. Structural cerebral anomalies: hydrocephalus, microcephalus, encephalocele, tuberous sclerosis (3%)
6. Obstetrical trauma: breech, forceps
7. Drugs: narcotics, phenothiazines, barbiturates, addiction and withdrawal, local anaesthetics
8. Pyridoxine dependency
9. Kernicterus
10. Aminoacidurias: phenylketonuria, maple syrup urine disease, hyperlysinuria, hyperglycinaemia, urea cycle disorders
11. Intrauterine infection: rubella, toxoplasmosis, CMV
12. Familial neonatal seizures (may be benign)

Table 74. Onset and type of seizures.

First 3 days:
1. Asphyxia: tonic or tonic/clonic, apnoea
2. Hypoglycaemia: clonic
3. Intraventricular haemorrhage: tonic, apnoea
4. Hypocalcaemia: tonic/clonic, multifocal
5. Inborn errors of metabolism: any type (see Chapter 20)
6. Congenital malformation: any type (see Chapter 23)
7. Meningitis: tonic, apnoea

After 3 days:
1. Meningitis: tonic, tonic/clonic, apnoea
2. Hypocalcaemia: clonic, multifocal
3. Hypomagnesaemia: clonic, multifocal
4. Kernicterus: tonic, apnoea, subtle
5. Drug withdrawal: clonic, jittery
6. Hypo- or hypernatraemia: clonic

should always be sought so that specific treatments may be used. Asphyxia is commonest cause accounting for 40%, followed by intracranial bleeding 30%, metabolic causes 12%, infection 8% and malformations 3%. The time of onset and type of seizure relate to both cause and outcome (Table 74). Seizures occurring in the first 3 days are usually more significant than those occurring later.

Investigation of neonatal seizures includes a full history and examination followed by investigation of possible underlying problems:

1. Glucose strip test and blood glucose
2. Serum calcium and magnesium
3. Electrolytes: Na^+, K^+, Cl^-, urea
4. Astrup: blood gases and pH
5. Urine examination for smell, culture and reducing substances (Clinitest and Clinistix)
6. Intrauterine infection (TORCH titres) and bacterial infection (blood culture, CSF examination and blood film)

7. Examine fundi
8. Ultrasound scan of brain
9. Transillumination of skull
10. EEG

The treatment of hypoglycaemia, hypocalcaemia and hypernatraemia has been fully discussed in Chapter 12. Seizures due to biochemical abnormalities usually tonic/clonic and multifocal in comparison to those caused by hypoxia or cerebral haemorrhage which are tonic and often asymmetrical.

If no underlying biochemical cause is found and seizures persist then anticonvulsant therapy should be started (Table 75). Phenobarbitone is probably safest and most effective drug. The loading dose is 20 mg/kg intravenously followed by 5 mg/kg/day in divided doses (usually every 8 hours).

Table 75. Treatment of neonatal seizures.

1. Correct underlying causes, e.g. hypoglycaemia or infection
2. Phenobarbitone 20 mg/kg loading dose intravenously then 5 mg/kg/day given 8 hourly
3. Phenytoin 5–10 mg/kg/day given 8 hourly intravenously
4. Diazepam 0.3 mg/kg iv single dose
5. Treat cerebral oedema (Table 72)

If seizures continue despite adequate serum levels of phenobarbitone (therapeutic range 15–20 μg/ml (100–140 μmol/l)), phenytoin may be added using a loading dose of 20 mg/kg followed by 5–10 mg/kg/day divided into 8 hourly doses (therapeutic serum levels 15–20 μg/ml (60–80 μmol/l)). Phenytoin must be given intravenously as it is poorly absorbed after oral and intramuscular administration. Cardiac arrhythmias are associated with intravenous use; infants should have ECG monitoring during infusion.

Phenobarbitone and phenytoin in combination are probably superior to diazepam or paraldehyde for the treatment of neonatal seizures. Diazepam may cause both respiratory depression and kernicterus from bilirubin displacement from albumin. In addition, the anticonvulsant action is short lived. Paraldehyde is inconvenient to administer. If plastic syringe is used, paraldehyde must be given within 1 min as contact with plastic denatures the drug. It is also malodorous and liable to cause sterile abscesses.

Duration of anticonvulsant treatment is often difficult to determine. Babies can be weaned from their treatment before discharge if seizures controlled and CNS examination normal. Some infants may need prolonged treatment: e.g. persistent seizures and/or EEG abnormality. More likely if CNS malformation, following meningitis or intraventricular haemorrhage. In these cases it is usual to treat for 3–6 months and then reassess.

Pyridoxine dependency is an uncommon cause of neonatal seizures and intravenous injection of 20 mg/kg of pyridoxine (vitamin B_6) will stop the seizures.

Prognosis of Neonatal Seizures

Outlook following neonatal seizures is influenced by several factors: underlying cause of seizures, type, severity and duration of seizures, and infant's potential for future intelligence (combination of genetic endowment, and social and environmental circumstances). Babies who have abnormal neurological signs at discharge or whose seizures were multifocal have a

Table 76. Prognosis of neonatal seizures.

Underlying cause	*Abnormal development*
Severe asphyxia	>50%
Subarachnoid haemorrhage	10%
Intraventricular haemorrhage	
Grade I/II*	10–20%
Grade III/IV	50–90%
Hypoglycaemia	50%
Meningitis	60%
Structural anomaly	100%
Hypocalcaemia	
early	50%
late	<10%

* Based upon ultrasound scan (Chapter 24 and Table 77)

poorer prognosis. Mortality is greatest if seizures due to intracranial haemorrhage (57%), followed by infection (33%) and asphyxia (27%). Of survivors overall, 43% have an abnormal outcome. Table 76 summarizes prognosis of neonatal seizures by cause.

JITTERY BABY

Shaking movements of the limbs that are not true seizures. When limbs are flexed, jitteriness disappears but seizures will continue. Exclude hypoglycaemia, hypocalcaemia or hypomagnesaemia and drug withdrawal (alcohol, benzodiazepines and narcotics). Some SGA infants remain jittery although no biochemical reason found. In this case treat by swaddling and avoid bright lights and loud noises. Only occasionally is sedation needed.

INTRAVENTRICULAR HAEMORRHAGE (IVH)

A common problem of the very low birth weight infant (up to 50% on ultrasound scan (USS)).

Incidence is increased following asphyxia and in the presence of RDS, and reduced after caesarean section delivery.

Capillaries in the germinal plate may be damaged during periods of hypotension. During hypoxia, hypertension occurs, and with hypercapnia increased cerebral blood flow leads to bleeding from these damaged capillaries. In the preterm infant or after asphyxia, cerebral autoregulation does not occur (i.e. when pressure increases, flow is not reduced to maintain even perfusion). Bleeding into the germinal plate or subependymal

Table 77. Grading of intraventricular haemorrhage (IVH) by ultrasound.

Grade	
I	Subependymal bleeding
II	Small intraventricular haemorrhage but no ventricular dilatation
III	Intraventricular haemorrhage and dilatation
IV	III and intracranial extension

matrix can be detected by ultrasound scanning (Chapter 24). Blood may rupture into one or both lateral ventricles causing infant to collapse at a later date.

IVH is graded according to ultrasound findings (Table 77).

Onset may be sudden with seizures and falling packed cell volume, or insidious with increasing head circumference. Diagnosis by ultrasound, CT scan, lumbar puncture or ventricular tap.

Prevention

Some evidence that large doses of vitamin E (p. 281) or ethamsylate (a platelet-stabilizing drug) may prevent or reduce incidence of IVH. Value of phenobarbitone and muscle relaxants is not convincingly proven. Prevention of asphyxia, increased use of caesarean section and surfactant replacement therapy lower incidence.

Treatment

Repeated lumbar punctures may lower CSF protein and remove blood to prevent hydrocephalus. Acetazolamide has been used to treat hydrocephalus (see p. 348) but electrolyte upsets occur. Ventriculoperitoneal shunting may be necessary if the ventricles progressively enlarge despite treatment, though this procedure carries the risks of sepsis, blocked shunt and seizures.

Prognosis

Depends upon extent of haemorrhage, but if symptomatic, 50% die; of survivors 20% severely abnormal, 20% mildly abnormal and 60% normal. Asymptomatic IVH is much more common, up to 50% of infants < 1500 g, with variable outlook (Table 76).

SUBARACHNOID HAEMORRHAGE

Subarachnoid haemorrhage may follow asphyxia or obstetric trauma. Presentation with seizures or initially asymptomatic with progressive hydrocephalus in a few. Diagnosis by lumbar puncture; ultrasound and CT scans exclude intracerebral bleeding. Prognosis is usually good with 90% having normal development.

SUBDURAL HAEMORRHAGE

Subdural haemorrhage is uncommon in newborn. Obstetric trauma and precipitate delivery predispose by tearing falx cerebri where the great cerebral vein enters the inferior sagittal sinus. May present with signs of raised intracranial pressure, focal seizures or subacutely with increasing head size, failure to thrive and bulging fontanelle. Diagnosis by ultrasound and CT scan or subdural taps (see p. 117). Treat by subdural tap which may need to be repeated, after consultation with neurosurgeon.

TRAUMATIC NERVE PALSIES

Trauma to facial nerve and brachial plexus not uncommon and may occur *in utero* or during birth. Forceps delivery increases risk of facial palsy and shoulder dystocia is associated with Erb's palsy.

Neurapraxia is commoner than axonotmesis so that recovery usually complete. Facial nerve can be damaged *in utero* by pressure against the sacral promontory. If unilaterally affected, when infant cries, the mouth is drawn to the side of the lesion and the eye cannot be fully closed. Methylcellulose drops provide lubrication and prevent corneal damage of exposed eye. The prognosis for facial palsy is usually good with the majority recovering within 1 month.

Erb's palsy is lesion of upper roots of brachial plexus. The arm is adducted and internally rotated at the shoulder to give 'waiter's tip' deformity. May also be sensory deficit over C5 distribution. Occasionally associated diaphragmatic paralysis on same side causing respiratory difficulty.

Klumpke's palsy from lesion of lower brachial plexus. Associated with wrist drop and difficult to distinguish from radial nerve palsy. Treatment with gentle passive physiotherapy and splinting of the wrists and fingers. Recovery should occur within 6 months (over 90%) but complete avulsion of lower nerve roots may occur in difficult deliveries. Presence of residual signs at 6 months carries poor prognosis for full recovery with two-thirds having long-term weakness.

FLOPPY BABY

Common causes of hypotonia in the newborn are outlined in Table 78, the commonest cause being birth asphyxia. Conversely, it should be remembered that a baby with muscle disease may present with birth asphyxia.

Investigations include: careful assessment of the family history, examination of the mother, muscle enzymes, urinary chromatogram, viral cultures, chromosome analysis, thyroid function tests, stool examination, EMG, muscle biopsy and test dose of edrophonium (p. 19).

Table 78. Causes of the floppy baby.

1. Hypoxic ischaemic encephalopathy
2. Prematurity
3. Intracranial haemorrhage
4. Sepsis, botulism, drugs
5. Down's syndrome, Prader–Willi syndrome
6. Metabolic: hypoglycaemia, hyponatraemia, inborn errors of metabolism
7. Endocrine: hypothyroidism
8. Spinal cord: transection, Werdnig–Hoffman syndrome, poliomyelitis
9. Muscle disorders: myasthenia gravis, congenital myopathies, myotonic dystrophy

CONGENITAL ANOMALIES

See Chapter 23.

NURSING POINTS

Nursing the 'cerebral baby':

1. Avoid stresses of noise, light and handling. Place baby in a

quiet incubator covered with a green towel and avoid excessive handling
2. Monitor heart rate, respiration, temperature, oxygen saturation
3. Carefully record fluid intake and output; test urine for specific gravity, protein and blood
4. Watch for seizures; these may be subtle, e.g. lip smacking, eye rolling, apnoeic periods
5. Encourage parents to visit and gently interact with the baby. Attend counselling sessions with senior medical staff

REFERENCES AND FURTHER READING

Bjerre, I., Hellstrom-Westas, L., Rosen, I. and Svenningsen, N. (1983). Monitoring of cerebral function after severe asphyxia in infancy. *Arch. Dis. Child* **58**: 997.

de Vries, L. S., Dubowitz, L. M. S., Dubowitz, V. *et al.* (1985). Predictive value of cranial ultrasound in the newborn baby: a reappraisal. *Lancet* **ii**: 137.

Dubowitz, L. and Dubowitz, V. (1981). *The Neurological Assessment of the Preterm and Fullterm Newborn Infant.* London: Spastics International Medical Publications and William Heinemann.

Eyre, J. A. and Wilkinson, A. R. (1986). Thiopentone induced coma after severe birth asphyxia. *Arch. Dis. Child* **61**: 1084.

Fernandez, F., Verdu, A., Quero, J. and Perez-Higueras, A. (1987). Serum CPK-BB Isoenzyme in the assessment of brain damage in asphyctic term infants. *Acta Paediatr. Scand.* **76**: 914.

Finer, N. N., Robertson, C. M., Peters, K. L. and Coward, J. H. (1983). Factors affecting outcome in hypoxic-ischemic encephalopathy in term infants. *Am. J. Dis. Child* **138**: 21.

Graham, M., Levene, M. I., Trounce, J. Q. and Rutter, N. (1987). Prediction of cerebral palsy in very low birthweight infants: prospective ultrasound study. *Lancet* **ii**: 593.

Levene, M. I., Wigglesworth, J. S. and Dubowitz, V. (1981). Cerebral structure and intraventricular haemorrhage in the neonate: a real-time ultrasound study. *Arch. Dis. Child* **56**: 416.

Lipp-Swahlen, A. E., Deonna, T., Micheli, J. L. and Calame, A. (1985). Prognostic value of neonatal CT scans in asphyxiated term babies: low density score compared with neonatal neurological signs. *Neuropediatrics* **16**: 209.

Pape, K. E. and Wigglesworth, J. S. (1979). *Haemorrhage, Ischaemia and the Perinatal Brain. Clinics in Developmental Medicine*, Vols. 69/70. London: Spastics International Medical Publications and William Heinemann.

Papile, L.-A., Burstein, J., Burstein, R. and Koffler, H. (1978). Incidence and evolution of subependymal and intraventricular hemorrhage. A study of infants with birthweights less than 1500 g. *J. Pediatr.* **92**: 529.

Sarff, L. D., Platt, L. H. and McCracken, G. H. (1976). Cerebrospinal fluid evaluation in neonates: comparison of high-risk infants with and without meningitis. *J. Pediatr.* **88**: 473.

Sarnat, H. B. and Sarnat, M. S. (1976). Neonatal encephalopathy following fetal distress. A clinical and electroencephalographic study. *Arch. Neurol.* **33**: 696.

Shankaran, S., Slovis, T. L., Bedard, M. P. and Poland, R. L. (1982). Sonographic classification of intracranial hemorrhage. A prognostic indicator of mortality, morbidity and short term neurologic outcome. *J. Pediatr.* **100**: 469.

Svenningsen, N. V., Blennow, G., Lindroth, M., Gaddlin, P. O. and Ahlstrom, H. (1982). Brain-orientated intensive care treatment in severe neonatal asphyxia. Effects of phenobarbitone protection. *Arch. Dis. Child* **57**: 176.

Tudehope, D. I., Harris, A., Hawes, D. and Hayes, M. (1988). Clonical spectrum and outcome of neonatal convulsions. *Aust. Paediatr. J.* **24**: 249.

Volpe, J. J. (1977). Neonatal intracranial hemorrhage. Pathophysiology, neuropathology and clinical features. *Clin. Perinatol.* **4**: 77.

Volpe, J. J. (1989). *Neurology of the Newborn*, 2nd edn. Philadelphia: W. B. Saunders.

Watkins, A., Szymonowicz, W., Jin, X. and Yu, V. V. Y. (1988). Significance of seizures in very low-birthweight infants. *Dev. Med. Child. Neurol.* **30**: 162.

17. Cardiovascular Problems

PERINATAL CIRCULATION

The fetal lung is fluid filled and receives only 5–10% of fetal cardiac output. Blood is shunted from the lungs to aorta across ductus arteriosus. Fetus also conserves oxygen for the brain by directing oxygenated blood from placenta through two further shunts: the ductus venosus, which bypasses liver, and the foramen ovale, which bypasses right ventricle and lungs.

At birth with onset of breathing, rapid changes in circulation take place. Pulmonary blood flow increases five-fold as pulmonary vascular resistance falls due to chemical effects of increasing P_aO_2 and decreasing P_aCO_2 and mechanical effect of inflation of lungs. When the three fetal shunts close, circulation is converted from parallel arrangement into series. The foramen ovale closes first as increased flow from lungs raises left atrial pressure. Removal of low resistance placental circulation increases systemic vascular resistance and raises blood pressure. The ductus venosus closes next, followed by the ductus arteriosus after about 24 hours in normal full-term infant. For 2–3 hours after birth blood may still flow R–L from pulmonary artery to aorta through the ductus arteriosus. Thereafter it flows L–R for up to 24 hours. During the first minutes the effects of increased oxygen, cold, mechanical stretching, and possibly vasoactive peptides such as bradykinin, cause marked constriction of the umbilical vessels. At birth the right ventricle is thicker than left but latter gradually increases in size to become twice as thick as the right by 6 months.

Some results of failure of normal adaptation of circulation at birth have already been discussed, e.g. persistent fetal circulation or persistent pulmonary hypertension (see p. 151), shock or hypovolaemia (see p. 31) and hypervolaemia with polycythaemia (see p. 282), and will not be dealt with further.

Table 79 lists some practical hints on neonatal heart disease.

Table 79. Some practical hints on neonatal heart disease.

1. Symptomatic heart disease without a murmur usually serious
2. An asymptomatic murmur often benign
3. Uncomplicated ventricular septal defect: no symptoms until about 3 weeks when pulmonary vascular resistance has fallen. May be no murmur at birth
4. If significant murmur heard during routine examination in first 24 hours likely to be due to PDA, stenosis of aortic or pulmonary valves, or AV valve regurgitation
5. A systolic ejection click after 12 hours is abnormal and suggests either a large pulmonary artery, large aorta or a true truncus arteriosus
6. Heart failure in first week of life usually due to hypoplastic left heart syndrome, fibroelastosis, multiple cardiac defects, supraventricular tachycardia

EXAMINATION OF THE CARDIOVASCULAR SYSTEM

1. History:
   - Feeding difficulty
   - Breathlessness
   - Cyanotic episodes
   - Vomiting
   - Family history
2. Inspection:
   - Colour: central cyanosis or pallor
   - Respiratory rate, resting/feeding
   - Active precordium
   - Any other malformation
3. Palpation:
   - All pulses: remember to palpate digital and femoral pulses
   - Precordium: locate apex beat, quality, thrills
   - Abdomen: liver size
4. Blood pressure: arms and legs (leg is higher than arm)
5. Auscultation:
   - *Heart sounds* { normal; increased/decreased; split or single }
   - *Murmur* { time: systolic/diastolic; type: ejection/pansystolic; grade of intensity; radiation }
   - *Lung fields*

SERIOUS NEONATAL HEART DISEASE

Serious neonatal heart disease may be divided into three major groups depending on aetiology and clinical findings (Table 80):

1. Cyanosis prominent
2. Cyanosis and respiratory distress
3. Low systemic cardiac output or shock

Any neonate with cyanotic heart disease or heart failure should be transferred immediately to specialized unit for investigation and treatment. Urgent consultation with paediatric cardiologist required.

Table 80. Serious neonatal heart disease.

	Cyanosis prominent	*Cyanosis and distress*	*Low cardiac output*
Cause	Hypoplastic right ventricle, severe Fallot's	Transposition of great arteries (TGA), anomalous pulmonary veins (TAPVD)	Hypoplastic left ventricle, complicated coarctation
Signs	Small, quiet heart, reduced pulmonary flow	Smallish, active heart, increased pulmonary flow	Large, active heart, increased pulmonary flow, venous congestion

CARDIAC FAILURE

There are three major signs of neonatal cardiac failure:

1. Tachycardia
2. Tachypnoea
3. Hepatomegaly

Oedema and neck vein engorgement may be absent or difficult to detect. Excessive weight gain is a late sign. Cardiomegaly and sweating may be prominent.

The causes of cardiac failure are:

1. Congenital heart disease
2. Asphyxia and acidosis
3. Hyperkalaemia or hypoglycaemia

4. Over-transfusion or anaemia:
   Placenta
   Rhesus
   Intravenous infusion
5. Arrhythmia, e.g. congenital heart block, paroxysmal atrial tachycardia
6. Myocarditis, intrauterine infection
7. Cardiomyopathy (infant of diabetic mother)

Management of the infant with cardiac failure requires determination of cause and digoxin and diuretic therapy. Digoxin should not be given to infants with suspected myocarditis, cardiomyopathy or some arrhythmias unless paediatric cardiologist has been consulted.

Note on Rapid Digitalization

The intravenous route may be used to administer digoxin in the ill infant. The total digitalizing dose is shown in Table 81. In preterm infant, total dose is 30 μg/kg. One-half of total digitalizing dose should be given stat., followed by one-quarter after 6 hours and final one-quarter after 12 hours. This means a stat. dose of 25 μg/kg for a term infant followed by 12.5 μg/kg at 6 hours and again at 12 hours. Daily maintenance digoxin dose is one-fifth of the total digitalizing dose (10 μg/kg/day) for a full-term infant and 6 μg/kg/day for a preterm infant. This daily maintenance dose is given in divided doses every 12 hours. Serum levels of digoxin measured if there is any doubt about the response of infant or if renal impairment or hypokalaemia (therapeutic range 1–2 ng/ml).

Table 81. Digitalization.

	Total loading dose (oral or im)	*Maintenance* (oral)
Preterm	30 μg/kg*	3 μg/kg b.d.
Term	50 μg/kg*	5 μg/kg b.d.

* Total digitalizing dose: give one-half stat., one-quarter at 6 hours and one-quarter at 12 hours. For intravenous digoxin use half total dose. If myocarditis or renal failure use half total dose and one-third to one-half maintenance dose. Measure serum levels to keep <2 ng/ml

INVESTIGATION OF A MURMUR

During the first day a soft murmur can be heard in about 60% of babies. This may be due either to PDA or turbulent pulmonary flow.

In a well infant with a short systolic murmur after the first 2 days of life the following should be done. Full clinical examination including palpation of all pulses, exclusion of heart failure (triad of tachypnoea, tachycardia and hepatomegaly) and measurement of blood pressure in arms and legs. If these are normal it is probably unnecessary to perform chest radiography and ECG, but infant must be examined again before discharge at 5–7 days and referred to the baby clinic at 2–3 weeks. The general practitioner should be told of murmur but the mother often only needs to know of an extra sound in the chest that will probably go away of its own accord. The word 'murmur' for some mothers instils unnecessary fear.

If, however, murmur is loud or long or the infant is unwell, full examination must be followed by investigation with chest radiography, ECG and echocardiography (Chapter 24). Murmurs that appear for the first time after the first week of life should also be fully investigated.

Chest Radiography

The heart of normal size should have a cardiothoracic (CT) ratio of less than 0.6. Heart size is increased in many cases of heart failure (p. 236), after birth asphyxia (p. 35), in the infant of the diabetic mother (p. 17) and during hypoglycaemia (p. 172). In some forms of congenital heart disease the heart has a characteristic shape, e.g. 'cottage loaf' in total anomalous pulmonary venous drainage (TAPVD) and 'egg-on-side' in transposition of the great arteries (TGA). Pulmonary vascularity is increased in large L–R shunts and decreased in pulmonary atresia or other types of right heart obstruction. Pulmonary venous obstruction causes mottling and thickened interlobular septa mimicking transient tachypnoea of the newborn (TTN) or RDS on occasions. The aortic arch is usually on the left but may be right-sided in Fallot's tetralogy and truncus arteriosus. If there is dextrocardia with situs inversus and right aortic arch then risk of congenital heart disease is low. With dextrocardia and situs solitus the incidence is high. Splenic anomalies are associated and bacterial infections can be life threatening.

ECG

Place electrodes as follows:

V_1, fourth ICS at right sternal edge (RSE)
V_2, fourth ICS at left sternal edge (LSE)
V_4, fifth left ICS in mid-clavicular line (MCL)
V_6, fifth ICS in mid-axillary line (MAL)
V_4R, as for V_4 on right

Mean frontal QRS axis is 135° with normal range of 110–180°. There is rapid change in the left in the first month (75°) and then more gradual change to adult values.

Right ventricular overload:

QR in V_1
R in $V_1 > 30$ mm
R in $V_4R > 20$ mm
S in $V_6 > 15$ mm
R/S ratio in $V_1 > 7$
RAD $> +180°$

Left ventricular overload:

S in $V_1 > \begin{cases} 20 \text{ mm term} \\ 26 \text{ mm preterm} \end{cases}$
R/S in $V_1 < 1.0$
R in $V_6 > 14$ mm
QRS axis $< 30°$
Q in $V_6 > 4$ mm

PATENT DUCTUS ARTERIOSUS (PDA)

Closure of ductus arteriosus is complex and involves raised $P\text{O}_2$, bradykinin and acetylcholine activity, and perhaps falling prostaglandin levels. As gestational age increases, the muscular wall of the ductus becomes more sensitive to these stimuli so that the ductus of preterm infants tends to close later and less effectively than term baby. During recovery from severe RDS the ductus may remain open and L–R shunting occurs when pulmonary vascular resistance falls below systemic. Increased mechanical ventilation may be needed and there may be raised $P\text{CO}_2$, metabolic acidosis or apnoea. Loud systolic or continuous murmur at the upper left sternal edge which may radiate under left clavicle or into back. The peripheral pulses (especially femorals) will be bounding and precordium hyperactive due to increased dimension and increased contraction of the left heart chambers. If L–R shunt is large there will be cardiomegaly, increased pulmonary vascularity and pulmonary oedema on chest radiograph. Increased left heart dimension on echocardiography. Left atrial to aorta ratio (LA/Ao) over 1.5:1 indicates large shunt (normal LA/Ao ratio = 1.1:1) (see p. 328). Fluid restriction and diuretic therapy may control symptoms until spontaneous closure of ductus occurs about 40 weeks postconceptional age. Continuous positive airways pressure may reduce pulmonary oedema. Some infants, however, have large L–R shunts and may have severe recurrent apnoea, intractable metabolic acidosis and need for prolonged mechanical ventilation. If they fail to respond to conservative therapy, then closure of the ductus either by surgical ligation or by prostaglandin synthetase inhibition with indomethacin. Surgical ligation carries low operative mortality in experienced hands but risk for tiny ill infants is increased and medical closure may be preferred provided no contraindications.

Indomethacin Therapy

This is effective in about 80% of cases. If infants with large PDA are treated early (within 10 days of birth), over 80% have satisfactory constriction or closure. After 14 days, response is reduced with 50% responding satisfactorily and rest requiring ligation. Reopening of PDA after treatment is relatively common, especially in babies < 1000 g. Response to repeated doses is often found so that ligation may not be necessary. Side-effects include decreased urinary output, raised serum creatinine and electrolyte disorders. Bleeding, especially gastric haemorrhage, can also occur. Indomethacin used only

Table 82. Indications for indomethacin treatment.

1. Large PDA (LA/Ao > 1.5). No response to conservative treatment
2. Adequate urinary output >2ml/kg/hour
3. Serum creatinine ⩽130 μmol/l (1.5 mg/dl)
4. Bilirubin <150 μmol/l (9 mg/dl)
5. Normal coagulation:
   platelets >100 000/mm^3
   prothrombin time <20 sec
   partial thromboplastin time <70 sec

when indicated (Table 82). The dose is 0.1–0.2 mg/kg orally or intravenously and this may be repeated at 12-hourly intervals until response is seen or total dose of 0.6 mg/kg. Urine output, serum creatinine, electrolytes and urea are monitored at least daily after therapy until return to normal. Favourable signs of ductus response are reduced intensity and shortening of murmur, decrease in precordial activity and peripheral pulses. Echocardiography shows diminution of LA/Ao ratio (see Chapter 24). Some infants show only partial improvement but symptoms will be controlled by fluid restriction and diuretics until spontaneous closure occurs later. Some infants, after apparently good response, reopen the ductus and together with the non-responders should be considered for surgical ligation. Second and third courses of treatment are worth trying in an attempt to prevent need for ligation.

CYANOTIC HEART DISEASE

Any infant with cyanosis must be treated as an emergency. Distinction from pulmonary (e.g. RDS) and pulmonary vascular (e.g. persistent fetal circulation) causes is sometimes difficult. Cyanosis in a term infant without asphyxia, which does not improve with oxygen, suggests cardiac disease. Table 80 lists four causes of cyanotic heart disease; others include pulmonary atresia, tricuspid atresia and Ebstein's anomaly.

Initial Management

1. ECG
2. Chest radiograph
3. Right radial blood gas, room air and 100% oxygen. If $P_aO_2 > 20$ kPa (150 mmHg) unlikely to be cyanotic heart disease
4. Blood pressure, arms and legs
5. Call paediatric cardiologist for echocardiography and catheterization
6. Prostaglandin infusion (see below)

Prostaglandin Infusion (PGE_2)

Used to dilate ductus arteriosus as a temporary measure (Table 83). If in doubt about its use consult paediatric cardiologist.

Table 83. Indications for prostaglandin infusion (PGE_2).

Possible indications
1. Transfer of infant with cyanotic heart disease
2. During cardiac catheterization
3. Awaiting surgical treatment
4. Postoperatively if shunt is inadequate
Specific cardiac anomalies
1. Pulmonary atresia with intact ventricular septum
2. Critical pulmonary valve stenosis with intact ventricular septum
3. Fallot's tetralogy with pulmonary atresia
4. Tricuspid atresia with small RV, or pulmonary stenosis
5. Double-outlet RV, single ventricle, and TGA if severe pulmonary stenosis also
6. Simple D-transposition prior to septostomy or when Rashkind's procedure has failed
7. Interrupted aortic arch or coarction of aorta

Dose. Each vial contains 0.5 mg PGE_2 in 0.5 ml (100 μg in 0.1 ml). Add 0.1 ml (100 μg) to 250 ml one-fifth normal saline/dextrose to obtain solution of 0.4 μg/ml. Infuse at 0.1 μg/kg/min.

Table 84. Complications and monitoring during prostaglandin infusion.

Complication	*Monitoring*
1. Hypotension	BP: Dinamap, urine output
2. Pyrexia	Core and skin temp.
3. Bradycardia	Cardiorespirograph
4. Apnoea	Cardiorespirograph + blood gases
5. Seizures	Observe for seizures

If there is a response (infant becomes pink and murmur gets louder) use maintenance infusion of one-quarter dose.

Look for complications and monitor infant as in Table 84.

NEONATAL HYPERTENSION

Defined as consistent blood pressure reading of over 90/50 mmHg in full-term infant. Normal blood pressure for preterm infants is given on p. 32. Measurement of blood pressure most accurate using indwelling aortic catheter connected to pressure transducer, but Doppler methods (Arteriosonde) and flush technique may be used. Dinamap instrument records heart rate and blood pressure on paper trace after intermittent inflation of cuff. This has been a major advance in non-invasive blood pressure measurement. Table 85 lists causes of neonatal hypertension and Table 86 lists drugs that have been used to treat it. We prefer hydralazine or methyldopa but have used diazoxide in the acute situation.

Table 85. Causes of neonatal hypertension.

1. Renal artery stenosis
2. Renal artery thrombosis: umbilical artery catheters
3. Renal failure (see p. 259): polycystic, dysplastic, urethral valve
4. Hypoplastic aorta, renal arteries and coarctation of aorta

Table 86. Drugs for neonatal hypertension.

1. Chlorothiazide 10–50 mg/kg/day orally
2. Frusemide 1–4 mg/kg/day iv or orally
3. Hydralazine 1–6 mg/kg/day iv or orally
4. Methyldopa 5–50 mg/kg/day iv or orally
5. Diazoxide 5 mg/kg/dose iv
6. Propranolol 0.5–2.0 mg/kg/day iv or orally
7. Nitroprusside 2.5–5.0 μg/kg/min iv infusion

CARDIAC ARRHYTHMIAS

May be diagnosed and in some cases treated antenatally (see below).

Sinus Bradycardia

Causes are:

1. Raised intracranial pressure
2. Hyperkalaemia
3. Hypothyroidism
4. β-Blocker drugs to mother

Correct underlying cause. Atropine occasionally used (see p. 348).

Congenital Heart Block

Causes are:

1. Complex congenital heart disease
2. Maternal collagen disease
3. Isolated finding

May need isoprenaline or cardiac pacing (Table 87).

Table 87. Indications for cardiac pacing in congenital heart block.

1. Previous sibling required pacing
2. Fixed heart rate <60 min
3. Frequent ventricular extrasystoles
4. Long QT interval
5. Presentation with heart failure (5%)

A/V Block

Causes are:

1. Digoxin therapy
2. Congenital heart disease
3. Isolated finding

No treatment usually; occasionally isoprenaline (see p. 350).

Sinus Tachycardia (160–200/min)

Causes are:

1. Blood loss or hypotension
2. Fever
3. Stress
4. Theophylline toxicity
5. Thyrotoxicosis

Correct underlying cause.

Supraventricular Tachycardia (200–300/min)

Causes are:

1. Accessory pathways, e.g. Wolff–Parkinson–White syndrome (20%)
2 Congenital heart disease
3. Isolated finding

Treat with vagal stimulation (ice pack on face) or digoxin, or DC conversion (see below).

Ventricular Tachycardia

Causes are:

1. Hypoxia
2. Electrolyte disturbance
3. Digoxin toxicity
4. Local injection of mepivacaine

Treat with lignocaine (1 mg/kg) or DC cardioversion (see below). Consult paediatric cardiologist urgently.

Ectopic Beats

Causes are:

1. Isolated finding
2. Digoxin toxicity
3. Myocarditis
4. Hypoxia
5. Electrolyte disturbance
6. Theophylline toxicity

Occasionally need treatment with lignocaine.

PAEDIATRIC CARDIOLOGIST SHOULD ADVISE ABOUT TREATMENT OF ALL CARDIAC ARRHYTHMIAS

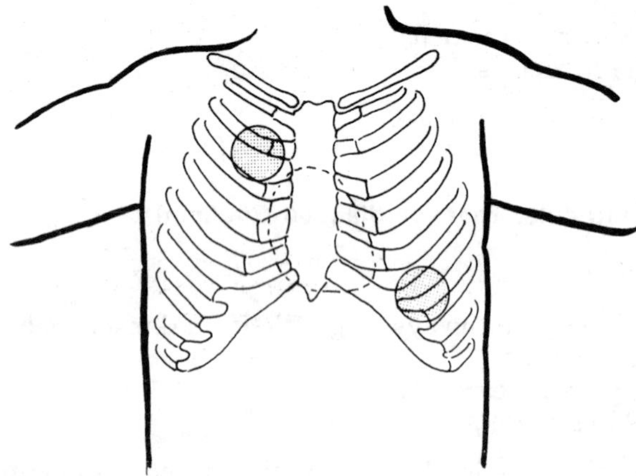

Fig. 50. DC cardioversion. Place paddles on chest wall as shown.

DC Conversion (Defibrillation)

Use 1–2 W sec/kg (1–2 J/kg) synchronized to downstroke of R wave. Place paddles at base and apex of heart (below right clavicle and fifth intercostal space in anterior axillary line (Fig. 50). Ensure good electrical conduction by putting saline-soaked gauze wipe beneath each paddle. Notify all assistants before discharging current. Defibrillation may be repeated after doubling the dose but burns can occur.

ANTENATAL DIAGNOSIS OF CARDIAC MALFORMATIONS

Now possible to examine heart by echocardiography at 18–20 weeks either as a routine screen or in selected high-risk pregnancies (family history of CHD, rubella infection or drug ingestion in early pregnancy, mother > 37 years). Four-chamber view, if normal, excludes about 70% of abnormalities. Arrythmias may be detected *in utero* with complete heart block due to maternal collagen disease and supraventricular tachycardia being commonest. Latter may be treated by giving digoxin or other drugs to mother to prevent cardiac failure and hydrops.

NURSING POINTS

1. Cardiorespiratory monitor, pulse oximetry
2. Blood pressure recorded in arms and legs
3. Careful fluid balance recording
4. Daily weighing
5. Nursing upright may help
6. Carefully check digoxin dosage; measure heart rate before administration
7. Indomethacin: watch urine output carefully and look for bleeding
8. Prostaglandin infusion: watch temperature, apnoeic spells, and seizures
9. Careful explanation and reassurance of parents. Need to be taught to administer drugs accurately at home

REFERENCES AND FURTHER READING

Gersony, W. M. (1986). Patent ductus arteriosus in the neonate. *Pediatr. Clin. North Am.* **33**: 545.

Halliday, H. L. (1988). Neonatal patent ductus arteriosus. *Pediatr. Rev. Commun.* **3**: 1.

Halliday, H. L., Hirata, T. and Brady, J. P. (1979a). Echocardiographic findings of large patent ductus arteriosus in the very low birthweight infant before and after treatment with indomethacin. *Arch. Dis. Child* **54**: 744.

Halliday, H. L., Hirata, T. and Brady, J. P. (1979b). Indomethacin therapy for large patent ductus arteriosus in the very low birthweight infant: results and complications. *Pediatrics* **64**: 154.

Parness, I. A., Yeager, S. B., Sanders, S. P. *et al.* (1988). Echocardiographic diagnosis of fetal heart defects in mid trimester. *Arch. Dis. Child* **63**: 1137.

Rowe, R. D., Freedom, R. M., Mehrizi, A. and Bloom, K. R. (1981). *The Neonate with Congenital Heart Disease*, 2nd edn. Philadelphia: W. B. Saunders.

Teitel, D., Heymann, M. A. and Liebman, J. (1986). The heart. In: *Care of the High-risk Neonate*, 3rd edition. (eds, Klaus, M. H. and Fanaroff, A. A.). Philadelphia: W. B. Saunders.

18. Gastrointestinal Problems

In the newborn gastrointestinal disorders may present as vomiting, diarrhoea, abdominal distension or passage of blood in the stools.

VOMITING

Defined as forceful expulsion of gastric contents through the mouth or nose. Important to distinguish between vomiting and possetting, which is common and benign. The causes of vomiting are listed in Table 88. The character of the vomitus may help in differentiating the causes of this symptom. Vomitus may be either frothy, bile stained or blood stained (Table 89).

Table 88. Causes of vomiting in the newborn.

1. Overfeeding
2. Infection: urinary tract, septicaemia, gastroenteritis
3. Intestinal obstruction: oesophageal atresia, ileal atresia, duodenal bands, annular pancreas, strangulated hernia, malrotation, volvulus, reduplication, meconium ileus, meconium plug, imperforate anus, Hirschsprung's disease, milk bolus obstruction
4. Functional ileus: sepsis, electrolyte imbalance, extreme preterm, severe RDS
5. Necrotizing enterocolitis
6. Hiatus hernia
7. Cerebral oedema, intracranial bleeding, meningitis
8. Adrenal insufficiency
9. Inborn errors of metabolism (Chapter 20)
10. Pyloric stenosis (very occasionally presents by 7–10 days)
11. Drugs: digoxin, oral antibiotics
12. Benign (possetting)
13. Biochemical disturbance, e.g. uraemia

Table 89. Nature of vomitus.

Frothy	Oesophageal atresia (secretions not really vomitus) (associated polyhydramnios)
Bile stained	Suggestive of intestinal obstruction (causes under Point 3, Table 88)
Blood stained	Haemorrhagic disease of newborn, swallowed maternal blood, feeding tube trauma, stress ulcers or hiatus hernia

Vomiting unlikely to be benign if blood or bile in the vomitus, associated watery or loose stools, abdominal distension and reluctance to feed or lethargy.

All vomiting babies should be carefully examined to exclude an underlying cause and to assess state of hydration. Signs of dehydration are:

1. Abnormal weight loss: > 10% of birth weight
2. Poor urinary output: < 1.5 ml/kg/hour
3. Loss of skin turgor
4. Depressed anterior fontanelle
5. Sunken eyes
6. Hypotension

Vomiting males occasionally have adrenal hyperplasia or posterior urethral valve with uraemia.

The following investigations may be indicated: electrolytes, pH, blood glucose, urine analysis, cultures, abdominal radiographs. Radiographs may suggest intestinal obstruction (air–fluid levels, double-bubble, p. 313), perforation (free peritoneal air), necrotizing enterocolitis (intramural air or pneumatosis intestinalis, p. 313) or ascites (uniform opaqueness in the flanks). Swallowed air reaches the intestine within an hour and should be present throughout the bowel to the rectum by 12–24 hours.

Management of vomiting depends upon severity and cause. If vomiting is persistent and dehydration present, feeding should be discontinued and intravenous fluids given. If shock present, fresh plasma or blood transfusion 15–20 ml/kg. To correct moderate dehydration (10% weight loss) about 100 ml/kg is deficit and 150 ml/kg/day maintenance.

DIARRHOEA

The frequent passage of watery or loose stools. Up to eight stools per day probably normal for bottle-fed baby but breast-fed infants may have as many as 16 stools each day. The normal stools of the breast-fed infant are not fully formed and may be green in colour. Table 90 lists the causes of neonatal diarrhoea.

Table 90. Causes of neonatal diarrhoea.

1. Gastroenteritis
2. Necrotizing enterocolitis
3. Breast-fed infants, maternal laxatives or diet, e.g. citrus fruits
4. Starvation stools: frequent small amounts of dark green material
5. Disaccharide intolerance
6. Urinary infection
7. Cystic fibrosis
8. Drugs: penicillin, iron, oral calcium. Phototherapy causes loose stools
9. Adrenal hyperplasia, thyrotoxicosis, maternal drug addiction, chloridorrhoea

Gastroenteritis

The chief dangers are dehydration, septicaemia and cross-infection. In some cases the stools may be watery and mistaken for urine; Uribag may be helpful and stool can be collected on polythene sheet. A bacterial pathogen is found in only 20–40% of cases: pathogenic *E. coli*, *Shigella*, *Salmonella* and *Campylobacter*. Many due to viral infection with rotavirus or astrovirus which can be detected by electron microscopy. In mild cases milk feeds should be discontinued and clear fluids given by mouth. Severe cases need intravenous fluids. Antibiotics should not be given unless septicaemia suspected. If hypernatraemia present (serum sodium over 150 mmol/l) danger of seizures if rehydration is too rapid. Half-normal saline or dextrose at 80–100 ml/kg/day for initial rehydration advised until the serum sodium is below 150 mmol/l.

Infected infants should be isolated: simply performed by

placing all infected infants in incubators in a room where all other infants are also in incubators. Scrupulous hand washing essential.

Some infants will have recurrence of diarrhoea after reintroduction of milk feeds; if the stools are acidic (pH < 5.5) and contain over 0.5% of reducing substances on Clinitest then secondary lactose intolerance is suspected and stools sent for sugar chromatogram. Symptoms can be relieved by using a lactose-free milk (Sobee, Pregestimil and Wysoy). Vitamin supplements should also be given.

Necrotizing Enterocolitis (NEC)

An inflammatory condition of both large and small bowel with presence of intramural air (pneumatosis intestinalis). Infants at risk of NEC are either very low birth weight or term infants with asphyxia, or following cardiac catheterization or exchange transfusion. Hypothermia and polycythaemia in SGA infants may also predispose. Underlying problem is ischaemia of bowel wall from asphyxia or shock, haemodynamic changes during exchange transfusion or arterial occlusion associated with umbilical arterial catheterization. Ischaemic damage to the bowel encourages bacterial invasion from the lumen with release of gas. Organism may be gas-producing anaerobe, e.g. *Clostridium*. Unusual for necrotizing enterocolitis to develop until feeding started. Colonization of intestine more likely after feeding and Gram-negative organisms more likely after artificial milk feeds. Intestine of breast-fed infants colonized primarily by lactobacilli which may partly explain lower incidence of necrotizing enterocolitis.

NEC may present with:

1. Vomiting
2. Increasing gastric aspirate
3. Bloody diarrhoea
4. Abdominal distension and ileus
5. Apnoeic attacks and lethargy
6. Temperature instability, skin mottling
7. Erythema of the anterior abdominal wall
8. Thrombocytopenia

Abdominal radiograph may show dilated bowel loops with thickened, oedematous walls. Later linear streaks of intramural gas appear (see p. 313) and perforation releases free peritoneal gas seen under the diaphragm in an erect film or under the umbilicus in a cross-table lateral radiograph. Gas may also be seen in portal venous system or within the hepatic veins.

Management of NEC includes prevention by careful placement of umbilical catheters and delay in feeding the very low birth weight and asphyxiated infant. Too long a delay before introducing feeds may also predispose because of intestinal mucosal atrophy; finding the ideal balance is not always easy. Expressed breast milk may also be beneficial in prevention of NEC. Oral antibiotics probably do not work but oral immunoglobulins may. Once signs are present, oral feeding must be stopped and parenteral nutrition started. Septicaemia is common so parenteral antibiotics given. If intramural gas present, cross-table lateral radiographs must be repeated 8 hourly to look for early bowel perforation. This diagnosis may be delayed if one relies on clinical signs alone. Only indication for surgery is perforation. At operation minimal resection of non-viable bowel and double-barrelled enterostomies made. Extensive resection leads to later problems of short bowel malabsorption. Platelet count is a useful indicator of severity of NEC. The inflammatory process in the bowel consumes platelets. Upon recovery, platelet count returns to normal. Later complications include malabsorption and stricture which may present with recurrent abdominal distension upon refeeding 2–6 weeks after the acute episode. Oral feeding is usually re-started, preferably with expressed breast milk, about 1 week after the signs of NEC have improved. Overall mortality is about 10% but this is higher in those with perforation.

ABDOMINAL DISTENSION

Causes of abdominal distension similar to those of vomiting (Table 88) plus pneumoperitoneum, bilateral pneumothoraces (liver and spleen pushed down), ascites (see p. 264), renal masses and disaccharide intolerance.

The causes of *paralytic ileus* are sepsis, asphyxia, drug withdrawal, necrotizing enterocolitis, hypermagnesaemia, hypothyroidism, adrenal insufficiency. Sometimes in the immature infant no cause can be found.

BLOOD IN THE STOOLS

Causes are listed in Table 91. Apt test for swallowed maternal blood described on p. 31.

Table 91. Causes of blood in the stools.

1. Swallowed maternal blood (do Apt test, see p. 31)
2. Haemorrhagic disease of the newborn
3. Rectal fissure from thermometer
4. Anal fissure due to thermometer, rectal examination or severe constipation
5. Necrotizing enterocolitis
6. Malrotation or volvulus
7. Reduplication of the bowel
8. Rarely gastroenteritis, shigellosis, intussusception, Meckel's diverticulum

SURGICAL PROBLEMS IN THE NEWBORN

These are discussed in Chapter 23 under congenital malformations (see p. 304).

REFERENCES AND FURTHER READING

Brown, E. G. and Sweet, A. Y. (1982). Neonatal necrotizing enterocolitis. *Pediatr. Clin. North Am.* **29**: 1149.

Clark, D. A. (1977). Times of first void and first stools in 500 newborns. *Pediatrics* **60**: 457.

Eibl, M. M., Wolf, H. M., Furnkranz, H. and Rosenkranz, A. (1988). Prevention of necrotizing enterocolitis in low-birth-weight infants by IgA–IgG feeding. *N. Engl. J. Med.* **319**: 1.

Kliegman, R. M. and Fanaroff, A. A. (1984). Necrotising enterocolitis. *N. Engl. J. Med.* **310**: 1093.

Lilien, L. D., Srinivasan, G., Pyati, S. P. *et al.* (1986). Green vomiting in the first 72 hours in normal infants. *Am. J. Dis. Child* **140**: 662.

Palmer, S. R., Biffin, A. and Gamsu, H. R. (1989). Outcome of neonatal necrotising enterocolitis: results of the BAPM/CDSC surveillance study, 1981–84. *Arch. Dis. Child* **64**: 388.

19. Genitourinary Problems

The fetal kidneys produce large quantities of dilute urine and have the major role of maintaining amniotic fluid volume. The placenta is the major excretory organ and maintains fetal homeostasis. The plasma urea and creatinine at birth will therefore be identical to those of the mother. A plasma creatinine of 70 mmol/l is common at birth and should fall to 30–40 mmol/l after the first week of life.

The neonatal kidney has normal number of nephrons (one million) but functional capacity is much less than the adult. Glomerular filtration and tubular reabsorption are reduced and there is a glomerulotubular preponderance. These characteristics of neonatal kidney resemble mild renal failure.

Urine of the neonate has reduced maximal osmolality due to low urea excretion.

Growth with its strong anabolic drive assists the neonatal kidney by reducing excretory load of sodium, water, phosphorus, hydrogen and nitrogen. Growth sometimes referred to as 'third kidney' of newborn. Under certain circumstances reduced renal function may be critical: ill or preterm infant, severe RDS, sepsis, severe asphyxia and after drugs (digoxin, muscle relaxants, aminoglycosides and tolazoline). Normal glomerular filtration rate and urine output is shown in Table 92. Thirty per cent of newborns pass urine during delivery, 90% within 24 hours and 99% within 48 hours of birth.

Presentation of a renal problem may be:

1. Antenatal ultrasound scan (see p. 8 and below)
2. Oligohydramnios (renal agenesis, posterior urethral valve)
3. Failure to pass urine (Table 93)
4. Non-specific symptoms, e.g. jaundice, lethargy, poor feeding, vomiting, weight loss, dehydration or temperature instability
5. Renal mass (Table 94); more than 50% of abdominal masses in the newborn are renal

Table 92. Normal renal function in the newborn.

<table>
<tr><th rowspan="2"></th><th colspan="2">Preterm</th><th rowspan="2">Full-term</th><th rowspan="2">At 2 weeks</th><th rowspan="2">At 8 weeks</th></tr>
<tr><th><32 weeks</th><th>>32 weeks</th></tr>
<tr><td>Glomerular filtration rate (ml/min/1.73 m^2)</td><td>7</td><td>18</td><td>23</td><td>50</td><td>75</td></tr>
<tr><td>Maximum concentrating ability (mosmol/l)</td><td colspan="2">480</td><td>800</td><td>900</td><td>1200</td></tr>
<tr><td>Urine output (ml/kg/hour)</td><td colspan="2">1–3*</td><td>1–3*</td><td>2–4*</td><td>2–4*</td></tr>
</table>

* May be less on first day
After Grupe (1979)

Table 93. Causes of failure to pass urine (oliguria).

1. Unnoticed urine passage in labour ward
2. Asphyxia and hypotension
3. Inadequate fluid intake
4. Increased fluid losses: phototherapy or radiant warmer
5. Renal agenesis
6. Acute tubular necrosis
7. Bilateral renal vein thrombosis
8. Congenital nephrosis or nephritis
9. Posterior urethral valve
10. Neurogenic bladder
11. Ureterocele
12. Inappropriate ADH secretion
13. Cardiac failure

Table 94. Causes of renal masses*.

1. Hydronephrosis
2. Polycystic kidneys
3. Multicystic kidneys
4. Horseshoe kidney
5. Ectopic kidney
6. Renal vein thrombosis
7. Retroperitoneal haematoma
8. Adrenal haemorrhage
9. Wilms' tumour

* Lower poles of normal kidneys may be palpable

Table 95. Causes of proteinuria.

1. Asphyxia
2. Cardiac failure
3. Large doses of penicillin
4. Dehydration
5. Fever
6. After IVP examination
7. Nephrotic syndrome: congenital syphilis, renal vein thrombosis, microcystic kidneys or Finnish type (see p. 264)
8. Urinary tract infection
9. Polycystic kidneys

6. Haematuria (see Table 97)
7. Visible abnormality: hypospadias, epispadias or ectopia vesicae (Chapter 23)

Investigation of infant with suspected renal problem should include history: family history, oligohydramnios, poor urinary output from birth, dribbling incontinence (neurogenic bladder or posterior urethral valve). Normal urine output in the newborn should be 2–4 ml/kg/hour after the first day (Table 92). Urine output of less than 1.0 ml/kg/hour should be considered as oliguria and a cause sought (Table 93). Measure urine output by Uribag which can be emptied by drawing into a syringe through a plastic mixing needle or accurate weighing of Gamgee pads placed under the infant.

Clinical examination of the abdomen may reveal a mass or a visible abnormality, e.g. exstrophy of the bladder (ectopia vesicae), hypospadias or epispadias. Remember it is frequently possible to palpate the lower pole of both kidneys in *normal* infants.

Examination of the urine performed after collection by Uribag or suprapubic aspiration (see Chapter 9). Urine examination may reveal presence of proteinuria, haematuria or pyuria. The causes of proteinuria are listed in Table 95. Presence of proteinuria on dip-stick should be confirmed by sending a timed sample of urine to laboratory for analysis.

INVESTIGATION OF THE BABY FOLLOWING ABNORMAL ANTENATAL ULTRASOUND SCAN

Not all babies will have abnormalities but do ultrasound scan of the urinary tract within first 24–48 hours. One of three findings:

1. Normal (no dilatation): repeat ultrasound at 1 month
2. Equivocal: do micturating cystogram (MCU) and if no reflux repeat ultrasound at 1 month; if reflux or infravesical obstruction needs treatment (surgery for posterior urethral valve, antibiotic prophylaxis)
3. Dilatation confirmed: do MCU and if reflux or infravesical obstruction then treat as above. If no reflux, must have supravesical obstruction and needs isotope scan (DTPA)

URINARY TRACT INFECTION (see also p. 201)

Quite common in the newborn; estimates vary from 0.1 to 1%. More common in males and blood-borne infection more likely than ascending. Lethargy, poor feeding, vomiting and increasing jaundice are signs. Coliforms are the usual organism. Clean-catch specimens or suprapubic aspiration should be performed. Significant growth more than 100 000 organisms/ml. Treatment will consist of appropriate antibiotic therapy, intravenous fluids and later radiographs (IVP and micturating cystogram) and ultrasound studies of the renal tract to exclude anomalies or ureteric reflux (50% of males and 35% of females).

ACUTE RENAL FAILURE

Probably more common than formerly realized. The causes are listed in Table 96.

Metabolic upsets are rising blood urea, serum creatinine, potassium and phosphate; metabolic acidosis and lowered serum sodium, calcium and magnesium. Clinically, may be difficulty in distinguishing prerenal from renal failure in the oliguric infant. Measure urine/plasma ratio of creatinine: > 14 in prerenal uraemia and < 10 in renal failure. Urine osmolality may also help (>400 mosmol in prerenal and <350 mosmol in

Table 96. Causes of acute renal failure.

1. Asphyxia
2. Hypovolaemia, haemorrhage
3. Dehydration: loss of fluid, inadequate fluid intake
4. Trauma, especially obstetrical
5. Renal artery thrombosis or embolism
6. Septicaemia
7. Heart failure, especially PDA
8. Drugs and toxins: gentamicin, tolazoline, indomethacin
9. Disseminated intravascular coagulation
10. Renal agenesis, polycystic kidneys, renal dysplasia
11. Congenital nephrotic syndrome
12. Nephritis
13. Obstructive uropathy: urethral valve, ureterocele, systemic candidiasis

renal). If plasma (P) and urine (U) electrolytes and creatinine (Cr) are available the fractional excretion of sodium (FE (Na)) or the renal failure index (RFI) may be calculated as follows:

$$FE(Na) = (UNa/PNa)/(UCr/PCr) \times 100$$
$$RFI = (UNa)/(U/PCr)$$

In prerenal failure FE(Na) is 0.8 ± 0.6 compared to 4.8 ± 1.4 in established renal failure while RFI is 1.0 ± 0.2 in prerenal failure and 7.2 ± 1.3 in established renal failure. If doubt exists try transfusion of blood or plasma (15–20 ml/kg). Mannitol increases renal medullary blood flow if given early in renal failure and frusemide increases renal cortical blood flow. Their value in the management of acute renal failure of the newborn has *not* been proved.

Hyperkalaemia may need urgent therapy. Arrhythmias unusual unless serum level over 8 mmol/l. Emergency treatment: 1–2 ml/kg of 10% calcium gluconate intravenously over 3 min with ECG monitoring. Insulin 0.2 units/kg with 0.5–1 g/kg of glucose and acidosis corrected with small doses (1 mmol/kg) of sodium bicarbonate. Calcium polystyrene sulphonate 1 g/kg/day in 10% dextrose rectally (see also p. 177).

Management

Look for underlying cause (see Table 96). Treat infection, stop nephrotoxic drugs, e.g. gentamicin.

Fluid and electrolytes

Fluids ordered on a day-to-day basis: the previous day's urinary output plus insensible water losses, which are in term infant 20 ml/kg/day in first week and in preterm 40–50 ml/kg/day. Catheterize bladder to measure urine output accurately. Protein restricted if blood urea high (3 g protein is catabolized to give 1 g urea). Limit sodium and potassium intake to < 0.3 mmol/kg/day. Correct hypoglycaemia, hypocalcaemia and acidosis.

Try effect (upon urine output) of 5 mg/kg frusemide. If response occurs then continue maintenance of 2 mg/kg 6 hourly. When diuretics fail dopamine infusion at 1 μg/kg/min may produce a diuresis by improving renal blood flow.

Dialysis

Only required in patients that cannot be managed conservatively by fluid balance and correction of metabolic abnormalities. Indications for dialysis are severe hyperkalaemia, metabolic acidosis or over-hydration with pulmonary oedema or congestive heart failure and intractable hypoglycaemia. Peritoneal dialysis is efficient because of the large peritoneal surface area/weight ratio and increased clearance of peritoneal urea and creatinine in newborn.

Technique of peritoneal dialysis. Under sterile conditions infant-sized peritoneal catheter (Pendlebury Neonatal Cannula-Medcomp) introduced percutaneously after injection of local anaesthetic. The dialysis fluid is delivered through a closed system (Paediatric Dialysis Set, Avon Medical R3370) in which a Y connection allows alternate filling and draining of the peritoneal cavity. The fluid should pass through a water bath to ensure delivery at 37 °C.

Volumes of 30–50 ml/kg are instilled in 30–60 min cycles until biochemistry or oedema corrected. Commercial dialysis fluids (Dialaflex 61, Boots) have similar electrolyte composition to plasma except for absence of potassium. A glucose concentration of 1.36% is usually employed but may be increased to 3–4% if satisfactory fluid removal is not achieved. When plasma potassium falls to 4 mmol/l, potassium chloride should be added to the dialysate to this concentration to prevent hypokalaemia. There is a major risk of peritonitis unless full aseptic technique is observed during fluid bag changes. Daily effluent cultures are necessary for early diagnosis and appropriate antibiotic treatment.

Haemodialysis may be performed in the newborn using continuous arteriovenous haemofiltration (CAVH) and is most effective in term infants where fluid overload is the main problem.

Technique of CAVH. The femoral or umbilical artery is catheterized and blood passed through a small hollow fibre ultrafilter. The blood flow required is about 20 ml/min and no pump is needed. The total extracorporeal volume of lines and filter (Gambro) is 20 ml. One disadvantage is the need for anticoagulation.

Prognosis

This is good if prerenal. For renal causes survival is 75% following birth asphyxia but 40% have neurological damage and 40% impaired renal function.

HAEMATURIA

Greater than three red cells per centrifuged high-power field. The causes are listed in Table 97.

This finding should always be taken seriously and needs further observation and investigation. Urinary urates can cause reddish-brown staining of urine.

PYURIA

Over five white cells per centrifuged high-power field. Causes are listed in Table 98.

This finding strongly suggests infection of genito-urinary system and full bacteriological assessment indicated.

Table 99 lists the indications for renal diagnostic imaging (intravenous urography (IVU), ultrasound scan (USS) or isotope scans (DMSA scan)).

Table 97. Causes of haematuria.

1. Asphyxia
2. Disseminated intravascular coagulation, haemorrhagic disease or thrombocytopenia
3. Urinary tract infection
4. Renal vein thrombosis
5. Congenital nephritis
6. Wilms' tumour or other tumours
7. Polycystic and dysplastic kidneys
8. Renal stones
9. Trauma to kidneys during delivery
10. Kanamycin or methicillin
11. After suprapubic aspiration
12. Focal genital lesions

Table 98. Causes of pyuria.

1. Urinary tract infection
2. Renal tubular acidosis
3. Interstitial nephritis, e.g. after methicillin
4. Dehydration
5. Bladder catheterization
6. After suprapubic aspiration

Table 99. Indications for renal diagnostic imaging. (IVU, USS or DMSA Scan)

1. After one urinary infection in either sex
2. Abdominal masses
3. Haematuria without obvious cause
4. Absent abdominal musculature (prune belly syndrome)
5. Single umbilical artery* or hypospadias and epispadias
6. Abnormal antenatal USS
7. Acute renal failure

* 25% of newborns with SUA have abnormalities: skeletal, gastrointestinal, skin, genitourinary, respiratory, cardiovascular or central nervous system

NEPHROCALCINOSIS

Nephrocalcinosis and renal stones have recently been reported in preterm babies on long-term frusemide therapy. The diagnosis is normally made by ultrasound scan but occasionally the babies also have clinical findings such as haematuria or obstructive uropathy. Chlorothiazide may be a safer diuretic for long-term use in the newborn.

CONGENITAL NEPHROTIC SYNDROME

Uncommon in the UK though seen frequently in Finland. Other important causes are congenital syphilis (responds to penicillin), renal vein thrombosis, cytomegalovirus infection and nail–patellar syndrome. Massive proteinuria and oedema are usual presenting features and ascites may be gross. Some babies present with failure to thrive and vomiting before oedema becomes obvious. Unless underlying cause is treatable renal failure ensues and dialysis and/or transplantation are only effective treatments. Initial therapy with diuretics and albumin infusions plus prevention of serious sepsis may allow survival until transplantation can be performed.

NEONATAL ASCITES

The causes are listed in Table 100 (see also hydrops, p. 60).

Table 100. Causes of neonatal ascites.

1. Haemolytic disease (hydrops)
2. Congenital nephrotic syndrome
3. Urinary tract obstruction
4. Peritonitis
5. Severe congestive heart failure
6. Congenital syphilis
7. Thoracic duct obstruction
8. Hepatoportal venous obstruction

CONGENITAL MALFORMATIONS OF RENAL TRACT

These are discussed in Chapter 23.

NURSING POINTS

Peritoneal dialysis:

1. Ensure absolutely aseptic technique for catheter insertion and all bag changes
2. Ensure dialysate is warmed to body temperature
3. Accurately record input and output cycles looking for negative balance in treatment of fluid overload
4. Monitor temperature, heart rate and respiration, and blood pressure
5. Check glucose strip test 4 hourly
6. Frequent weighing
7. Watch for signs of peritonitis or bacteraemia
8. Change tubing every 48 hours and send daily sample of fluid for culture and sensitivities

REFERENCES AND FURTHER READING

Brocklebank, J. T. (1988). Renal failure in the newly born. *Arch. Dis. Child* **63**: 991.

Engle, W. D. (1986). Evaluation of renal function and acute renal failure in the neonate. *Pediatr. Clin. North Am.* **33**: 129.

Jacinto, J. S., Modanlou, H. D., Crade, M., Strauss, A. A. and Bosu, S. K. (1988). Renal calcification incidence in very low birth weight infants. *Pediatrics* **81**: 31.

Thomas, D. F. M. and Gordon, A. C. (1989). Management of prenatally diagnosed uropathies. *Arch. Dis. Child* **64**: 58.

Vanpee, M., Herin, P., Zetterstrom, R. and Aperia, A. (1988). Postnatal development of renal function in very low birthweight infants. *Acta Paediatr. Scand.* **77**: 191.

20. Metabolic and Endocrine Problems

Inborn errors of metabolism are rare disorders but should be suspected in any newborn with an unexplained illness. The presenting features may be abnormal neurological signs, acidosis, jaundice, vomiting, hypoglycaemia, odd odour or by mimicking sepsis (Table 101).

A urine sample taken at the onset of symptoms is a useful screening test for the more common disorders: galactosaemia, urea cycle defect, hyperglycinaemia, maple syrup urine disease and organic aciduria. Investigate suspected inborn errors of metabolism by taking a careful family history; look for metabolic acidosis and send plasma and urine samples for amino acid and sugar chromatography, organic acid determination and blood ammonia levels. Once samples have been taken treatment should be started: correct dehydration and acidosis, infuse dextrose, avoid protein and, in the event of continued deterioration, give high-dose vitamins which act as coenzymes. If the baby should die, a skin biopsy for fibroblast culture and enzyme assays should be performed. Table 102 summarizes treatment and outcome for some metabolic disorders of the newborn.

SOME NOTES ON SPECIFIC METABOLIC DISORDERS

Phenylketonuria

Incidence 1 in 10 000 to 1 in 15 000 newborns but more common in Irish communities (about 1 in 4000). Due to a deficiency of enzyme phenylalanine hydroxylase and inherited as autosomal recessive. The presentation in older infants of delayed development, seizures, severe eczema and musty odour is no longer seen since screening introduced. Blood phenylalanine is measured once milk feeds established, usually on seventh day, and high levels confirmed by plasma amino acid analysis.

Table 101. Presentation of metabolic disorders.

Acidosis Propionic acidaemia (Organic) Methylmalonic acidaemia (Organic) Isovaleric acidaemia (Organic) Maple syrup urine disease Congenital lactic acidosis Renal tubular acidosis Von Gierke's disease	*Coma* Hyperglycinaemia Maple syrup urine disease Methylmalonic acidaemia Propionic acidaemia Carbamyl phosphate synthetase deficiency (Urea cycle defects) Ornithine carbamyl transferase deficiency (Urea cycle defects) Argininosuccinate synthetase deficiency (citrullinaemia) (Urea cycle defects) Argininosuccinase deficiency (argininosuccinic aciduria) (Urea cycle defects) Arginase deficiency (hyperargininaemia) (Urea cycle defects)	*Seizures* Hyperglycinaemia Maple syrup urine disease Hyperlysinuria β-Alaninaemia	*Hypoglycaemia* Maple syrup urine disease Methylmalonic acidaemia Galactosaemia Hereditary fructose intolerance Von Gierke's disease
Vomiting Congenital adrenal hyperplasia Urea cycle abnormalities (see coma) Organic acidaemias (see acidosis) Hypervalinaemia Phenylketonuria Galactosaemia Hereditary fructose intolerance	*Jaundice* Galactosaemia Hypothyroidism Tyrosinaemia α_1-antitrypsin deficiency Hereditary fructose intolerance	*'Sepsis'* Galactosaemia Organic acidaemias (see acidosis) Tyrosinaemia	*Odd odour* Isovaleric acidaemia (sweaty feet) Maple syrup urine disease Phenylketonuria Tyrosinaemia

Table 102. Treatment and outcome of metabolic disorders.

Disorder	*Enzyme deficiency*	*Treatment*	*Outcome*
Galactosaemia	Galactose-1-phosphate uridyl transferase	Lactose free milk	Good if treated promptly
Phenylketonuria	Phenylalanine hydroxylase	Aminogram	Good if treated promptly
Tyrosinaemia	Many	50 mg vitamin C daily for 1 week	Good
Maple syrup urine disease	Branched chain keto acid decarboxylase	Intravenous fluids, exchange transfusion, dialysis, thiamine	Good if treated promptly
Non-ketotic hyperglycinaemia	Brain glycine cleavage enzyme	Exchange transfusion, dialysis, strychnine	Poor: death or handicap
Propionic acidaemia (ketotic hyperglycinaemia)	Propionyl-CoA carboxylase	Intravenous fluids, HCO_3^-, exchange transfusion, dialysis, biotin 5 mg/day, low protein diet	Poor
Methylmalonic acidaemia	Methylmalonic-CoA mutase	As for propionic acidaemia except vitamin B_{12} 1 mg/day instead of biotin	Variable
Isovaleric acidaemia	Isovaleric dehydrogenase	Intravenous fluids, HCO_3^-, low leucine diet	Good
Urea cycle disorders	Many	Intravenous fluids, exchange transfusion, dialysis, low protein diet, oral neomycin	Poor

Treatment is dietary, restricting natural protein and phenylalanine intake to that necessary for normal growth and maintaining levels between 125 and 375 μmol/l.

All infants with hyperphenylalaninaemia should be screened routinely for deficiency of tetrahydrobiopterin. This disorder cannot be treated by diet and causes rapid neurological deterioration unless neurotransmitter deficiency is corrected.

Galactosaemia (see also p. 190)
Incidence about 1 in 50 000 and is inherited as autosomal recessive. Due to deficiency of galactose-1-phosphate uridyl transferase which results in accumulation of galactose and galactose-1-phosphate which damages the lens of the eye, liver, brain and ovary. Antenatal detection and neonatal screening is possible. Presents acutely with prolonged jaundice, vomiting, lethargy, weight loss, hepatosplenomegaly, sepsis and early development of cataracts. The sepsis is often due to coliforms and may be associated with hypoglycaemia and severe haemolysis. If the baby is being fed, urine testing will show reducing sugars (Clinitest tablets) but no glucose (Clinistix reagent strip). The diagnosis may be confirmed by sending urine for chromatography, plasma for elevated galactose-1-phospate and red cells for enzyme assay (galactose-1-phosphate uridyl transferase). This should be done before blood transfusion to correct anaemia.

Treat with intravenous fluids to stabilize and then feed lactose-free milk. With a known family history, subsequent babies should have lactose-free diet from birth which will prevent illness but not affect red cell enzyme assay. Heterozygote mothers shoud have a lactor-free diet in subsequent pregnancies.

Tyrosinaemia
Transient tyrosinaemia is relatively common in preterm infants especially if high protein intake. Previously thought to be detrimental but not confirmed on follow-up studies. Presents with jaundice, lethargy and poor feeding and responds to vitamin C 50 mg daily for 1 week.

Hereditary tyrosinaemia is much less common and presents either as an acute illness with progressive liver dysfunction or more chronically as cirrhosis. Hypoglycaemia and renal tubular defects may also occur. Urinary succinylacetone is raised and treatment is with low tyrosine and phenylalanine milk.

Urea cycle disorders

A series of five hepatic enzymes (Table 101) are needed to synthesize urea from ammonia, released from the deamination of amino acids. Absence of a urea cycle enzyme or suppression of urea cycle function by various organic acidaemias results in the accumulation of ammonia.

The commonest defect is ornithine transcarbamylase deficiency which is X-linked dominant. Usually lethal in boys but girls may present later with milder symptoms. Presentation includes vomiting, seizures, tachypnoea and respiratory alkalosis. Blood ammonia is high and orotic acid is present in urine. Treatment is by protein restriction, arginine supplements and removing excess nitrogen with sodium benzoate and α-keto analogues of amino acids. Peritoneal dialysis or exchange transfusion may help the acutely ill baby.

The other enzyme defects of urea synthesis are autosomal recessive and present with varying degrees of severity. All except carbamyl phosphate synthetase deficiency may be diagnosed antenatally.

Organic acidaemias

Methylmalonic, propionic, isovaleric and lactic acidaemia result from defects in the catabolism of isoleucine, leucine and pyruvate. All conditions are autosomal recessive and rare, occurring in less than 1 in 100 000 births. Often a past history of early neonatal deaths. Presentation soon after birth with vomiting, lethargy, coma, peculiar odour and hypotonia. Ketoacidosis is common and may be accompanied by hypoglycaemia, hyperammonaemia and hyperglycinaemia. Untreated these conditions progress to coma and death. Treatment consists of stopping all milk feeds, erecting intravenous fluids, giving glucose, correcting acidosis, providing plasma to correct coagulation disorder, exchange transfusion or peritoneal dialysis to lower serum levels of toxic metabolites and specific vitamin therapy: B_{12}, biotin, thiamine in pharmacological doses to act as coenzymes (Table 102). Prognosis is variable.

ENDOCRINE DISORDERS

Endocrine disorders of the newborn are uncommon, although with recent introduction of screening for congenital hypothyroidism many subclinical cases have been detected. Apart from disorders of thyroid metabolism, disorders of the adrenal gland are probably the next most common and like inborn errors of metabolism make a significant contribution to morbidity and mortality in childhood.

Thyroid Disorders

Congenital hypothyroidism

With neonatal screening, incidence of this is now about 1 in 3000. At recall most have minor symptoms but probably only 5% have clinical signs. Before screening was introduced the clinical diagnosis was often delayed until 6 months (clinical signs described on p. 190) and the longer the delay in starting replacement treatment the greater the effect on intelligence. Transient hypothyroidism can occur so a short period off treatment after 2 years of age will confirm the need for lifelong treatment. Most cases of hypothyroidism are sporadic due to ectopic, hypoplastic or absent thyroid glands. About 10% result from enzyme defects in thyroxine synthesis which may cause goitre and have autosomal recessive inheritance.

At diagnosis most infants appear well but some have non-specific symptoms from birth: lethargy, slow feeding, poor weight gain or prolonged jaundice. A radiograph of knee shows delayed maturation of upper tibial or lower femoral epiphysis.

Screening measures T_4 and TSH or TSH alone (normal values of 5 days: $T_4 > 6 \mu g/dl$ in preterm, $> 9 \mu g/dl$ in term; TSH $< 20 \mu U/ml$). If T_4 remains low and TSH high then treatment is begun with l-thyroxine 25 μg daily in term babies increasing to 100 $\mu g/m^2/day$ as the baby grows (p. 352).

Neonatal goitre may be due to maternal ingestion of iodides or antithyroid drugs (p. 21) or to one of the inherited forms of hypothyroidism.

Neonatal thyrotoxicosis (see also p. 18)

This is a serious disorder with a significant mortality. May occur in the baby of a mother with Grave's disease. The infant may present after a few days with signs of acute thyrotoxicosis: tachycardia, heart failure, thirst, irritability, weight loss, goitre and collapse. Serum thyroxine concentrations will be increased. Urgent treatment is required to prevent the development of heart failure and collapse. Adequate nutrition and hydration for increased metabolic demand. Heart rate controlled by propranolol and serum thyroxine lowered by potassium iodide drops and antithyroid drugs (p. 18). Treatment needed for at least 8 weeks but in one-third of babies disorder lasts for 2–6 months or longer.

Intersex

Urgent investigation is needed when the sex (gender) of an infant is in doubt. Do not guess the gender but reassure the parents that this will be determined as quickly as possible. It is best to delay the announcement and registration of the birth until investigations are complete. The most important aspect of clinical examination is to determine if a gonad is palpable. The most important laboratory investigation is serum 17α-hydroxyprogesterone to diagnose virilizing congenital adrenal hyperplasia. Radiological and ultrasound examination help to identify internal genitalia. Chromosome analysis helps to determine aetiology but should not necessarily dictate the sex of rearing which will depend on the appearance of the external genitalia and the likely effect of puberty. The causes of intersex presenting in infancy are shown in Table 103.

Male pseudohermaphrodites have a normal male karyotype and well-differentiated testes but abnormal male genital development. There are two main causes: firstly, impairment of fetal testosterone biosynthesis caused by an enzyme deficiency or hypoplasia of Leydig cells leading to androgen deficiency;

Table 103. Causes of intersex presenting in infancy.

Male pseudohermaphrodite (poorly virilized male):
Disorders of Leydig cell activity
Impaired androgen activity in peripheral tissues
Others
Female pseudohermaphrodite (virilized female):
Congenital adrenal hyperplasia
Maternal androgens
Iatrogenic
Others
Abnormal gonadal differentiation:
Mixed gonadal dysgenesis
True hermaphroditism

secondly, impaired androgen activity in peripheral tissues, androgen insensitivity syndrome, may vary from complete (totally female) to incomplete forms (variable degrees of masculinization). Incomplete virilization may also occur in some dysmorphic syndromes and renal anomalies.

Female pseudohermaphrodites have a normal female karyotype with normally developed ovaries and Mullerian structures but a masculine appearance of external genitalia. Congenital adrenal hyperplasia due to 21-hydroxylase deficiency is commonest and most important cause (see below). Other causes include maternal androgen-secreting tumours and progesterone or androgen ingestion during pregnancy.

Abnormal gonadal differentiation usually presents with absence of pubertal development rather than genital anomalies (eg Turner's Syndrome). Exceptions are mixed gonadal dysgenesis and true hermaphroditism. The former is usually caused by 46XY/45XO mosaicism. Some testicular tissue is present causing variable virilization. There is an increased risk of malignancy in the testis or streak gonad. True hermaphrodites have both testicular tissue with seminiferous tubules and ovarian tissue with primary follicles. The karyotype is variable but 46XX is the most common.

Congenital Adrenal Hyperplasia

This group of disorders has an incidence of about 1 in 10 000 births but this varies greatly in different populations. Autosomal recessive inheritance with presentation depending on site of enzyme deficiency in the synthesis of cortisol and aldosterone.

More than 90% are due to 21-hydroxylase deficiency. Wide spectrum of presentation but in neonate may cause virilization of external genitalia in females and acute salt-losing crisis in males at 2–3 weeks of age. The diagnosis may be confirmed by elevation of 17α-hydroxyprogesterone ($<$ 18 nmol/l) in serum 48 hours after birth and glucocorticoid and mineralocorticoid replacement therapy will prevent adrenal crises.

An acute adrenal crisis is managed with intravenous normal saline, glucose to avoid hypoglycaemia and physiological replacement of hydrocortisone. When oral fluids can be taken, hydrocortisone is given in a dose of 20 mg/m^2/day divided into three doses, and 9α-fludrocortisone 0.1–0.2 mg once daily as mineralocorticoid replacement. Continued salt loss over the first few months may require 2–3 g of salt supplements daily. Replacement therapy is needed for life and parents should be warned that increased dose of hydrocortisone will be needed for infections or other stress. Long-term follow up should be shared by a paediatric endocrinologist. Females present earlier and adrenal crises can usually be prevented. Clitoroplasty may be needed in later infancy.

About 5% of congenital adrenal hyperplasia is due to deficiency of 11β-hydroxylase and this causes virilization of female infants. Salt-losing crises do not occur so males are not recognized in infancy. Diagnosis is confirmed by increased 11-deoxycortisol levels in serum.

Hypoglycaemia

See also p. 57 and Chapter 12. Undoubtedly prolonged or recurrent symptomatic hypoglycaemia leads to permanent neurological damage. The most common reason for recurrent hypoglycaemia outside the immediate perinatal period is an endocrine disturbance such as hyperinsulinism due to nesidioblastosis or congenital panhypopituitarism.

Signs of hyperinsulinism include macrosomia and the need for high glucose infusion rates to maintain normoglycaemia. Serum insulin is elevated and β-hydroxybutyrate is low in the presence of hypoglycaemia. Initial treatment of nesidioblastosis is with diazoxide and chlorothiazide but if unsuccessful a somatostatin infusion may be a helpful short-term measure before surgical exploration. If an adenoma is not found then > 90% pancreatectomy should be performed.

Congenital panhypopituitarism may be suspected if prolonged conjugated hyperbilirubinaemia, small external genitalia in males, midline facial defects or optic atrophy. Serum growth hormone and cortisol are inappropriately low for the degree of hypoglycaemia.

For severe or recurrent hypoglycaemia, investigations should be performed during an episode of hypoglycaemia: glucose, insulin, cortisol and growth hormone. Also helpful, are

β-hydroxybutyrate, amino acids, glycerol, lactate and pyruvate which may be abnormal in the less common disorders.

NURSING POINTS

1. Routine neonatal screening tests for PKU, hypothyroidism and cystic fibrosis (immune reactive trypsin) are done on fifth day after feeds established
2. Preterm baby not established on feeds has Guthrie test for PKU delayed but important to do hypothyroid screening on fifth day so that appropriate action can be taken early
3. Remember that mother of a baby with unexplained microcephaly may have undiagnosed or untreated PKU
4. Parents of baby with an intersex problem need much support and explanation

REFERENCES AND FURTHER READING

Brook, C. G. D. (1989). *Clinical Paediatric Endocrinology*, 2nd edn. Oxford: Blackwell.

Burton, B. K. and Nadler, H. L. (1978). Clinical diagnosis of the inborn errors of metabolism in the neonatal period. *Pediatrics* **61**: 398.

21. Haematological Problems

Normal haematological values in newborn differ from adult standards and also vary with gestational and postnatal age. Typical normal values by gestational age are shown in Table 104. Nucleated red cells may be present soon after birth – 500/mm^3 in term infants and 1500/mm^3 in preterm – but disappear after 48 hours. They may cause erroneous increases in white cell counts, especially if automated Coulter counter is used. Corrected white cell counts should always be given after looking at blood film.

Normal values for white cell count are:

Day 1	6000–30 000/mm^3
Day 2	6000–25 000/mm^3
Day 3	6000–20 000/mm^3
Day 4 onward	6000–18 000/mm^3

ANAEMIA

Anaemia in Early Neonatal Period (First Week)

Defined as haemoglobin < 13 g/dl (packed cell volume (PCV) < 40%).

The causes are listed in Table 105. History may reveal obvious reasons, e.g. antepartum haemorrhage or early cord clamping in preterm infant. With acute blood loss there may be tachycardia and tachypnoea but pallor may not be present (p. 31). When chronic intrauterine anaemia has been present there may be congestive heart failure, hepatosplenomegaly and a relatively undistressed baby. Where explanation not obvious full investigation carried out:

1. Maternal Kleihauer test
2. Blood film
3. Coombs' test, indirect bilirubin, reticulocyte count

If these are negative and cause still unclear:

Table 104. Normal neonatal haematological values.

	At birth			*At 24 hours*	*At 72 hours*	*Range at term*
	28 weeks	34 weeks	40 weeks			
Haemoglobin (g/dl)	14.5	15.0	16.8	18.4	17.8	15–20
Packed cell volume (%)	45	47	53	58	55	48–60
Red cells (millions/mm^3)	4.0	4.4	5.3	5.8	5.6	4.0–6.5
MCV (fl)	120	118	107	108	99	96–112
MCHC (%)	31	32	32	33	33	30–35
Reticulocytes (%)	10	10	7	7	3	3–10
Platelets (thousands/mm^3)	180	230	290	192	213	160–360
Total white cells (thousands/mm^3)	16.8	13.0	18.1	18.2	12.2	6–30
Segmented neutrophils (thousands/mm^3) 54%	9.1	7.2	9.4	9.4	4.7	3–13
Band forms (thousands/mm^3) 7%	1.2	1.0	1.6	1.6	0.8	0–4
Lymphocytes (thousands/mm^3) 30%	5.0	3.9	5.5	5.5	5.0	2–11
Monocytes (thousands/mm^3) 6%	1.0	0.7	1.0	1.0	1.1	0.4–3.1
Eosinophils (thousands/mm^3) 2%	0.3	0.3	0.4	0.4	0.5	0.2–0.9
Basophils (thousands/mm^3) 1%	0.2	0.1	0.1	0.1	0.05	0–0.6
ESR (mm/hour)	1–6	1–6	1–3	1–3	1–8	1–8

	0–96 hours	*>96 hours*
Absolute neutrophil count	<14 000	2000–4700
Absolute band count	<1400	<500
Band/neutrophil ratio*	<0.17	<0.14

* Increased in sepsis, infants of diabetic mothers, meconium aspiration, respiratory distress syndrome, hypoglycaemia and asphyxia

After Manroe *et al*. (1976, 1977)

Table 105. Anaemia in the early neonatal period.

1. Fetal haemorrhage: vasa praevia, placenta praevia, abruption, amniocentesis, incision of placenta at caesarean section
2. Fetomaternal transfusion (check Kleihauer)
3. Twin-to-twin transfusion
4. Fetoplacental transfusion at delivery: early cord clamping — failure of normal placentofetal transfusion, and fetoplacenatal transfusion if baby held above mother
5. Acute or chronic fetal haemolysis: rhesus, α-thalassaemia, intrauterine infection
6. Neonatal haemorrhage: ruptured liver or spleen, fractures, breech, intracranial, pulmonary, gastrointestinal, from umbilical cord, subaponeurotic
7. Repeated blood sampling

1. Exclude intrauterine infection
2. Exclude bleeding disorder
3. Red cell enzymes, haemoglobin electrophoresis

Later Onset Anaemia

This is defined as anaemia occurring after the first week of life. Table 106 shows the normal haematological values during the first year for two groups of preterm babies. Table 107 lists the causes of late anaemia.

Usual cause iron-deficiency anaemia but iron stores rarely depleted before 12 weeks (Fig. 51). For first 8 weeks transferrin > 30% saturated so iron supplementation not needed. Iron may be disadvantage as saturated transferrin loses antibacterial effect. Also iron accentuates haemolysis from vitamin E deficiency.

Vitamin E deficiency likely to occur in infants < 1500 g. Vitamin E has antioxidant properties and protects red cell membrane from oxidants such as oxygen or iron. Give all infants < 1500 g vitamin E 10 mg daily from seventh day. Recent studies have suggested that much larger doses of vitamin E, e.g. 50–100 mg/kg/day from birth, may prevent or reduce incidence of intraventricular haemorrhage, retinopathy of prematurity and bronchopulmonary dysplasia. This work needs to be confirmed.

Table 106. Normal haematological values during the first year of life.

	Age (weeks)								
	3 days	3	6	9	12	18	24	36	54
Haemoglobin (g/dl)									
28–32 weeks									
Mean	17.9	13.1	9.9	10.3	11.3	11.6	11.9	12.3	12.6
Lowest	12.6	10.0	8.1	8.1	8.5	9.6	10.2	10.9	11.2
33–36 weeks									
Mean	18.4	14.1	11.9	11.6	11.9	11.9	12.3	12.8	12.5
Lowest	13.2	9.2	9.2	8.5	8.8	10.3	10.5	10.9	10.1
Ferritin (μg/l)									
28–32 weeks									
Mean	265	280	213	165	179	118	64	37	26
Lowest	110	123	78	78	82	11	10	11	11
33–36 weeks									
Mean	296	276	245	178	163	118	86	30	31
Lowest	65	164	131	49	53	11	11	11	11
Iron (μmol/l)*									
28–32 weeks									
Mean	10(59)	24(132)	17(95)	17(94)	18(99)	18(103)	17(97)	14(80)	20(114)
Lowest	4(20)	6(35)	7(40)	11(60)	11(60)	9(50)	7(40)	7(40)	8(45)
33–36 weeks									
Mean	11(61)	25(138)	19(105)	18(100)	13(75)	16(89)	17(94)	17(93)	19(106)
Lowest	5(30)	9(50)	11(60)	9(50)	7(40)	7(40)	7(40)	7(40)	8(45)

Table 106. Normal haematological values during the first year of life (continued).

	Age (weeks)								
	3 days	3	6	9	12	18	24	36	54
Transferrin (μmol IBC/l)†									
28–32 weeks									
Mean	33(131)	41(165)	49(195)	60(241)	63(253)	77(309)	70(279)	72(286)	89(355)
Highest	68(270)	61(244)	68(270)	90(360)	85(340)	98(390)	98(390)	78(310)	130(520)
33–36 weeks									
Mean	35(138)	40(158)	50(201)	68(271)	69(277)	67(266)	73(292)	75(299)	94(375)
Highest	54(214)	76(304)	83(330)	98(390)	100(400)	98(390)	95(380)	103(410)	140(560)
Transferrin saturation (%)									
28–32 weeks									
Mean	37	59	37	30	29	24	24	20	23
Lowest	11	22	14	14	19	10	11	10	12
33–36 weeks									
Mean	34	72	36	32	21	24	24	23	21
Lowest	12	19	23	11	11	12	10	14	12

IBC = Iron-binding capcity
* Numbers in parentheses indicate μg/100 ml
† Numbers in parentheses indicate mg/100 ml
From Halliday *et al.* (1984) with kind permission of S. Karger AG, Basel

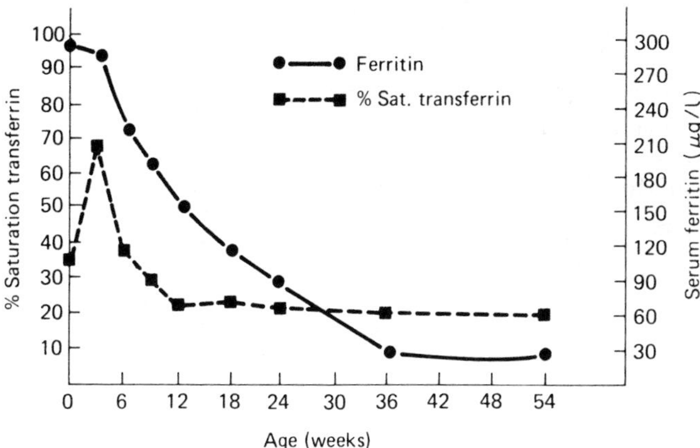

Fig. 51. Depletion of iron stores (serum ferritin) and percentage saturation of transferrin in the preterm infant.

Table 107. Causes of late anaemia.

1. Excessive blood-letting (iatrogenic)
2. Chronic haemolysis: rhesus, ABO, red cell defects, enzyme defects, haemoglobinopathies and sepsis
3. Sepsis
4. Bleeding: vitamin K deficiency, DIC, intraventricular haemorrhage
5. Physiological anaemia of prematurity (early anaemia), deficient erythropoiesis and reduced red cell survival
6. Late anaemia of prematurity: iron-deficiency (usually after 8 weeks)
7. Vitamin E deficiency: haemolytic anaemia
8. Possible folate and vitamin B_{12} deficiency
9. Bone marrow failure or replacement

Treatment

Look for underlying cause and correct it. If infant is shocked give blood transfusion at once. In other infants haemoglobin raised by using packed cells. The amount of packed cells to raise PCV is calculated from following formula:

$$\frac{(\text{desired PCV} - \text{actual PCV}) \times \text{weight (kg)} \times 90}{\text{donor PCV (about 60–70\%)}} = \text{ml of donor blood}$$

The 90 refers to estimated blood volume at birth (i.e. 90 ml/kg). In practice, transfusion of 10 ml/kg packed cells will raise PCV by 10%.

Transfusion is given to infants with:

1. RDS, apnoeic attacks and chronic lung disease if PCV < 45% (haemoglobin <14 g/dl).
2. Haemolytic disease if haemoglobin < 9 g/dl (PCV <28%).
3. Physiological anaemia with haemoglobin <7 g/dl (PCV <25%), unless symptoms of anaemia such as tachycardia, tachypnoea, poor feeding or poor weight gain when transfusion is given at higher levels.

POLYCYTHAEMIA

Arbitrarily defined as venous PCV > 65% (haemoglobin >22 g/dl) in newborn. Blood viscosity is related to haematocrit and fibrinogen levels. Blood viscosity usually increases linearly with increasing PCV until latter reaches 65–70% and thereafter viscosity increases in logarithmic fashion (Fig. 52). Normal

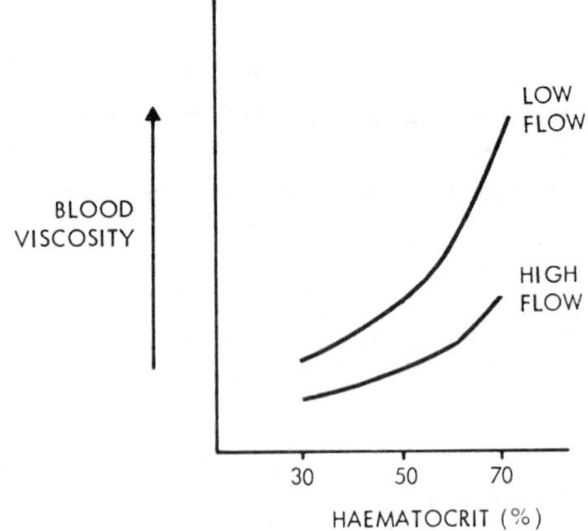

Fig. 52. Increase in blood viscosity with packed cell volume at low and high blood flows. From Phibbs *et al.* (1977) with kind permission of the authors and Appleton-Century-Crofts.

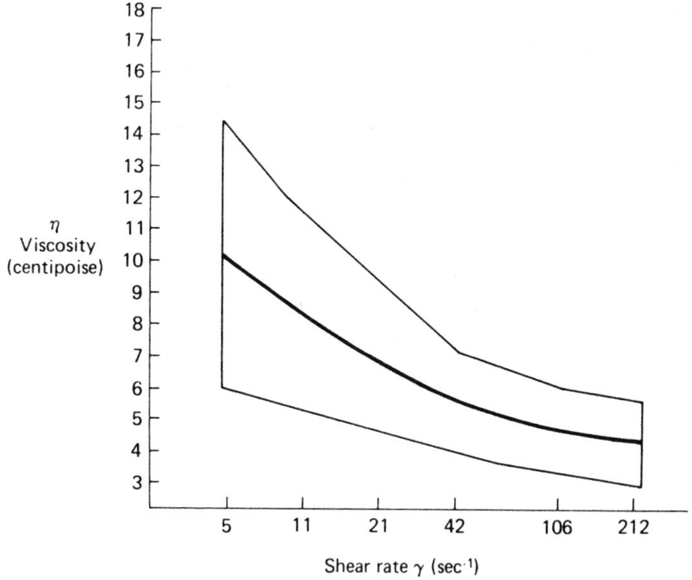

Fig. 53. Viscosity of cord blood at different shear rates for healthy fullterm AGA infants (±2 sd). From Gross *et al.* (1973) with kind permission of the publishers C. V. Mosby.

neonatal blood viscosity at different shear rates is shown in Fig. 53. Hyperviscosity associated with decreased flow both in the microcirculation and in large veins. May cause cerebral, renal or inferior vena caval thrombosis. There is decreased oxygen transport. Clinical features are cerebral hyper-excitability and seizures, apathy, vomiting, abdominal distension, congestive heart failure, cyanosis, persistent fetal circulation, hypoglycaemia and jaundice. The causes of polycythaemia are listed in Table 108. Most are due to either chronic intrauterine hypoxia or excessive placentofetal transfusion at birth. In the infant of the diabetic mother insulin stimulates erythropoietin.

Check PCV on all ill infants, infants of diabetic mothers, SGA infants and twins. If over 65% on initial capillary sample then check venous sample (capillary PCV may be 20% above venous values, less if heel is warmed). If venous PCV $>$ 65% and infant

Table 108. Causes of polycythaemia.

1. Delayed cord clamping and milking of umbilical cord
2. Intrauterine growth failure: smoking, altitude
3. Diabetic mother
4. Twin-to-twin transfusion
5. Maternofetal transfusion
6. Others: Down's syndrome, maternal thyrotoxicosis, congenital adrenal hyperplasia, Beckwith's syndrome

has any symptoms attributable to polycythaemia then carry out partial exchange transfusion with albumin or plasma. If PCV is > 70% (haemoglobin >24 g/dl) then partial exchange also performed even if symptoms absent. Aim to lower PCV to about 55% and this usually achieved by exchanging with about 20 ml/kg 5% salt-poor albumin or plasma. The formula below used to calculate exact amount:

$$\frac{\text{actual PCV} - \text{desired PCV}}{\text{actual PCV}} \times 90 = \text{volume of exchange (ml/kg)}$$

Often large peripheral vein is suitable and umbilical vessel catheterization should be avoided unless indicated for other reasons.

It is now possible to measure blood viscosity rapidly so that need for dilutional exchange transfusion can be based on high viscosity levels (normal values in Fig. 52).

HAEMORRHAGIC DISEASE OF THE NEWBORN

Due to accentuation of coagulation defects found in all newborns. Needs differentiation from disseminated intravascular coagulation (Table 109). Major defect is deficiency of prothrombin and other vitamin-K-dependent factors. Vitamin K required for hepatic synthesis of factors II (prothrombin), VII, IX and X. Cow's milk contains four times as much vitamin K as breast milk so that haemorrhagic disease normally seen only in breast-fed infants. Vitamin K deficiency also in chronic diarrhoea, prolonged broad-spectrum antibiotic therapy,

Table 109. Comparison of haemorrhagic disease and disseminated intravascular coagulation (DIC).

	Haemorrhagic disease	*DIC*
Clinical associations	Well infant: vitamin K not given	Ill infant: sepsis, hypoxia, acidosis, obstetrical accidents
Capillary fragility (Hess test)	Normal	Abnormal
Bleeding time	Normal	Prolonged
Clotting time	Prolonged	Variable
Prothrombin time	Prolonged	Prolonged
Partial thromboplastin time	Prolonged	Prolonged
Thrombin time	Normal	Prolonged
Fibrin degradation products	Absent	Present
Factor V	Normal	Reduced
Fibrinogen	Normal	Reduced
Platelets	Normal	Reduced
RBC fragmentation	Absent	Present
Response to vitamin K	Yes	No

prematurity, especially if having parenteral nutrition, and maternal drug therapy (phenytoin, phenobarbitone, salicylates, warfarin and dicoumarol). It should be possible to prevent haemorrhagic disease by routine administration of vitamin K to all babies in the labour ward or with the first feed. Bleeding into the skin, umbilical cord, mucous membranes, or viscera. There may be catastrophic intracranial or gastrointestinal haemorrhage. Usual onset is third to seventh day. Prothrombin time prolonged and treatment with intravenous or intramuscular vitamin K_1 (Konakion) 1–2 mg. Dose may be repeated once if necessary and for continued or life-threatening bleeding, fresh frozen plasma or fresh whole blood transfused at 10 ml/kg. Local bleeding from umbilical cord may stop after pressure or topical coagulants (thrombin gauze). Normal coagulation values are shown in Appendix XII. Partial thromboplastin time (PTT) measures all the intrinsic clotting system, especially factors VIII and IX. Prothrombin time (PT) measures factors II, V, VII, X and fibrinogen (I). Thrombin time (TT) measures fibrinogen (I), antithrombins including heparin, and fibrin degradation products (FDP). Reptilase time (RT) measures same as TT but excludes heparin.

DISSEMINATED INTRAVASCULAR COAGULATION (DIC)

Probably more common in neonatal period than previously recognized. Table 110 lists the causes of DIC. Thrombin formation is stimulated by bacterial endotoxin or thromboplastin released from damaged tissues. This causes intravascular coagulation with consumption of platelets, factors II, V, VIII, XIII and fibrinogen. The fibrinolytic system is also stimulated causing increase in fibrin degradation products (FDP) which may exacerbate bleeding.

Table 110. Causes of DIC.

1. Septicaemia, shock and birth asphyxia (acidosis and hypothermia)
2. Tissue release of thromboplastins: placental abruption, IUD of twin, hypoxia (RDS) or neoplasm
3. Giant haemangioma
4. Necrotizing enterocolitis
5. Renal vein thrombosis

Any severely ill infant may develop DIC

Blood films shows fragmented red cells and treatment first aimed at finding and removing underlying cause. Controversy over whether heparin and/or steroid therapy of benefit in newborn. Usual practice to give fresh blood and plasma infusion and consider exchange transfusion in critically ill infant, especially if sepsis suspected as underlying cause.

Appendix XII shows normal coagulation values for the newborn.

INHERITED BLEEDING DISORDERS

1. Haemophilia: factor VIII activity deficient; males
2. Christmas disease; factor IX deficient; males

3. von Willebrand's disease; factor VIII deficient and platelet function reduced; both sexes
4. Dysfibrinogenaemia; factor I abnormal; both sexes
5. Others; uncommon; autosomal recessive

NEONATAL THROMBOCYTOPENIA

Usually defined as platelet count < 150 000/mm^3 in term infant and < 100 000/mm^3 in preterm infant. Underlying causes are listed in Table 111. Table 112 lists drugs causing thrombocytopenia. Most causes of thrombocytopenia in newborn are serious and full investigation indicated. This should include careful history of contact with rubella or infection during pregnancy, maternal illness, e.g. idiopathic thrombocytopenia (ITP) or DLE, and drugs taken during pregnancy. If infant is ill, sepsis, DIC, necrotizing enterocolitis are the most likely.

Table 111. Causes of thrombocytopenia.

1. Autoimmune
2. Isoimmune (maternal ITP)
3. DIC
4. Haemolytic disease (erythroblastosis)
5. Maternal DLE
6. Infections: septicaemia, herpes simplex, candidiasis, toxoplasmosis, CMV, rubella, syphilis
7. Drugs: thiazides, sulpha drugs (see Table 112)
8. After exchange transfusion
9. Necrotizing enterocolitis
10. Aplastic anaemia (with limb deformity)
11. Congenital leukaemia
12. Down's syndrome
13. Letterer–Siwe disease
14. Giant haemangioma
15. Wiskott–Aldrich syndrome
16. Associated with osteogenesis imperfecta

Table 112. Drugs causing thrombocytopenia.

Acetazolamide	Phenytoin
Aspirin	Potassium perchlorate
Carbamazepine	Primidone
Carbimazole	Propylthiouracil
Chloramphenicol	Quinidine
Chloroquine	Quinine
Cytotoxic drugs	Rifampicin
Ethambutol	Sulphonamides
Ethosuximide	Tetracyclines
Indomethacin	Thiazide diuretics
Novobiocin	Tricyclic antidepressants
Penicillin	Troxidone
Phenothiazines	

Therapy to correct the underlying cause and occasionally platelet transfusions or fresh blood given to correct life-threatening bleeding or platelet counts $< 20\,000/mm^3$. At this level cerebral haemorrhage more likely. Platelets in transfusions, however, have half-life of < 12 hours so only temporary relief. Immunoglobulin infusions may help in ITP, perhaps acting as a blocking antibody. Steroids sometimes used to treat thrombocytopenia secondary to maternal ITP but benefit not proved. They may act by improving capillary wall integrity and so lessening risk of life-threatening haemorrhage. Dose of prednisone 2 mg/kg/day initially, rapidly reducing if there is response. Response, however, may take many days (see also p. 18).

INVESTIGATION OF BLEEDING NEWBORN

1. History: family history, maternal drugs, obstetrical history
2. Examination:

   Ill infant: suspect DIC, infection, severe liver disease

   Well infant: suspect platelet defect, haemorrhagic

disease, clotting factor deficiency
Petechiae: suspect thrombocytopenia
Ecchymoses: suspect DIC, haemorrhagic disease, liver disease, clotting defects

3. If gastrointestinal bleeding: do Apt test (see p. 31)
4. Other investigations: platelet count, prothrombin time, partial thromboplastin time, bleeding time, fibrin degradation products (urine and blood), fibrinogen

Thrombocytosis

Platelet count > 400 000/mm^3. Occurs during growth and after fat infusions. Commonest at 2–4 months of age but not associated with morbidity.

NURSING POINTS

1. Signs of anaemia are important as they indicate reduced oxygen delivery to the tissues: look out for tachycardia, tachypnoea, poor feeding and poor weight gain in addition to pallor in an otherwise well preterm baby
2. Avoid early iron supplementation as this increases risk of haemolysis from vitamin E deficiency and may also increase risk of infection
3. Check that vitamin K (Konakion) has been given in labour ward: preterm babies can miss out and need intramuscular or intravenous injection in NICU
4. Look for excessive bleeding from venepuncture sites as this may indicate a developing coagulopathy
5. Local measures to stop bleeding include pressure with sterile gauze wipe and local thrombin-containing material such as Oxycel. Medical staff should be alerted

REFERENCES AND FURTHER READING

Gross, G. P., Hathaway, W. E. and McCaughey, H. R. (1973). Hyperviscosity in the neonate. *J. Pediatr.* **82**: 1004.

Halliday, H. L., Lappin, T. R. J. and McClure, G. (1983). Do all preterm infants need iron supplements? *Ir. Med. J.* **76**: 430.

Halliday, H. L., Lappin, T. R. J. and McClure, G. (1984). Iron status of the preterm infant during the first year of life. *Biol. Neonate* **45**: 228.

Manroe, B. L., Brown, R., Weinberg, A. G. and Rosenfeld, C. R. (1976). Normal leukocyte (WBC) values in neonates. *Pediatr. Res.* **10**: 428.

Manroe, B. L., Rosenfeld, C. R., Weinberg, A. G. and Brown, R. (1977). The differential leukocyte count in the assessment and outcome of early-onset neonatal group B streptococcal disease. *J. Pediatr.* **91**: 632.

Oski, F. A. and Naiman, J. L. (1982). *Hematologic Problems in the Newborn*, 3rd edn. Philadelphia: W. B. Saunders.

Phibbs, R. H. (1987). Neonatal Polycythaemia. In: *Pediatrics*, 18th edn (eds, Rudolph, A. M. and Hoffman, J. I. E.). New York: Appleton-Century-Crofts.

22. The Very Low Birth Weight Infant

The very low birth weight infant is one whose birth weight is 1500 g or less. Infants <1500 g (<30–32 weeks gestation) comprise only 1% of liveborn population, but account for 70% of all neonatal deaths not due to congenital anomalies. Table 113 shows survival of very low birth weight infants admitted to the Royal Maternity Hospital, Belfast, in 1982–83. Figure 54 shows outcome with and without major handicap over the same

Table 113. Survival of very low birth weight infants (%).

Gestational age (weeks)	*Approx. birth weight* (g)	*RMH** (1982–83)
23	550	0
24	600	10
25	700	33
26	850	87
27	950	83
28	1100	87
29	1200	87
30	1300	91
31	1400	94
32	1500	94

* RMH = Royal Maternity Hospital, Belfast. Survival to discharge from hospital

Table 114. Causes of death in very low birth weight infant.

1. *Pulmonary hypoplasia and asphyxia*	At birth with sustained respiration not acquired
2. *Intrauterine bacterial infection*	Associated with prolonged rupture of membranes
3. *Respiratory distress syndrome*	Or its sequelae including pneumothorax, patent ductus arteriosus, intraventricular haemorrhage and bronchopulmonary dysplasia
4. *Delayed death*	From apnoea, late infection, necrotizing enterocolitis, hydrocephalus

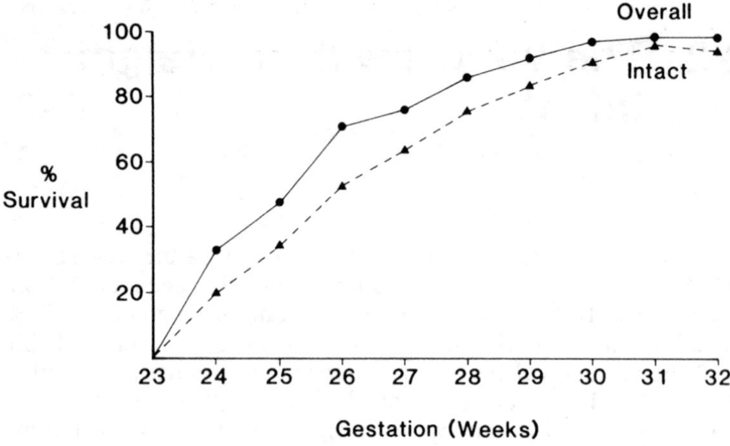

Fig. 54. Percentage survival by gestational age for babies <1500 g birth weight and ⩽32 weeks gestation, born in Royal Maternity Hospital Belfast 1981–85. Overall survival means alive at discharge from hospital and intact survival means absence of major handicap at age 2 years.

period. These results can only be achieved in centres where neonatal intensive care is available. There are now reports of babies of 22 and 23 weeks gestation surviving after intensive care in UK, USA, Australia and Japan. There are four common causes of death in very low birth weight infants (Table 114). In practice these are interrelated; severe asphyxia and intra-uterine infection often occur together. Respiratory distress syndrome leading to respiratory failure and death is now unusual because of mechanical ventilation. Deaths after 7 days (beyond perinatal period) and 28 days (beyond neonatal period) are common (20% of all deaths) with many due to sepsis (about 30% of deaths) or bronchopulmonary dysplasia or sequelae of intraventricular haemorrhage. Table 115 gives the incidence of morbidity in very low birth weight infants. The very low birth weight infant suffers from physiological immaturity like the larger preterm infant but has additional special problems which require specific management. These special problems include asphyxia, temperature control, over-handling, respiratory distress, fluid balance, nutrition and electrolyte problems, fluid retention, apnoeic attacks, patent ductus arteriosus, chronic

Table 115. Morbidity of very low birth weight infants admitted to Royal Maternity Hospital, Belfast, 1982–83.

	Birth weight	
	< 1000 g	< 1500 g
Respiratory distress syndrome	95%	63%
Needed IPPV	73%	45%
Needed CPAP alone	5%	5%
Pneumothorax	18%	10%
Intraventricular haemorrhage		
clinical	36%	12%
ultrasound	55%	23%
Patent ductus arteriosus (needing ligation or indomethacin)	19%	13%
Necrotizing enterocolitis	12%	8%
Bronchopulmonary dysplasia	18%	17%
Retrolental fibroplasia	3%	1%
Subglottic stenosis	—	3%
Cerebral palsy	9%	6%

pulmonary disease, anaemia, infection, necrotizing enterocolitis, subcapsular haematoma of liver and problems with parent/infant interaction.

ASPHYXIA

Especially important that experienced personnel conduct delivery and resuscitate the infant. Really a prime example of perinatal intensive care at its best. For very short gestation pregnancies (22–24 weeks) it is important to talk to the parents during labour to find out their views on how best to proceed. To do this they need simple and sympathetic counselling with a realistic estimate of chances of survival and potential handicap. After birth adverse prognostic signs are firmly fused eyelids, marked bruising and birth weight <500 g. After endotracheal intubation, if the lungs are very non-compliant, a decision to proceed to mechanical ventilation with or without surfactant replacement should be taken by a senior doctor after parental discussion if possible.

For more mature babies endotracheal intubation is often required, small doses of sodium bicarbonate helpful (1 mmol/kg). Remember asphyxia shuts off early pathway of surfactant production increasing the severity of RDS and risk of subsequent IVH.

TEMPERATURE CONTROL

Resuscitate and stabilize under servo-controlled radiant warmer. Important to obtain baby's weight and erect intravenous fluids. After stabilization remove to incubator to reduce high insensible water losses; incubator may need to be 37–38 °C during first hours of life. Heat shield or bubble wrap may be used to reduce heat losses but often high humidity is required in the incubator.

OVER-HANDLING

All handling is poorly tolerated. All procedures should be assessed as to relative benefit versus risk. Even simple procedures such as weighing infant, starting scalp vein infusion and placing monitor leads carry risk but benefit outweighs risk. Use of pulse oximeter to control oxygen needs reduces handling. Blood gases and packed cell volume can be checked at 30 min. Constant observation required in first 30 min.

RESPIRATORY DISTRESS

Respiratory problems and their sequelae are the major causes of death and management of these infants is very difficult. When problems occur, diagnosis and treatment should be carried out rapidly and gently. Treatment is otherwise essentially the same as for larger infants but the margin of tolerance is narrower. Respiratory assistance from birth is often needed for babies weighing <1000 g (Table 115). Surfactant replacement has certainly improved the outcome for these immature babies (see Chapter 10).

Careful control of oxygen therapy to keep P_aO_2 in range of 7-10 kPa (50-70 mmHg) or oxygen saturation 90-94% with pulse oximeter. If arterialized capillary samples used keep oxygen tension at 5-7 kPa (40-50 mmHg). Often only 30% oxygen required initially unless severe asphyxia. Watch for increased oxygen needs after 3 days when thoracic gas volume decreases and breathing becomes periodic.

INTRAVENTRICULAR HAEMORRHAGE

IVH and periventricular leucomalacia (ischaemic damage) are not uncommon in very immature babies. Related to immaturity, asphyxia, sudden stresses such as pneumothorax and hyper- and hypotension. Important to maintain physiology as close to normal as possible; keep blood pressure in normal range. Regular ultrasound scans to monitor progression and help with prognosis (see Chapters 16 and 24).

FLUIDS AND NUTRITION

Fluid and electrolyte balance in these babies is so labile that they can only be prescribed for 8-12 hour periods based upon a knowledge of serum and urinary electrolytes, fluid input and output, and body weight. Most need intravenous fluids of 5 or 10% dextrose at 80-100 ml/kg/day on first day. If radiant warmers or phototherapy used, insensible water loss may increase by 50-100% and an extra 30-60 ml/kg/day needed. The very immature baby with thin shiny skin may have massive insensible water losses and have fluid requirements up to 250-300 ml/kg/day for first 3 days. Electrolytes are usually not needed during this time. The more mature baby, if clinically well, can be started on oral milk feeds. Parenteral nutrition is often required so that one can gradually increase oral milk feeds (expressed breast milk if possible) by end of first week. Watch for abdominal distension, increasing gastric aspirates and reducing substances or blood in stool. Breast milk feeds are deficient in protein, iron, phosphorus, sodium and chloride and supplementation may be necessary unless specially prepared milk used (Table 40). Expected weight gain is 1-1.5% of body weight per day, i.e. for 750 g infant, 7.5–10 g daily (see Appendix VIII).

ELECTROLYTE PROBLEMS

Acid–base and electrolyte balance may be upset. Early hypernatraemia is common due to high insensible water losses; electrolytes are usually not needed for first 2–3 days. Hyponatraemia often follows due to inappropriate ADH secretion and renal sodium losses. This should be treated with fluid restriction and increased sodium supplements (up to 6–8 mmol/kg may be needed).

Later metabolic acidosis may occur because the kidney is unable to excrete an increased acid load related to high protein intake. Oral sodium bicarbonate may be required to keep pH >7.3. Other causes of metabolic acidosis include sepsis, hypovolaemia, PDA, anaemia, necrotizing enterocolitis and IVH.

Hypercapnia may develop at end of first week and is associated with hypoventilation. Carbohydrate intolerance may also occur and is exaggerated by illness and sepsis. Five per cent dextrose is given to avoid hyperglycaemia which causes hyperosmolarity, osmotic diuresis and cerebral depression. High blood urea almost constant feature during the first 3 days because of catabolism from inadequate nutrition and renal immaturity. Once growth established blood urea levels fall.

FLUID RETENTION

Caused by combination of excessive fluid intake and renal immaturity. Also associated with patent ductus arteriosus and bronchopulmonary dysplasia. Fluid retention can be prevented by limiting fluid to less than 150 mg/kg/day during the first week of life.

May occasionally require diuretic therapy (frusemide 0.5 mg/kg or chlorothiazide 20 mg/kg/day). Fluid intake can be limited by using modified, relatively high-calorie milks (Table 40).

APNOEIC ATTACKS

Common from 3 days to 2 weeks of age, usually associated with bradycardia. Over 90% of babies < 1000 g and 60% from 1000 to 1500 g have these. Early intervention by continuous stimulation reduces the need for resuscitation. Heart and respiration rate monitors must be used on all infants less than 32 weeks gestation, until apnoea-free for at least 1 week. Always look for predisposing factors, especially infection. Start with simple therapies first, but drugs are often unsuccessful and mechanical ventilation is frequently needed (Table 66).

PATENT DUCTUS ARTERIOSUS (PDA)

Systolic or continuous murmur usually has onset at 3–5 days when pulmonary vascular resistance declines to allow increased L–R shunt. Aortic run-off causes bounding pulses and pulmonary congestion. Echocardiogram used to measure left atrial and left ventricular dimensions (p. 326). Most ominous clinical sign is apnoea because this may mean decreased cerebral blood flow. Initial treatment is conservative with fluid restriction and diuretics. Blood transfusion given to maintain haemoglobin above 14 g/dl (PCV 45%). Digoxin reserved for those not responding or when echocardiogram shows decreased left ventricular contraction. If conservative measures fail then either prostaglandin inhibition with indomethacin or surgical ligation.

CHRONIC PULMONARY DISEASE

Probably many separate entities with different aetiologies but Wilson–Mikity syndrome perhaps best known. Infant usually has not had severe RDS and at 7–10 days develops progressive respiratory distress and oxygen need of about 30%. Chest radiograph shows streaky infiltrations and later cystic changes. This chronic condition tends to improve after 4–8 weeks of age. Fluid overload, mineral and vitamin deficiencies have been suggested, though weak muscular chest wall and chronic deficiency of surfactant may also be causes. Treatment with oxygen given to maintain normal blood gases and CPAP to stabilize the alveoli. Fluid restriction, diuretics and dietary supplements may be helpful.

RETINOPATHY OF PREMATURITY

Increasingly commonly seen in the very immature baby, with acute changes more common than chronic ones which lead to impaired vision. Oxygen is only one factor in aetiology and disease may not be preventable in very immature babies. Important to examine fundi at 6 weeks to detect changes that might benefit from cryotherapy (see p. 65).

ANAEMIA

Earlier onset and greater severity than in more mature baby. Reasons are lower initial haemoglobin (12–14 g/dl), decreased red cell survival and increased losses from blood sampling. Also relative growth rates greater so that 900 g infant may treble birth weight in 10 weeks. Delay oral iron supplements until 8 weeks. Anaemia occurring before this is due to haemolysis or blood loss and should be treated by blood transfusion. Vitamin E deficiency is discussed on p. 281.

INFECTION

Beware of pregnancy complicated by prolonged ruptured membranes. This may lead to pulmonary hypoplasia, and pneumonia and septicaemia are also common (5–10%). After culture of infant, antibiotics are started if infant has any symptoms or mother is ill and febrile, or Gram stain of gastric aspirate shows organisms or pus cells (see p. 24). Anaerobic infections not uncommon, especially if the baby is 'smelly', and drug of choice is metronidazole (dose: 7.5 mg/kg every 8 hours infused over 30 min). Babies with congenital infection may suffer from bouts of bacteraemia later, perhaps as a result of immune depression or altered bacterial flora secondary to antibiotic therapy. These latter bacteraemias may be due to *Staphylococcus albus*; or fungaemia due to candidiasis (see Chapter 14).

NECROTIZING ENTEROCOLITIS

Predisposing events are extreme immaturity, birth asphyxia, hypotension, polycythaemia, hypothermia, umbilical vessel catheterization, exchange transfusion, patent ductus arteriosus and early milk feeding. Careful introduction of milk feeds essential. Any distension of the bowel with increased gastric aspirate means that feeding should be stopped at least temporarily. Surgery reserved for infants with evidence of perforation, i.e. free peritoneal air or cellulitis of anterior abdominal wall.

SUBCAPSULAR HAEMATOMA OF LIVER

Uncommon condition almost exclusively seen in babies < 1000 g birth weight and commoner in assisted breech deliveries. Chest drain insertion is a postnatal risk factor. May present as shock and collapse, or less dramatically as unexplained thrombocytopenia and abnormal ultrasound scan. Sometimes the diagnosis is only made at autopsy. If suspected during life abdominal ultrasound scan and paracentesis are indicated and volume replacement with correction of coagulation disorder should be urgently begun. Surgical intervention has been successful on a few occasions.

PARENT–INFANT BONDING PROBLEMS

Being the parent of a 23–25 week premature infant can be one of the most emotionally draining experiences of a lifetime. The infant seems to pass from one crisis to another and it may be only after several weeks that the parents realize that their infant may survive. Parents should be encouraged to visit their infants and caress them. Visits by siblings should also be encouraged and as soon as feasible babies should be dressed in nice clothes. Photographs to keep are very important, especially if the parents live far away and are unable to visit often or use parental accomodation within the hospital. Providing expressed breast milk allows mother to take part in baby's care. All the good news should be conveyed at each visit and only serious setbacks notified by telephone. Infrequent visiting by parents is an early warning sign of future mothering problems so that all visits by the parents should be noted in the chart (see also Chapter 25).

NURSING POINTS

1. Before handling a tiny baby have a good reason: benefit must outweigh the cost
2. Maintain a stable environment at all times
3. Encourage parent–infant relationships
4. Dress baby in suitable clothes as soon as feasible

REFERENCES AND FURTHER READING

Halliday, H. L. (1988). Care of preterm babies in the first hour. *Care Crit. Ill* **4**: 7.

Ryan, C. A. and Finer, N. N. (1987). Subcapsular hematoma of the liver in infants of very low birth weight. *Can. Med. Assoc. J.* **136**: 1265.

Whitelaw, A. and Cooke, R. W. I. (1988). The very immature infant: less than 28 weeks gestation. *British Medical Bulletin*, Vol. 44. Edinburgh: Published for British Council by Churchill Livingstone.

23. Congenital Malformations

These are important as they account for 40% of neonatal or perinatal deaths. They are also a major cause of handicap in childhood and later life. For effect of congenital malformation on the family see p. 333. It is difficult to establish true incidence of congenital abnormalities at birth: some are obvious, e.g. meningomyelocele, while others are diagnosed much later in life, e.g. atrial septal defect. Some minor abnormalities, e.g. mild hypospadias, extra digits and accessory auricles, are often not included in surveys. It is believed that the overall incidence of congenital abnormality is about 2% (Table 116). There is a geographical variation in the incidence of abnormalities, especially neural tube defects which tend to have a high incidence in the western part of the British Isles. At present the incidence of neural tube defects is dramatically decreasing, but it is uncertain whether this has been due to therapeutic intervention, such as termination of pregnancy or vitamin supplementation, or whether the phenomenon is unexplained.

Causes of congenital malformations are largely unknown. Some are due to genetic disorders, chromosomal disorders,

Table 116. Incidence of congenital malformations at birth per 1000 births (1979).

	England and Wales	*Northern Ireland*
Limbs and skeleton	8.5	12.7
Central nervous system	2.5	8.2
Cardiovascular system	1.2	6.3
Gastrointestinal	0.7	5.6
Genitourinary	1.9	3.8
Face and palate	2.0	1.7
Chromosomal	1.0	1.6
Other multiple anomalies	1.5	3.0
All anomalies	21	46

rubella, radiation and drugs. The trisomy abnormalities are associated with increased maternal age and there is a higher incidence of abnormalities in maternal diabetes. Lower socioeconomic classes have a higher incidence of neural tube defects.

Some congenital malformations require urgent assessment and treatment from birth (Table 117). Antenatal diagnosis or suspicion of congenital abnormality is now made by ultrasound scan at 18–20 weeks or later (Chapter 1). Management of cardiac (Chapter 17) and renal (Chapter 19) abnormalities diagnosed antenatally have already been discussed.

Table 117. Congenital malformations needing urgent assessment at birth.

Tracheo-oesophageal fistula ± oesophageal atresia
Diaphragmatic hernia
Choanal atresia
Pierre Robin syndrome
Omphalocele
Gastroschisis
Myelomeningocele
Encephalocele
Imperforate anus

PREPARATION FOR SURGERY

Surgery should be carried out at a regional children's hospital and this will often necessitate transfer of the infant. The baby should be stabilized before transfer being sure to obtain parental consent (p. 39). Always explain very carefully to the parents why surgery is needed and what will be done. In addition to providing intravenous fluids, ensure that cross-matched blood is available before surgery and that the baby has been given prophylactic vitamin K. Postoperatively, fluid and electrolyte balance needs careful management which should be performed in a specialist ICU. All abnormal fluid losses, e.g. continuous gastric aspiration, must be replaced in addition to basic requirements. Metabolic abnormalities are common after surgery, e.g. hypo- or hyperglycaemia, hypocalcaemia, hypothermia and acidosis. Infection may also be a major problem and this may occur as pneumonia, septicaemia or urinary infection.

MALFORMATIONS OF THE CNS

The CNS is the most frequent site of congenital malformation; about 1/1000 births have anencephaly and similar numbers for meningomyelocele. Microcephaly is less common. Assessment of neural tube defects is essential to determine those infants who would benefit from surgical closure. Surgery is probably contraindicated if any of Lorber's adverse features are present:

1. Total paraplegia
2. Kyphoscoliosis
3. Hydrocephalus: head circumference 2 cm greater than 90th centile
4. Large thoracolumbar lesion, greater than four segments
5. Associated anomalies

Microcephaly is an abnormally small head, i.e. more than three standard deviations below the normal. Infants are usually severely retarded. Intrauterine infection, inborn errors of metabolism and severe intrauterine hypoxia may be underlying causes. Maternal phenylketonuria is an important cause to exclude. There is also a sex-linked familial type.

Hydrocephalus is due to excessive CSF within the cerebral ventricles and usually results in increased occipitofrontal circumference. May be caused by meningomyelocele, intrauterine infection, or after cerebral haemorrhage or meningitis. Occasionally due to aqueduct stenosis or the Dandy–Walker syndrome. Other causes of a large head are benign familial macrocephaly, chronic subdural haematoma and hydranencephaly. Ultrasound and CT scan are used in investigation of these patients (see also Chapter 24).

CARDIOVASCULAR ABNORMALITIES

These are discussed in Chapter 17.

GASTROINTESTINAL ABNORMALITIES

These include exomphalos, gastroschisis, intestinal atresia, Hirschsprung's disease, imperforate anus and tracheo-oesophageal fistula (Table 118).

Table 118. Gastrointestinal anomalies requiring surgery.

1. *Tracheo-oesophageal fistula*	1/3500 births. 50% other malformations. Presents with polyhydramnios, frothy secretions or aspiration pneumonia
2. *Diaphragmatic hernia*	1/4000 births. 90% left sided. Presents with asphyxia, shift of heart beat and respiratory distress. Abdomen is scaphoid. In two-thirds there is pulmonary hypoplasia and death is likely
3. *Exomphalos or omphalocele*	Herniation of abdominal contents into umbilical cord. Coils of intestine and liver covered by peritoneal membrane unless this has ruptured. Over 30% have associated abnormalities of gastrointestinal, genitourinary and cardiovascular systems. Beckwith's syndrome of visceromegaly, macroglossia, omphalocele and hypoglycaemia. Immediate treatment: cover the lesion with warm, sterile saline dressings (and if available a polythene 'poly bag') and aspirate stomach to prevent distension
4. *Gastroschisis*	Similar to omphalocele except that coils of intestine herniated through defect in anterior abdominal wall near umbilicus. No covering peritoneal membrane and associated abnormalities, except ileal atresias, uncommon. Intestinal circulation often impaired causing ischaemia of bowel with frank gangrene. Lesion should be covered with warm saline soaks before transfer, large protein losses need replacement with intravenous plasma
5. *Intestinal atresia*	Presentation with vomiting, abdominal distension and delayed passage of meconium. Duodenal obstruction (double-bubble on radiograph) associated with other abnormalities in 70% (Down's syndrome, malrotation and congenital heart disease). Higher obstructions present earlier. In ileal atresia with obstruction below the ampulla of Vater bile-stained vomiting occurs. Even in complete obstruction small amounts of 'stool' passed in first 24 hours
6. *Malrotation*	Often associated with duodenal bands (of Ladd). Associated abnormalities include duodenal atresia or stenosis and exomphalos. Obstruction may be

Table 118. Gastrointestinal anomalies requiring surgery (continued).

	incomplete so diagnosis may be missed. Bile-stained vomiting and bloody stools or failure to thrive. Intestinal ischaemia can lead to necrosis with shock and sepsis
7. *Meconium ileus*	In 10% of infants with cystic fibrosis. Pancreatic enzyme deficiency associated with production of thick, inspissated meconium. Ischaemia, perforation and peritonitis. Meconium peritonitis in utero but as meconium is sterile effects not recognized for some time after birth. Radiological densities in abdomen. Radiograph shows granular appearance inside distended bowel (hornet's nest)
8. *Hirschsprung's disease*	Aganglionic segment of bowel from rectum proximally. Short segment disease more common in males but long segment has equal sex distribution. May be familial. Barium enema usually required for diagnosis: narrow aganglionic segment distal to dilated bowel. Diagnosis confirmed by rectal biopsy
9. *Imperforate anus*	Lesion high or low. *High*: a fistula from upper rectal pouch to bladder, urethra or vagina usual. Large bowel obstruction only if fistula not patent. *Low*: anus may be obstructed by membrane at level of anal valves. Lateral abdominal radiographs with baby inverted distinguishes these two types. A radio-opaque marker placed over anus. If air in upper rectal pouch below a line from pubis to sacrococcygeal junction then lesion is low. Associated with tracheo-oesophageal fistula and Vater syndrome (V = ventricular septal defect and vertebral anomalies, A = anal atresia, TE = tracheo-oesophageal fistula, R = radial and renal anomalies)
10. *Others*	Meconium plug: preterm, diabetic mother (also small left colon), Hirschsprung's disease Appendicitis: rare Annular pancreas: duodenal obstruction Pyloric stenosis: occasionally in first week

GENITOURINARY ABNORMALITIES

Antenatal diagnosis is now possible as a result of improved ultrasound imaging (see Chapter 19). After antenatal diagnosis, mother should be transferred to a regional perinatal centre for evaluation and delivery.

Renal Agenesis

Relatively common affecting about 1/4000 births with male preponderance. Oligohydramnios usually present and stillbirth or early neonatal death occur often. Prenatal diagnosis is possible by ultrasound (see Chapter 1). Placenta shows amnion nodosum. Characteristic Potter's facies with low-set ears, prominent skinfold below eyes, small flattened or upturned nose, small chin and redundant scalp skin found. May be abnormal bowing of legs and flattened hands and feet (spade-like). In renal agenesis stillbirth or early neonatal death is inevitable. Common cause of death: pulmonary hypoplasia with pneumothoraces after resuscitation.

Polycystic Kidneys

Either sporadic or autosomal recessive. Neonatal, infantile and adult types: both kidneys involved and become enlarged while keeping normal shape (unlike multicystic kidneys). Polycystic changes may also be present in liver leading to cirrhosis. Early death is common unless renal dialysis and transplantation. Prognosis is somewhat better in adult type.

Multicystic Kidney

Also called dysplastic or hypoplastic kidney. Associated anomalies common: absent ureter, cardiovascular and gastrointestinal anomalies. Progressive pyelonephritis can occur.

Posterior Urethral Valve

Only in male infants. Hypertrophy and trabeculation of bladder with bilateral ureteric reflux and hydronephrosis. May be recurrent infections and progressive renal damage unless obstruction relieved. Urine passed by constant dribbling and diagnosis should be made in neonatal period.

Every male infant should be observed passing urine with normal stream before discharge.

FACE AND PALATAL ABNORMALITIES

Cleft lip with or without cleft palate occurs in about 1/1000 births, and cleft palate alone in 1/2000 births. Genetic factors are important. The risk of having another affected baby is about 4% if both parents are normal and 10% if one parent has a cleft lip. Occasionally there may be other abnormalities, e.g. Patau's syndrome (see below).

CHROMOSOMAL ABNORMALITIES

The trisomy syndromes are the commonest (Table 119). Incidence tends to increase with maternal ageing with logarithmic increase after age 37 years (Table 120). Other

Table 119. Trisomy syndromes.

	Down's	*Edwards'*	*Patau's*
Trisomy:	21	18	13
Incidence:	1/600	1/2000	1/5000
Features:	Flat head, epicanthic folds, Brushfield's spots, low-set ears, small nose, prominent, fissured tongue, broad short neck, simian crease, clinodactyly, ventriculoseptal defect (VSD) or endocardial cushion defects	Long narrow head, extended neck, short palpebral fissures, micrognathia, flexed overlapping fingers, Rocker bottom feet, renal anomalies, VSD, atrial septal defect (ASD)	Holoprosencephaly, micro-ophthalmia, low-set ears, bilateral cleft lip and palate, flexed overlapping fingers, omphalocele, renal anomalies, VSD, persistent ductus arteriosus, dextrocardia

Table 120. Incidence of Down's syndrome by maternal age.

Maternal age (years)	*Incidence of Down's syndrome*
20	1/1200
25	1/1100
30	1/1000
35	1/400
40	1/100
45	1/40

chromosomal abnormalities include cri du chat syndrome and sex chromosome abnormalities such as Turner's syndrome or Klinefelter's syndrome. More sophisticated methods of chromosome analysis, e.g. banding, have led to more minor abnormalities being detected as the explanation for babies with abnormal facial features.

OTHER MULTIPLE ANOMALIES

These include babies with syndromes such as Smith–Lemli–Opitz, Vater (see p. 305), Cornelia de Lange, Aarskog, Apert, Zellweger, Robinow, and the fetal alcohol syndrome. These syndromes often have typical features so the diagnosis is possible after reference to standard textbooks (e.g. Smith, 1982). There are no definitive confirmatory investigations.

REFERENCES AND FURTHER READING

Chittmittrapap, S., Spitz, L., Kiely, E. M. and Brerton, R. J. (1989). Oesophageal atresia and associated anomalies. *Arch. Dis. Child* **64**: 364.

Lorber, J. (1972). Spina bifida cystica. Results of treatment of 270 consecutive cases with criteria for selection for the future. *Arch. Dis. Child* **47**: 854.

Smith, D. W. (1982). Recognizable patterns of human malformation: genetic, embryologic and clinical aspects. In: *Major Problems in Clinical Pediatrics*, 3rd edn. Philadelphia: W. B. Saunders.

24. Imaging Techniques

The following imaging techniques have been used in neonatal care:

1. Radiography
2. CT scan
3. Ultrasound
4. Magnetic resonance spectroscopy
5. Near infrared spectroscopy

Many of these techniques have been developed only recently and portable equipment allows investigation of the baby at the bedside.

RADIOGRAPHY

Used for many decades to investigate the newborn. Ionizing radiation, however, has the potential disadvantage of mutagenicity, especially after repeated investigation. Risk is usually offset by benefit. Table 121 lists the regions of the body that may be investigated by straight radiography. Figures 55–64 show schematic representations of some common neonatal radiographs.

COMPUTER-ASSISTED TOMOGRAPHY (CT SCANNING)

Used prior to ultrasound for investigation of neonatal brain. CT scan has the following advantages over ultrasound.

1. Better imaging of posterior fossa and frontal areas. This means that haemorrhages there and in subdural space are more easily detected
2. Parenchymal lesions, e.g. periventricular leucomalacia, and focal ischaemic lesions are better seen
3. Vascular abnormalities and solid lesions are more easily seen

Table 121. Radiography of the newborn.

Straight radiography	
Chest:	Respiratory distress syndrome Transient tachypnoea of the newborn Pneumothorax Pulmonary interstitial emphysema Pneumopericardium Pleural effusion Congenital pneumonia Aspiration pneumonia Meconium aspiration syndrome Bronchopulmonary dysplasia Wilson–Mikity syndrome Congenital heart disease Positioning of endotracheal tubes, pleural drains
Abdomen:	Necrotizing enterocolitis Intestinal obstruction: duodenal or ileal atresia meconium ileus Hirschsprung's disease malrotation Ascites Meconium peritonitis Pneumoperitoneum Vertebral anomalies Positioning — transpyloric tubes
Skull, pelvis and limbs:	Down's syndrome Short-limbed dwarfism Rickets Craniostenosis Hydrocephalus Intrauterine infection
Contrast radiography	
Intravenous pyelography:	Renal masses Hypospadias Urinary infection Single umbilical artery
Barium meal:	Hiatus hernia Pyloric stenosis H-type tracheo-oesophageal fistula Vascular rings
Barium enema:	Hirschsprung's disease Malrotation Intussusception
Venography:	IVC obstruction

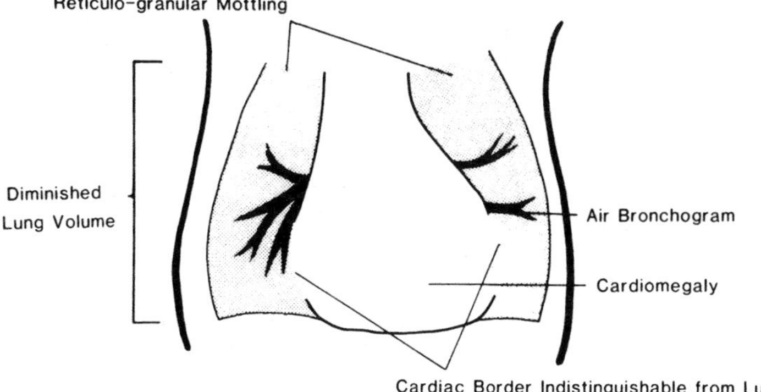

Fig. 55. Schematic representation of chest radiograph of a baby with respiratory distress syndrome. Note the generalized reticulogranular mottling and presence of air bronchogram.

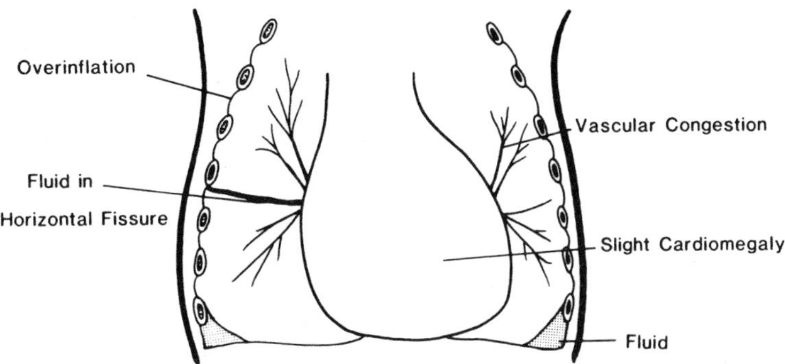

Fig. 56. Schematic representation of chest radiograph from a baby with transient tachypnoea of the newborn. Note the fluid in the horizontal fissure and at the costophrenic angles. There is also over-inflation of the chest and prominent vascular markings radiating from each hilum.

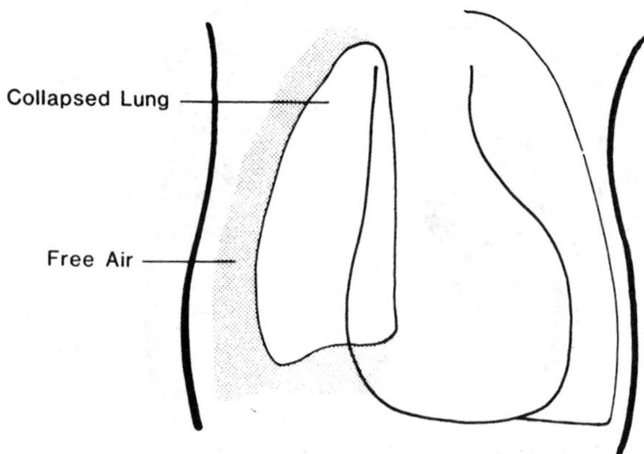

Fig. 57. Schematic representation of chest radiograph from a baby with a right-sided pneumothorax. Note collapse of the affected lung and shift of the mediastinum to the opposite side.

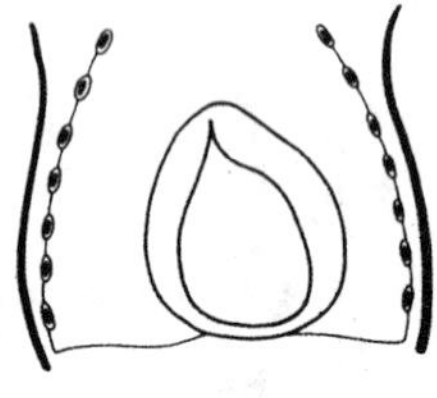

Fig. 58. Schematic representation of chest radiograph from a baby with pneumopericardium. The heart is outlined by a ring of air which may cause compression and reduce heart size.

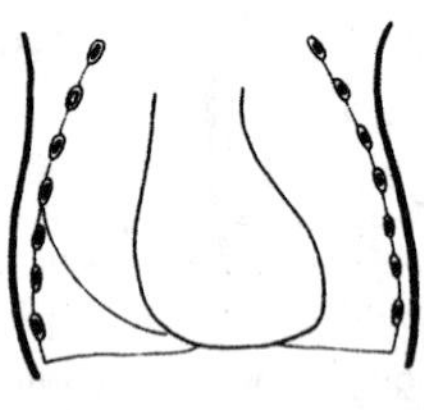

Fig. 59. Schematic representation of chest radiograph from a baby with a right-sided pleural effusion.

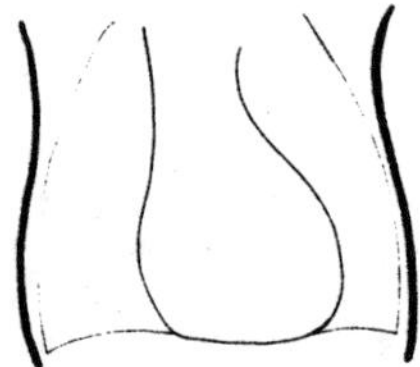

Fig. 60. Schematic representation of chest radiograph from a baby with meconium aspiration syndrome. There is patchy streaking with opacity throughout both lung fields and relative over-inflation of the lungs.

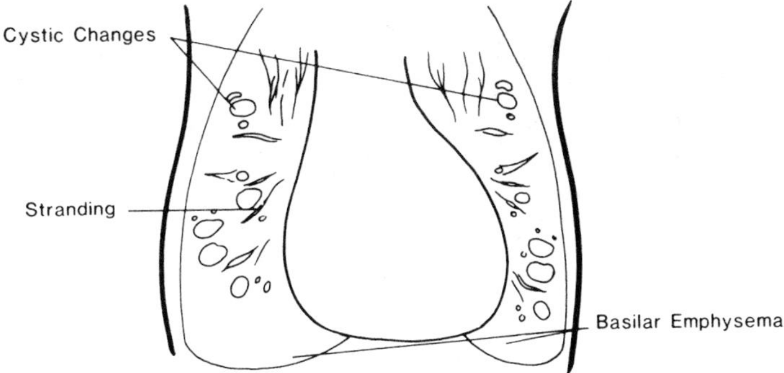

Fig. 61. Schematic representation of chest radiograph from a baby with bronchopulmonary dysplasia. Note the over-inflation of the lungs with basilar emphysema. There is also some coarse stranding and cystic changes.

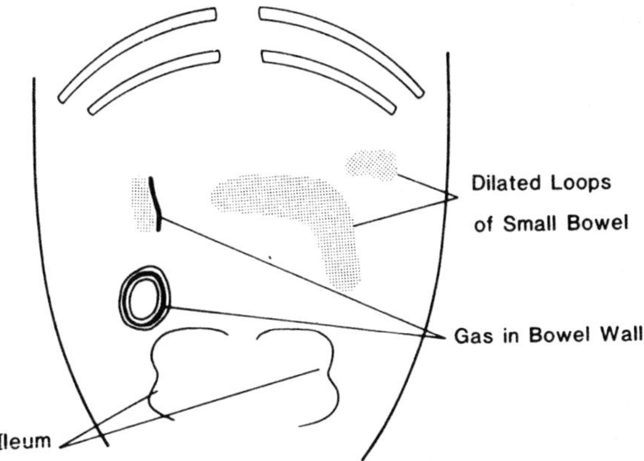

Fig. 62. Schematic representation of an abdominal radiograph in a baby with necrotizing enterocolitis. There are dilated loops of small bowel and intramural air is seen in the bowel both longitudinally and circumferentially.

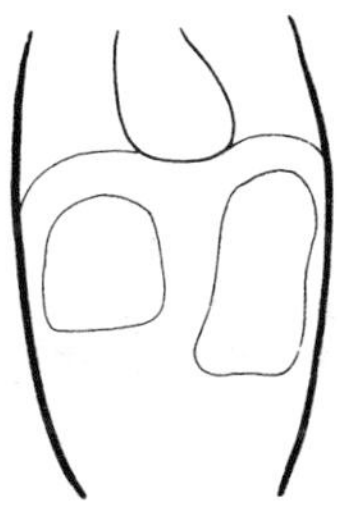

Fig. 63. Schematic representation of abdominal radiograph from a baby with duodenal atresia. This is the so-called double-bubble radiograph.

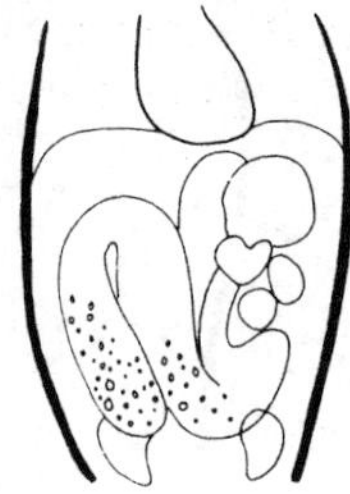

Fig. 64. Schematic representation of abdominal radiograph from a baby with meconium ileus. Note the dilated bowel and the speckled appearance which is often described as 'hornet's nest'.

The disadvantages of CT scanning, however, outweigh its advantages and are:

1. Not portable
2. Expensive
3. Infant must lie still: sedation sometimes needed
4. Poor definition of small intracranial haemorrhages

Papile and others in 1978 used CT scan to grade intraventricular haemorrhage (Table 122).

Table 122. Grading of intraventricular haemorrhage by CT scan.

Grade	*CT features*
0	No haemorrhage
I	SEH or IVH < ½ of one or both lateral ventricles, no distension
II	IVH, unilateral or bilateral > ½ of lateral ventricle, no distension
III	IVH distending any part of lateral ventricle
IV	Haemorrhage extending into parenchyma

IVH = intraventricular haemorrhage
SEH = subependymal haemorrhage
From Papile *et al.* (1978) with kind permission of the publishers C. V. Mosby.

ULTRASOUND

A-mode and B-mode ultrasonography now rarely used in neonatal investigation. M-mode ultrasonography used to examine heart (see later) and real-time ultrasonography used to examine neonatal brain and heart. In real-time scanning the probe or transducer contains many piezoelectric crystals activated in sequence. Linear array real-time scanning uses a row of crystals giving a rectangular image. The disadvantage of linear array scanning is that only the central region of the brain may be visualized through the anterior fontanelle. However, this type of ultrasound may be used transaxially through the skull in the parietal region. Real-time mechanical sector scanning uses crystals that rotate giving a wedge-shaped image. Real-time scanning has considerable advantages:

1. Mobile: bedside technique
2. Relatively inexpensive
3. Instantaneous image: patient movement is irrelevant
4. Probe easily moved to select planes of scanning and determine continuity of cerebral structure
5. Moving image shows vascular pulsations, helping to define normal anatomy

There have been no adequately documented hazardous effects of ultrasound in animals or humans. Ultrasound images of the skull appear as dense white echoes, and the CSF as black echo-free areas. The cerebellum and choroid plexus are relatively vascular and appear white, while the thalamus is darker than the caudate nucleus. Access to the brain in the newborn is through the anterior or posterior fontanelle or through the relatively thin parietal bones, allowing measurement of the size of the lateral ventricles.

Technique

Transducers of 5 or 7.5 MHz should be used. A 3.5 MHz probe gives inadequate parenchymal detail and may miss small haemorrhages. The transducer should be placed in the coronal plane over the anterior fontanelle and angled first towards the face and then towards the occiput (Fig. 65). To obtain the sagittal view the transducer is rotated through 90° and both lateral ventricles may be seen by angling the probe first to the right and then to the left (Fig. 66). Finally, the probe should be placed over the parietal bone above the ear with the baby's head laterally positioned. This gives the transaxial view and allows measurement of ventricular size. This may be recorded as the

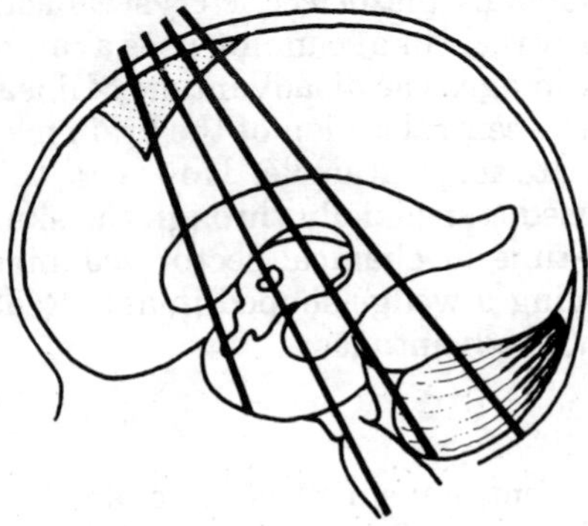

Fig. 65. Coronal planes obtained through the anterior fontanelle with the ultrasound probe.

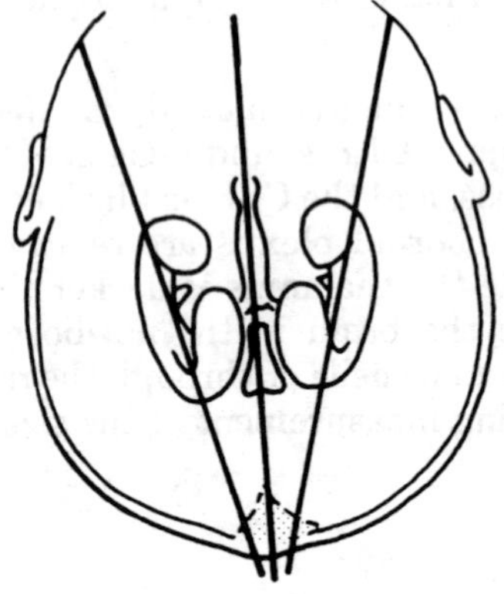

Fig. 66. Sagittal planes obtained through the anterior fontanelle with the ultrasound probe.

V/C ratio (ventriculocerebral hemisphere) (Fig. 67). The width of the lateral ventricle is measured at the level of the mid-body and the cerebral hemisphere as the distance from the midline echo to the inner table of the skull. The normal V/C ratio is less than 35% (see below).

Normal Anatomy

Coronal plane

With the scanner head angled anteriorly, the interhemispheric fissure is seen as a clear echo-free region in the midline.

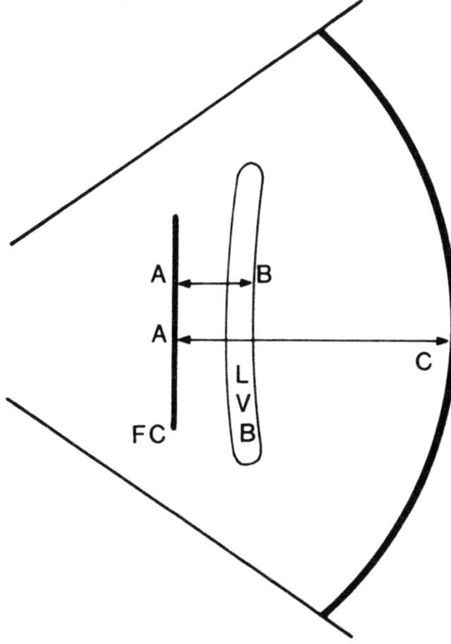

Fig. 67. Measurement of the ventriculocerebral ratio (V/C). The normal ratio is the distance AB divided by AC and should be less than 35%. LVB = lateral ventricular body, FC = falx cerebri.

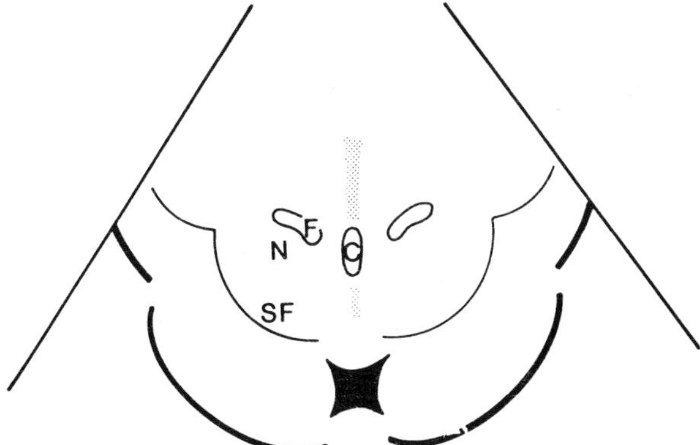

Fig. 68. Normal anatomy in the coronal plane. F = frontal horn, N = caudate nucleus, C = cavum septum pellucidum and SF = sylvian fissure.

Laterally the anterior horns of the lateral ventricles can be seen as echo-free crescents, concave laterally, and below is the cavum septum pellucidum (Fig. 68).

As the scanner head is rotated posteriorly the head of the caudate nucleus and then the thalamus form the lateral walls of the ventricles (Figs 69, 70). The choroid plexus is echo-dense and is first seen superior and medial to the caudothalamic notch in the floor of the lateral ventricle. As the scanner head is rotated posteriorly, the choroid plexus can be seen to widen and deepen and to swing downward and laterally hugging the ventricular wall to the temporal horn (Fig. 70). As the scanner is rotated following the choroid plexus, the third ventricle may be seen as an echo-free slit in the midline inferior to the lateral ventricle.

With the scanner head rotated posteriorly, parts of the cerebellum may be seen, although good views of this structure are unusual. Below the cerebellum the cisterna magna is occasionally seen.

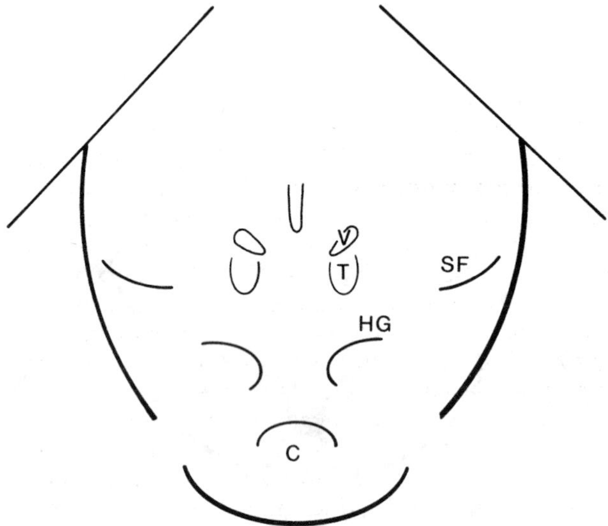

Fig. 69. Normal anatomy in the coronal plane. V = lateral ventricle, T = Thalamus, SF = sylvian fissure, HG = hippocampal gyrus, C = cerebellum.

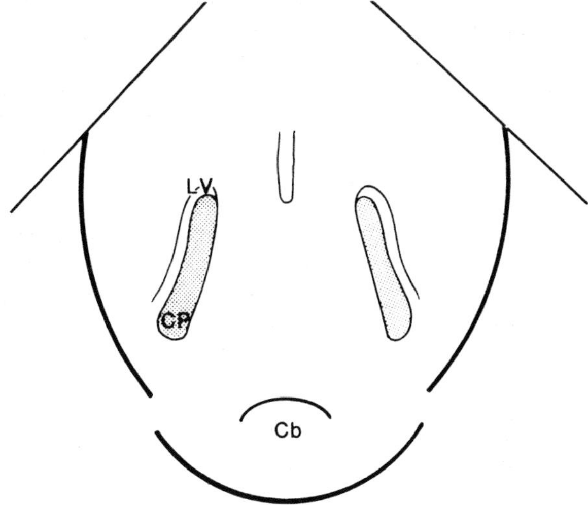

Fig. 70. Normal anatomy in the coronal plane. LV = lateral ventricle, CP = choroid plexus, Cb = cerebellum.

Sagittal plane

With the scanner head angled obliquely it is usually possible to see all of the lateral ventricle (Fig. 71) especially if the scanner head is rocked slightly to bring lateral areas into view. The corpus callosum is seen as an echo-dense curvilinear structure sweeping posteriorly. Below it, in the midline, the cavum septum pellucidum is seen and more laterally, the lateral ventricle. Anteriorly, the anterior horn is usually easily visualized and extends backwards over the head of the caudate and thalamus. The angle between the caudate and thalamus is important as the choroid plexus begins here and it is the site of origin of intraventricular haemorrhages (Fig. 71).

The lateral ventricle can be seen beyond this point to swing posteriorly with the choroid plexus in its floor until it finally turns back to form the inferior horn. It is sometimes possible to see the third ventricle as a rather ill-defined echo-free structure inferior to the lateral ventricle in the midline, and very occasionally the fourth ventricle can also be seen (Fig. 72).

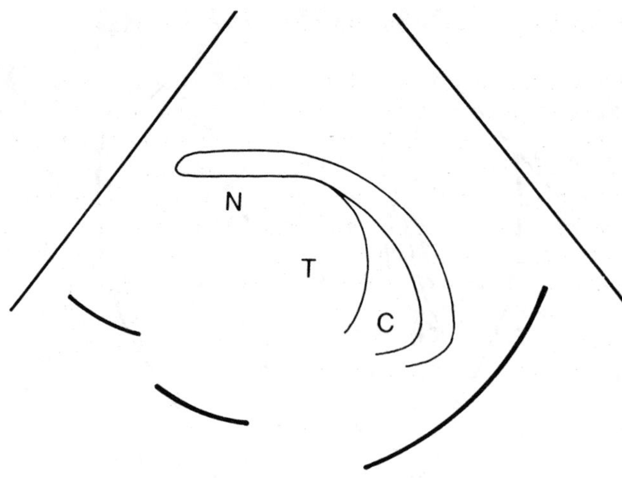

Fig. 71. Normal anatomy in the sagittal plane. N = caudate nucleus, T = thalamus, C = choroid plexus.

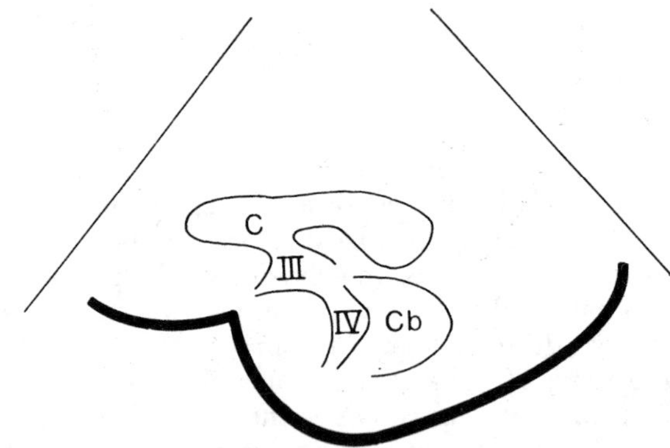

Fig. 72. Sagittal view in midline showing the cavum septum pellucidum (C), third and fourth ventricles (III, IV) and cerebellum (Cb).

Periventricular and Intraventricular Haemorrhage

Blood is echo-dense on ultrasonic examination and the usual first appearance of intraventricular haemorrhage is a bright spot either in the caudothalamic notch or in the head of the caudate nucleus (Fig. 73). This is classified as a grade I haemorrhage. Blood in the ventricular space appears white (grade II haemorrhage) and may obstruct the ventricular foramina causing dilatation (grade III haemorrhage). If blood extends into the cortical substance, often into an ischaemic area, this is termed grade IV haemorrhage (Table 123). Following grade III or IV intraventricular haemorrhage, hydrocephalus is relatively common.

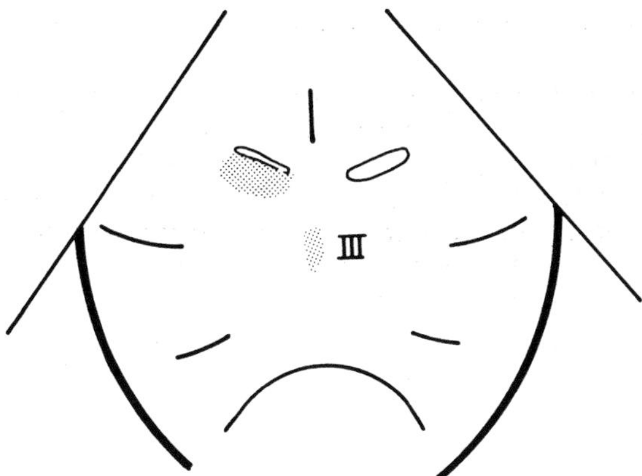

Fig. 73. Coronal view of the brain showing sub-ependymal haemorrhage. This is seen compressing the left lateral ventricle with some dilatation of the contralateral ventricle. The third ventricle (III) contains blood.

Coronal scan

Subependymal haemorrhage (SEH) may appear as a round area of increased density below and lateral to the frontal horn of the body of the lateral ventricle (Fig. 73). Often bulges into the ventricle and the commonest site is the head of the caudate nucleus at the caudothalamic notch. Even small SEHs should be detected if the transducer is slowly swept in the coronal plane towards the frontal horns. The presence of haemorrhage must always be confirmed by examination in the sagittal plane, as a common cause of false positive scan is asymmetry causing one choroid plexus to appear larger than the other. Figure 73 demonstrates blood in the third ventricle after more extensive haemorrhage.

Sagittal view

Choroid plexus normally tapers to a small anterior portion. However, if SEH is present, it will appear as a bulge in the choroid (Fig. 74). Intraparenchymal extension of the haemorrhage into the caudate nucleus and thalamus (Fig. 75) appears initially as a very echogenic density, but after 10–14 days may become cystic, and after a further 3–4 weeks may retract allowing the edges of the haematoma to separate from the brain. Complete resolution of an intraparenchymal haemorrhage may take many weeks or months.

When intraventricular haemorrhage (IVH) has occurred, a densely echogenic clot may fill or obscure the lateral ventricle. Clots may also be seen attached to the choroid or in the occipital horns. Sometimes a unilateral caudate nucleus haemorrhage may be seen, with dilatation of the contralateral ventricle. Grading of IVH has been based upon the size and site of the

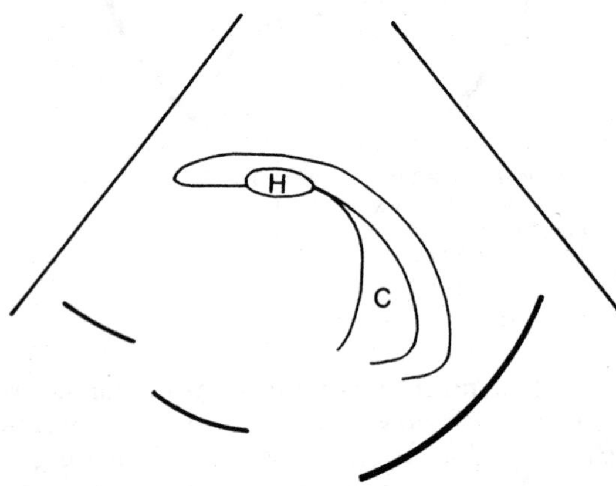

Fig. 74. Subependymal haemorrhage in the sagittal view. H = haemorrhage, C = choroid plexus.

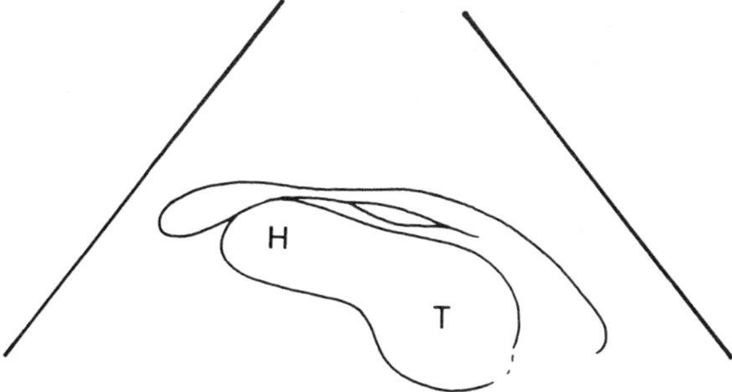

Fig. 75. Sagittal view showing extension of the subependymal haemorrhage into the parenchyma. H = haemorrhage, T = thalamus.

haemorrhage and the presence of ventricular dilatation or on the degree of haemorrhage after evolution of about 2 weeks (Table 123).

Up to 70% of IVH may be detected within 6 hours of birth and very few new haemorrhages occur after 7 days. IVH can be detected for much longer on ultrasound scan than by CT scan. Most parenchymal haemorrhages on CT scan are isodense by 5–10 days. Subarachnoid haemorrhage may be diagnosed by using a water bath (surgical glove filled with water) placed against the baby's head to reduce reverberation artefact. If subdural fluid is present, the brain appears separated from the cranial vault and the gyri and sulci appear more prominent. The differential diagnosis is cerebral atrophy, but head growth is slow, while in the presence of subdural haemorrhage the head normally grows more rapidly than usual.

Table 123. Grading of intraventricular haemorrhage (IVH) and outcome.

Mild	SEH alone or small IVH, normal sized ventricles
Moderate	Intermediate sized IVH and ventricular dilatation
Severe	Gross IVH, cast within ventricle ± parenchymal extension
Moderate to severe	44% handicaps
Severe	75% mortality if ventricular cast 70% handicapped if parenchymal extension

Other unusual cerebral haemorrhages can occur in caudate nucleus, thalamus and posterior fossa, especially cerebellum, but these are difficult to diagnose by ultrasound and can often be seen by CT scan.

Periventricular Leucomalacia

The cause is unclear, but may be due to ischaemia or to venous infarction, leading to cystic areas and developmental problems later. The first appearance, which is most easily demonstrated with a 7.5 MHz transducer, is of periventricular flare often triangular shaped with the apex pointing medially. This may resolve or progress over a few weeks to cyst formation which if large or persistent carries a poor prognosis.

Hydrocephalus

Dilatation of the ventricles can be diagnosed by measuring the V/C ratio in the trans-axial plane (Fig. 76). The normal V/C ratio

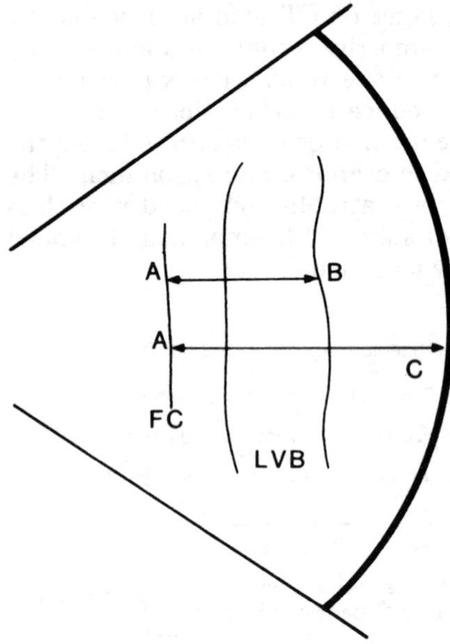

Fig. 76. Trans-axial view showing the V/C ratio in hydrocephalus. V/C ratio = AB/AC = 60%. FC = falx cerebri, LVB = lateral ventricular body.

in the full-term infant is 28% (range 24–30%) and in the preterm infant 31% (range 24–34%).

Good correlation between ultrasound and CT scan. V/C ratio may be used for diagnosis and to measure the effects of therapy such as repeated lumbar puncture or shunting.

The earliest sign of dilatation of the ventricles is loss of the lateral curvature and widening of the frontal horn. Conversely, the response of the ventricular system to shunting is seen first in the body of the lateral ventricle and last in the occipital horn. Following IVH there may be acute dilatation of the ventricles due to obstruction of the aqueduct or foramen of Monro and when this occurs, there is a high mortality. The lateral ventricle will be enlarged in both coronal and sagittal views (Fig. 77). The third ventricle may also be enlarged. Later dilatation is due to communicating hydrocephalus, secondary to obliterative arachnoiditis. In many cases this resolves spontaneously, with only 20–30% requiring shunting.

Other causes of hydrocephalus include the Arnold–Chiari malformation in which there is herniation of the fourth ventricle into the spinal canal causing dilatation of the third and lateral ventricles with pointing of the frontal horns and markedly enlarged occipital horns. It is possible also to diagnose Dandy–Walker syndrome.

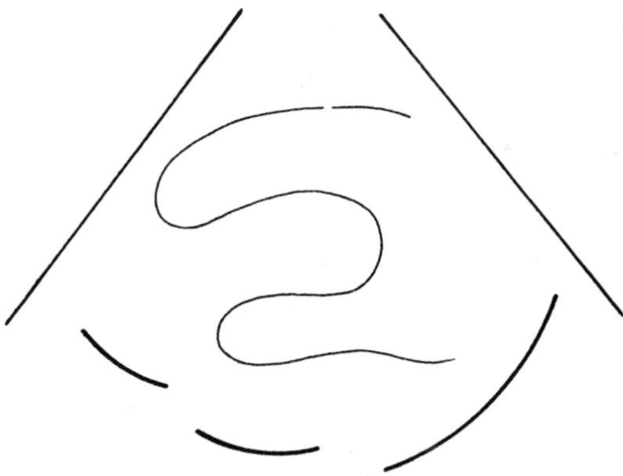

Fig. 77. Sagittal view showing marked hydrocephalus. Note the dilatation of the entire ventricular system.

Other Lesions

1. *Cystic.* Porencephaly, hydranencephaly (an extreme form of porencephaly or hydrocephaly), arachnoid cysts, ependymal cysts and Dandy–Walker cysts. Cystic lesions are easy to diagnose, solid ones more difficult
2. *Periventricular and cortical infarction.* Irregular periventricular echoes of about 2 mm in diameter and enhanced arterial pulsations. There may be progressive ventricular dilatation as a result of cerebral atrophy, with widening of the inter-hemispheric fissure
3. *Cerebral oedema.* Decreased ventricular size, generalized increased echodensity, and decreased pulsation in the circle of Willis
4. *Ventriculitis.* Subependymal pseudocysts
5. *Other cerebral anomalies.* For example, holoprosencephaly and Aicardi's syndrome (absent corpus callosum)

Suggested indications for ultrasound examination in the newborn are shown in Table 124. Routine scanning of all newborns is not recommended. CT scanning is to be preferred if there are persistently abnormal neurological signs in the presence of normal ultrasound scan, or for infants > 6 months.

Table 124. Indications for cerebral ultrasound.

	Time from birth
All infants <32 weeks	End of first week
>32 weeks + CNS signs	Onset of CNS signs
Intracranial haemorrhage (ICH) found	Repeat weekly
Dysmorphic syndromes	At birth
Rapidly growing head	At diagnosis
Ventriculomegaly found	Repeat weekly
Abnormal development (<6/12)	When diagnosed

Ultrasound of the Heart (M-mode Echocardiography)

Discussion will be limited to M-mode echocardiography and exclude real-time scanning, which has recently become available to the paediatric cardiologist. M-mode echocardiography

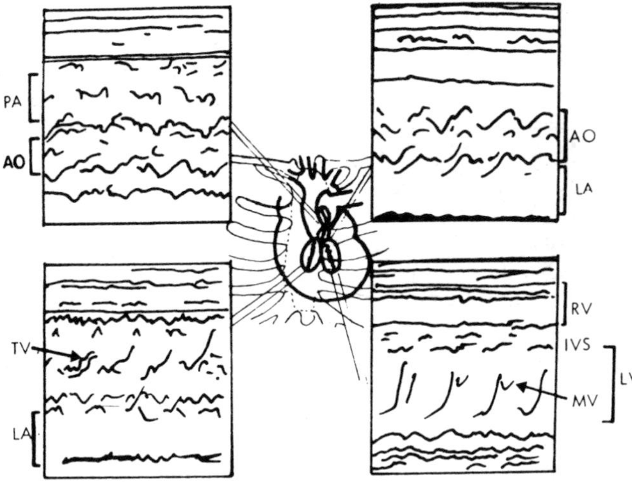

Fig. 78. Schematic representation of the heart as seen at M-mode echocardiography in four standard views. PA = pulmonary artery, AO = aorta, TV = tricuspid valve, LA = left atrium, RV = right ventricle, IVS = inter-ventricular septum. MV = mitral valve, LV = left ventricle.

has been available for some time and allows direct, accurate measurements of left heart chamber sizes which reflect indirect degree of L–R shunting in PDA. May be performed at cotside and helps with decisions about treatment with indomethacin or ligation. For M-mode echocardiography, a 5 MHz focused transducer should be used and traces recorded on moving paper for hard copy. Figure 78 is a schematic representation of the neonatal heart, in frontal view showing the four standard positions for echocardiographic recordings. The mitral valve serves as a good landmark in echocardiography and is normally found to the left of the tricuspid valve. It is in fibrous continuity with the posterior aortic cusp and posterior margin of the aorta. This allows easy identification of mitral valve and left ventricle which is usually recorded from directly overhead, placing the transducer in the third left intercostal space beside the sternum and directing its beam inferiorly and posteriorly.

Figure 79 shows a sagittal section of the heart with three transducer positions. In transducer position 1, left ventricular

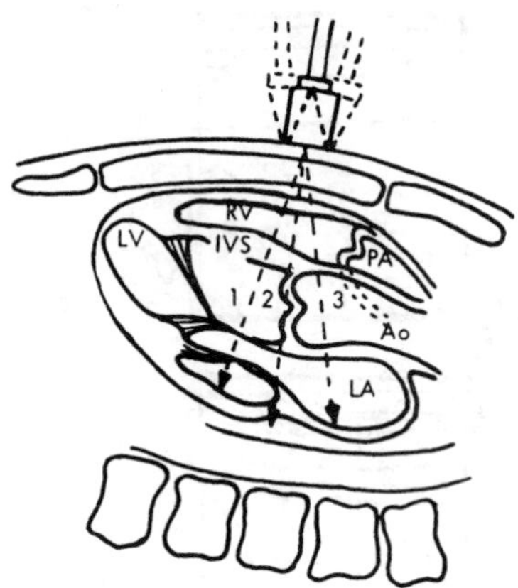

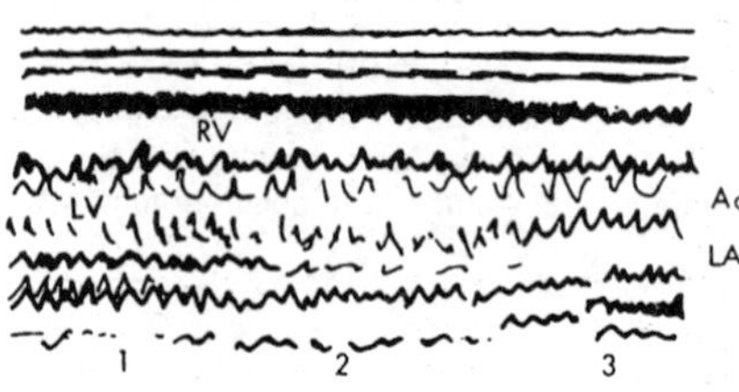

Fig. 79. Schematic representation of the heart in sagittal view showing the three transducer positions. RV = right ventricle, LV = left ventricle, IVS = inter-ventricular septum, PA = pulmonary artery, AO = aorta, LA = left atrium.

dimensions may be measured. Figure 80 shows the heart in sagittal section with sweep of transducer from apex towards left atrium; in this position aortic and left atrial dimensions may be measured. If left atrium becomes enlarged, its ratio to aortic root size will also increase (LA/Ao). The normal LA/Ao ratio is about 1.1:1 (Fig. 81, Appendix VI). In the presence of large PDA, LA/Ao ratio increases to above 1.5:1 and there is also increase is size of the left ventricle (Fig. 82).

Ultrasound of Other Organs

Ultrasound has been used to investigate cystic lesions of kidney, liver or spleen and to look for the presence of localized areas of pus, e.g. subphrenic abscess. The hips may also be examined by ultrasound which clearly outlines the anatomy of

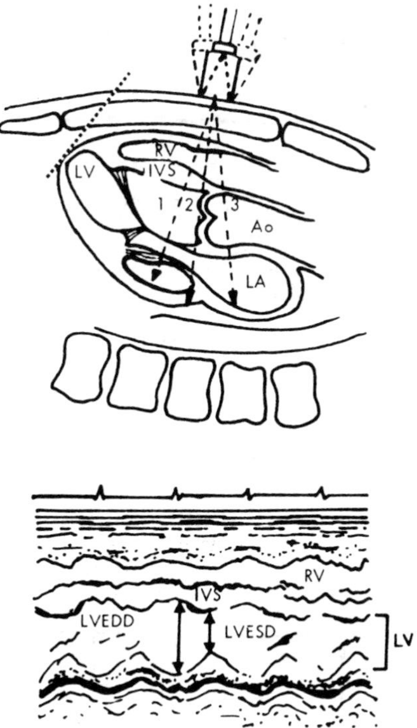

Fig. 80. Schematic representation of the heart in sagittal view concentrating on position 1 where the left ventricle is clearly seen. RV = right ventricle, IVS = interventricular septum, LV = left ventricle, LVEDD = left ventricular end-diastolic dimension, LVESD = left ventricular end-systolic dimension.

the acetabulum and femoral head. Further description of these techniques is beyond the scope of this book.

MAGNETIC RESONANCE SPECTROSCOPY

This technique is used to measure the concentrations of phosphorus compounds involved in brain energy metabolism. Intracellular pH can also be measured. Abnormalities are seen following asphyxia after a delay of up to 12 hours and these are predictive of long-term outcome. Disadvantages are that the equipment is bulky and expensive.

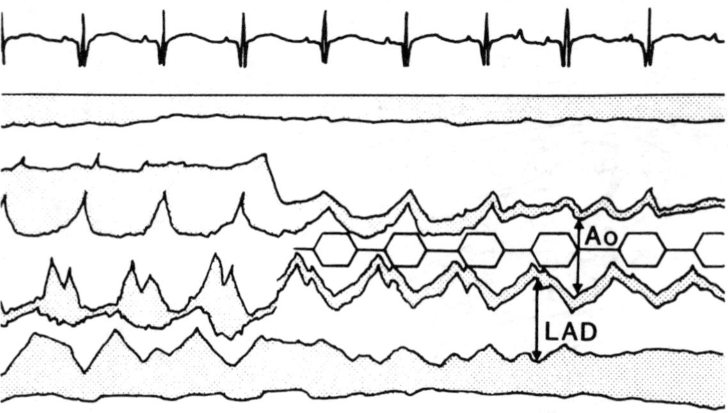

Fig. 81. Schematic representation of echocardiographic scan from left ventricle to aorta and left atrium to demonstrate measurement of normal left atrium to aortic root ratio (LA/Ao). The normal LA/Ao ratio is about 1:1.

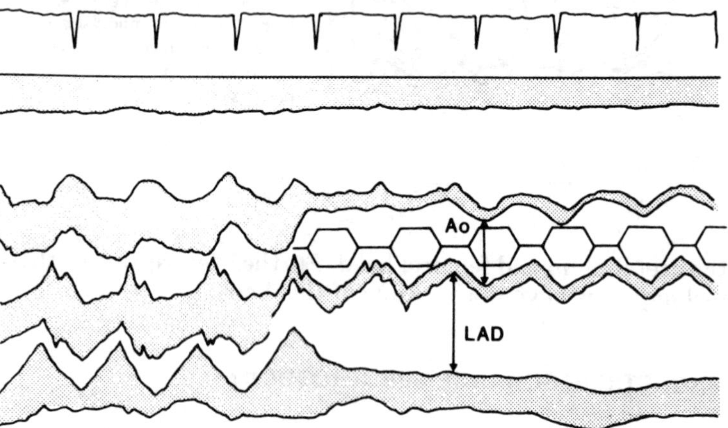

Fig. 82. Echocardiogram corresponding to that in Fig. 81 for a baby with a large patent ductus arteriosus. Note that the left atrial dimension is enlarged, that the LA/Ao ratio is about 1.5:1.0.

NEAR INFRARED SPECTROSCOPY

This is another new technique that has been used to measure cerebral oxygenation and blood flow. May be applied at the cotside and is less expensive than magnetic resonance spectroscopy. Experience is limited to a few centres worldwide.

REFERENCES AND FURTHER READING

Levene, M. I., Williams, J. L. and Fawer, C.-L. (1984). *Ultrasound of the Infant Brain*. London: Spastics International Publications and Heinemann Medical.

Meyer, R. A. (1977). *Pediatric Echocardiography*. Philadelphia: Lea and Febiger.

Reynolds, E. O. R., Wyatt, J. S., Azzopardi, D. *et al.* (1988). New non-invasive methods for assessing brain oxygenation and haemodynamics. *Br. Med. Bull.* **44**: 1052.

Swischuk, L. E. (1980). *Radiology of the Newborn Young Infant*. Baltimore: Williams and Wilkins.

25. Parental Attachment

In 1907 Pierre Budin wrote in *The Nursling*:

> Unfortunately a certain number of mothers abandon the babies whose needs they have not had to meet, and in whom they have lost all interest. The life of the little one has been saved, it is true, but at the cost of the mother.

It is possible that this tragic situation may be avoided by encouraging the natural mother–infant bonding process. Klaus and Kennell (1982) suggested that there was a critical or sensitive period in the first minutes or hours during which interaction between mother (and father) and infant should occur for ideal later development of the baby. Parental anxiety about the baby on the first day may cause long-lasting concern about future development.

A combination of present-day knowledge of high-risk obstetrics, neonatology and mother–infant attachment suggests that a home-like birth in hospital might be the ideal situation. Medical intervention may be necessary only in high-risk pregnancies and in the low-risk pregnancy in labour when an unexpected complication arises. The delivery of a mother with a low-risk pregnancy and labour in a special 'bedroom' in a maternity hospital has great potential benefits. After birth, father, mother and infant can be together. This can take place once the infant has been examined and the cord clamped. Touching the baby and eye-to-eye contact appear to be important parts of the early attachment process.

If the infant is *premature* the mother will often expect that her baby will die. She may grieve in anticipation of this so that bonding to her infant will be delayed. It is especially important that the mother of a premature baby sees her infant soon after birth, even if only for a brief moment. When babies are being transported for intensive care always provide a Polaroid photograph for the mother to use in 'bonding'. Free visiting of premature babies by their parents is a relatively new phenomenon, but frequent contact with the baby may be beneficial. Gentle touching and fondling may reduce the number of apnoeic attacks, increase weight gain, decrease the daily number of stools and improve some higher CNS functions. Visits by siblings should also be encouraged once the initial high-risk situation has improved. Relatives should always be given a friendly welcome by nursing and medical staff, allowing time for regular discussion of the baby's condition at each visit.

Pessimistic remarks about the chances of a baby's survival are not helpful to a mother unless the baby's condition is hopeless. If the baby survives, the mother's grief in anticipation may be heightened and bonding with her infant delayed. One should always use cautious optimism without quoting statistics. All queries must be honestly and optimistically answered. Disturbances of brain function should not be specifically mentioned to the parents unless they ask or the outcome can be accurately predicted, e.g. in chromosomal trisomies. The pattern of parental visiting and telephone calls is predictive of the ability of the mother to cope with the stresses of premature birth. If she visits fewer than three times in 2 weeks the probability of mothering disorder increases and failure to thrive, child abuse or giving the baby up for adoption increase.

It is especially helpful for the mother to make some tangible contribution to her infant's care, such as providing breast milk. Mothers of babies of 32 weeks and less should be encouraged to express their milk. As the baby grows and no longer needs intensive care he/she should be dressed in attractive clothing such as that produced by companies who manufacture doll's clothes. The more attractive a tiny preterm baby appears to the mother the easier it is for her to grow attached.

PATTERN OF GRIEF

Parents who have an infant with a congenital malformation or one who subsequently dies will pass through five phases in their grief. These are:

1. *Shock.* Often overwhelming, characterized by crying, feelings of helplessness and irrational behaviour. There may also be physical symptoms such as choking, shortness of breath, sighing, lethargy and 'empty' feeling
2. *Disbelief.* This form of denial serves to cushion the blow but should be of short duration

3. *Sadness, anger and anxiety.* The anger may be directed at nurses, doctors, the baby who has died or is malformed and nearby mothers who have had normal babies. This stage needs to be dealt with in an understanding manner
4. *Equilibrium.* Gradual lessening of both anxiety and emotional reactions, the parents able to cope with the situation; may take a few weeks in the case of a malformed infant or many months after the death of an infant. This process may be eased if parents talk over their problems, meet with the paediatrician for counselling and visit the graveside on occasions
5. *Reorganization and acceptance.* Parents are now able to deal with the malformed infant and are reassured that the baby's problems were not due to their own neglect. In the case of an infant who has died the parents are able to resume fairly normal living

It usually takes about 6–9 months for this normal grief response to be completed. If the process becomes fixed at any stage, pathological grief can occur. It may be helpful to allow a mother whose infant has died to see and handle him/her and a simple family funeral may also help to ease the grieving. It is important for the paediatrician to see the parents as soon as postmortem examination has been carried out, and discuss all the problems that the parents are likely to meet. It is unhelpful for them to hide their feelings ('bottle things up') and parents should be told that many of their friends will not know how to react to the death of their baby and that some will even appear to be rather off-hand. The parents are seen again after about 3 months so that their progress can be assessed and any further questions dealt with. The autopsy results and the risks of recurrence in future pregnancies can be discussed. Parents should be advised against a 'replacement pregnancy' until the grieving process has been completed. Once grieving has run its course, another pregnancy can be considered.

NURSING POINTS

1. Important to have good liaison between medical and nursing staff so that information given to parents is

consistent. Counselling jointly by doctors and nurses is helpful.
2. Father's position should not be forgotten and he should be encouraged to participate as much as possible in the care of his baby. This is especially important in multiple births
3. Talk to parents at each visit; make them feel at home; show common purpose and get to know their views, religious beliefs, family support, etc.
4. Use parent support groups for premature and abnormal babies; useful lists of names and addresses below:

The Association of Breastfeeding Mothers
71 Hall Drive London SE26 6XL Tel. 01-788 4381

Association of Paediatric Nurses
c/o Miss D. MacCormack Children's Hospital Western Bank Sheffield S10 2TH Tel. 0742 7111

Association for Spina Bifida and Hydrocephalus
Tavistock House North Tavistock Square London WC1 9HJ Tel. 01-388 1382

BLISS (Baby Life Support System) (a charity raising money for neonatal units),
Chairman: Susanna Cheal 50 Sumatra Road London NW6 1PR Tel. 01-435 6867

British Heart Foundation
57 Gloucester Place London W1H 4DH Tel. 01-935 0185

British Paediatric Association
5 St. Andrews Place Regents Park London NW1 4LB Tel. 01-486 6151

Cystic Fibrosis Research Trust
5 Blyth Road Bromley Kent BR1 3RS Tel. 01-464 7211

Down's Babies Association
Queenbourne Community Centre Ridgacre Road Quinton Birmingham B32 2PW Tel. 021-427 1374

Foundation for the Study of Infant Deaths
5th Floor, 4-5 Grosvenor Place London SW1X 7HD Tel. 01-235 1721 or 01-245 9421

Gingerbread (for one-parent families)
35 Wellington Street London WC2E 7BN Tel. 01–240 0953

Haemophilia Society
16 Trinity Street London SE1 1DB Tel. 01–407 1010

Invalid Children's Aid Association
126 Buckingham Palace Road London SW1W 9SB Tel. 01–730 9891

La Leche League of Great Britain (for help with breast feeding)
BM 3424 London WC1V 6XX Tel. 01–404 5011

National Association for Deaf/Blind and Rubella Children
164 Cromwell Lane Coventry Tel. 0203 23308

National Association for Hospital Play Staff
Thomas Coram Foundation 40 Brunswick Square London WC1 Tel. 01–278 2424

National Association for Maternal and Child Welfare
1 South Audley Street London W1Y 6JS Tel. 01–491 1315

National Association for the Welfare of Children in Hospital (NAWCH)
Argyl House, Euston Road London NW1 Tel. 01–261 1738

National Childbirth Trust (education for parenthood)
9 Queensborough Terrace London W2 3TB Tel. 01–221 3833

National Deaf Children's Society
45 Hereford Road London W2 5AH Tel. 01–229 9272

National Society for Brain-damaged Children
35 Larchmere Drive Hall Green, Birmingham

National Society for Mentally Handicapped Children
123 Golden Lane London EC1Y 0RT Tel. 01–253 9433

National Society for Phenylketonuria and Allied Disorders
58A Burton Road, Melton Mowbray Leicester LE13 1DJ

Prenatal Diagnosis Group
Dr Alan McDermott (Editor of Newsletter) S. W. Regional Cytogenetics Centre Southmead Hospital Bristol

Royal National Institute for the Blind
224 Great Portland Street London W1N 6AA Tel. 01–388 1266

Royal National Institute for the Deaf
105 Gower Street London WC1 6AH Tel. 01–387 8033

Spastics Society
12 Park Crescent London W1N 4EQ Tel. 01–636 5020

Stillbirth and Neonatal Death Society (SANDS)
Argyle House 29–31 Euston Road London NW1 Tel. 01–833 2851

The Stillbirth and Perinatal Death Association
37 Christchurch Hill London NW3 1LA Tel. 01–794 4601

Many of these Associations have local branches in provincial cities and their address should be available in the NICU.

REFERENCES AND FURTHER READING

Davis, J. A., Richards, M. P. M. and Roberton, N. R. C. (1983). *Parent–Baby Attachment in Premature Infants*. Beckenham: Croom Helm.

Drotar, D., Baskieuriez, A., Irvin, N. *et al.* (1975). The adaption of parents to the birth of an infant with a congenital malformation: a hypothetical model. *Pediatrics* **56**: 710.

Klaus, M. H. and Kennell, J. H. (1989). *Parent–Infant Bonding*, 3rd edn. St Louis: C. V. Mosby.

O'Connor, S., Vietze, P. M., Sherrod, K. B. *et al.* (1980). Reduced incidence of parenting inadequacy following rooming in. *Pediatrics* **66**: 176.

Sluckin, W., Herbert, M. and Sluckin, A. (1984). *Maternal Bonding*. Oxford: Blackwell.

26. Infant Follow Up

There are five major reasons why infants that are treated in special care nurseries should be closely followed up. These are:

1. To assess growth and development
2. To detect complications associated with abnormal perinatal period, e.g. asphyxia, prolonged mechanical ventilation
3. To reassure parents and give continuing advice on infant rearing
4. To collect data relating to perinatal problems and their management, with outcome – the neonatologist's feedback
5. To detect early the emergence of groups of problems that might be attributable to some recently adopted form of therapy

NORMAL GROWTH AND DEVELOPMENT

At each visit the infant should have weight, height and head circumference measured and plotted on appropriate growth

Table 125. Normal development.

6 weeks	Aware of stimuli, start of head control, ventral suspension: head momentarily horizontal. Moro present, smile to mother's voice or face
6 months	Primary reflexes absent, firm head control, turns to stimuli, no squint, reaches out, palmar grasp, transfers objects, responds to strangers
10 months	Mobile, crawls, pulls to stand, mature finger–thumb grasp, imitates sounds, discriminates people
18 months	Toddler, builds two or three blocks, verbal comprehension, speaks few words. Slightly obstructive.
24 months	Independent toddler, runs, climbs stairs, mimics, more words and short sentences

chart (see p. 358). In general, birth weight of full-term infant is doubled by 4 months, trebled by 12 months and quadrupled by 24 months. Developmental screening is best assessed at 6 weeks, 6 months, 10 months, 18 months and 2 years. Always make allowances for prematurity in assessment of growth and development. Corrected ages should be used for the first 18–24 months of life. Consider developmental assessment in four main areas: locomotion and posture, vision and fine manipulation; hearing, language and speech; and everyday skills and social environment. Table 125 summarizes normal infant development, but for a fuller discussion other texts should be consulted (Egan *et al.*, 1971; Illingworth, 1989).

DETECTION OF COMPLICATIONS

The most important long-term problems are those associated with delayed or abnormal neurological development: 5–15% of infants who have received intensive care will suffer from some long-term neurological deficit, though evidence suggests that the incidence of spastic diplegia is much less than 30 years ago. Recent increases are due to survival of very immature infants who formerly would have died.

Chronic lung disease (see Chapters 10 and 22) may be seen in low birth weight infants, especially those who have received assisted ventilation. Apart from the recognized syndromes of chronic lung disease, these infants are also more likely to need hospital admission for respiratory infections in the first year of life. Up to 30% of very low birth weight babies are rehospitalized in the first year. For a discussion on home oxygen management see p. 150.

Diseases with an iatrogenic element are fairly common (around 10%) in infants who survive intensive care. The most important of these are retinopathy of prematurity associated with excessive oxygen therapy and hearing loss from aminoglycoside antibiotics. Follow-up clinics must have ready access to ophthalmological and audiological assessment. Some of these complications, including small areas of skin necrosis from extravasated intravenous fluid therapy and scars from repeated arterial sampling are unavoidable and not due to carelessness or negligence.

REASSURANCE AND FURTHER GUIDANCE

This is part of the well-baby clinic service provided for mothers whose babies were admitted to the nursery and is similar to the service provided by family doctors and community paediatricians. Advice often concerns feeding, possetting, rashes and constipation. Be on the look out for two interesting conditions: the persistent vomiter who has hiatus hernia or the mother who is having genuine mothering difficulty and may need special help.

DATA COLLECTION

This is a system of feedback to provide information regarding long-term effects of intensive care. Comprehensive follow-up service and accurate record keeping are needed. Follow up includes developmental testing, neurological examination and assessment of vision and hearing. Standardized developmental testing skills, e.g. Denver and Bayley, may be administered by trained psychologist or developmental paediatrician. For older children, assessment of IQ by Stanford–Binet or WISC. Factors associated with high incidence of abnormal development are intracranial haemorrhage, severe asphyxia (Apgar score 0–3 at 5 min), seizures and neonatal meningitis. It is important to obtain close to 100% follow up and help is often needed from general paediatricians, general practitioners, community paediatricians and health visitors.

NEW PROBLEMS

In the past, neonatologists have been too ready to accept and use new drugs and treatments before complete evaluation of their effects. This has led to a series of 'neonatal disasters' from which no one can derive any credit; for example, uncontrolled oxygen and retinopathy of prematurity, sulphonamides and kernicterus, chloramphenicol and grey-baby syndrome, hypothermia for asphyxia, nikethamide in resuscitation and thalidomide as a sedative in pregnant women (this is really an obstetric disaster). These therapeutic misadventures can be avoided in future by exhaustive evaluation of all new drugs and therapies before they are applied to the human newborn. The use of properly designed randomized controlled trials are essential for this purpose and failure to carry these out is unethical. Long-term effects of drugs may be missed unless there is careful follow up, e.g. diethyl stilboestrol causing vaginal carcinoma in the offspring of mothers given the drug to prevent recurrent abortion.

Risk of Sudden Infant Death Syndrome (SIDS)

This is increased in very low birth weight babies or those that needed neonatal intensive care. Other risk groups include babies of drug-addicted mothers, near-miss episodes and babies with bronchopulmonary dysplasia (Table 126).

When a preterm infant with recurrent apnoea is being discharged from hospital, consideration of home monitoring is necessary. One should wait until no apnoeas have been recorded for 10 days before discharge, or home monitor should be advised (p. 111). Criteria for home monitoring are shown in Table 127. Not all siblings of previous SIDS should be offered monitoring and often reassurance of the mother, encouragement of breast feeding, frequent health visitor follow up and regular weighing are just as effective.

Table 126. Infants at increased risk of SIDS.

Risk	*Incidence of SIDS/1000 births*
Very low birth weight infant	12
Needed neonatal intensive care (all weights)	4
Drug-addicted mother	20
Sibling who died of SIDS	20
Twin of SIDS	42
Near-miss episode	32
Bronchopulmonary dysplasia	113
General population	2–3

Adapted from Brady and Gould (1984)

Table 127. Criteria for home apnoea monitoring.

1. Good indication (see Table 126)
2. Mother has asked for monitor or shown genuine interest if approached
3. Full explanation of monitor's capability — operation, false alarms, possible unreliability — no simple monitor is 100% reliable
4. Mother and father instructed in resuscitation techniques, including stimulation of the infant and mouth-to-mouth resuscitation
5. Family practitioner and health visitor notified by telephone prior to discharge and show general agreement with plan
6. Card typed up with patient's details and monitor number. Nursery telephone number with 24-hour-a-day cover for emergency advice given to the parents
7. Full letter of explanation to family practitioner after discharge
8. Regular review at follow-up clinic

We have found that the major benefit of home apnoea monitoring has been reassurance of the anxious parent. Mothers say they feel less likely to check their baby's breathing regularly when the monitor is attached. There are many types of monitor ranging from those that detect abdominal movement (MR 10) to those that measure heart rate and oxygen saturation in addition to respiration rate. These latter monitors may be more effective but are expensive and rather cumbersome.

REFERENCES AND FURTHER READING

Brady, J. P. and Gould, J. B. (1984). Sudden infant death syndrome. In: *Advances in Paediatrics*, Vol. 31 (ed., Barness, L. A.). Chicago: Year Book Medical Publishers.

Egan, D. F., Illingworth, R. S. and McKeith, R. C. (1971). Developmental Screening 0–5 years. *Clinics in Developmental Medicine*, Vol. 30. London: Spastics International Medical Publications and Heinemann Medical.

Illingworth, R. S. (1982). *Basic Developmental Screening 0–4 Years*, 3rd edn. Oxford: Blackwell.

Illingworth, R. S. (1989). *The Normal Child: Some Problems of the Early Years and their Treatment*, 9th edn. Edinburgh: Churchill Livingstone.

Silverman, W. A. (1980). *Retrolental Fibroplasia: A Modern Parable*. London: Academic Press.

Silverman, W. A. (1985). *Human Experimentation: A Guided Step into the Unknown*. Oxford: Oxford University Press.

Appendix I. Siggaard–Andersen nomogram

The Siggaard–Andersen nomogram is used for calculating the bicarbonate and base excess from pH and $P\text{CO}_2$ when haemoglobin is known. Use a ruler to read off the unknowns.

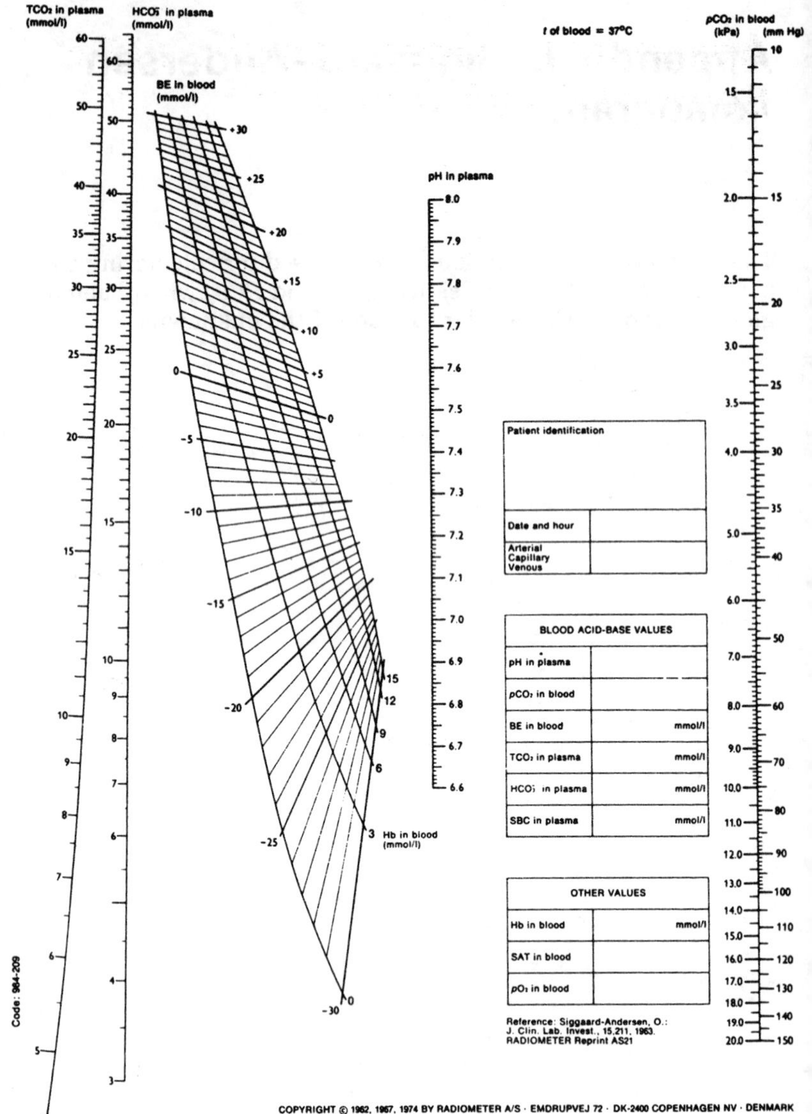
TCO₂ in plasma (mmol/l)
HCO₃⁻ in plasma (mmol/l)
BE in blood (mmol/l)
pH in plasma
t of blood = 37°C
pCO₂ in blood (kPa) (mm Hg)
Hb in blood (mmol/l)
Patient identification
Date and hour
Arterial
Capillary
Venous
BLOOD ACID-BASE VALUES
pH in plasma
pCO₂ in blood
BE in blood mmol/l
TCO₂ in plasma mmol/l
HCO₃⁻ in plasma mmol/l
SBC in plasma mmol/l
OTHER VALUES
Hb in blood mmol/l
SAT in blood
pO₂ in blood
Reference: Siggaard-Andersen, O.: J. Clin. Lab. Invest., 15,211, 1963. RADIOMETER Reprint AS21
Code: 984-209
COPYRIGHT © 1962, 1967, 1974 BY RADIOMETER A/S · EMDRUPVEJ 72 · DK-2400 COPENHAGEN NV · DENMARK

Appendix II. Operating circuit for Bourns BP 200 ventilator

BOURNS BP 200 CIRCUIT

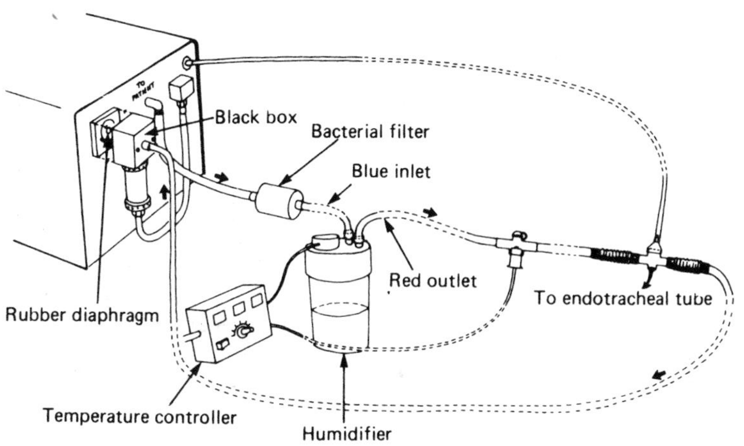

Appendix III. Operating circuit for Draeger baby log

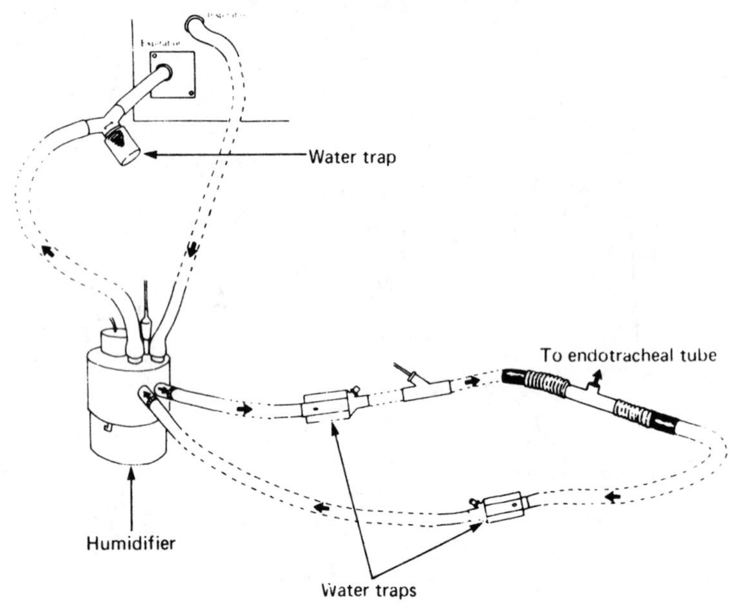

Appendix IV. Drug dosages

The following table gives details of drugs which may be used in the newborn baby.

Drug	*Dose* (mg/kg/day unless otherwise stated)	*Interval* (hours)	*Route*	*Comments*
Acetazolamide	20–50	8	Oral	Hydrocephalus treatment
Adrenaline (1:10 000)	0.1–0.3 ml/kg*	—	iv, endotracheal tube	Use by endotracheal tube
Albumin 5%	1 g/kg*	—	Slow iv	Can cause heart failure
Aldosterone	1	12	im or iv	Use in adrenal hyperplasia
Aminophylline	5 mg/kg load then 4 (maintenance dose)	6	iv	Use in intractable apnoea
	7.5 mg/kg/day	8	Rectal	
Amphotericin B	0.25–1.0	—	Infusion over 6 h	In 5% dextrose, protect from light
Atropine	0.03 mg/kg*	—	sc or iv	Use in some bradycardia
Calcium gluconate (10%)	0.2 ml/kg*	—	Slow iv	Bradycardia caused and potentiates digoxin, tissue necrosis
Carbimazole	0.5–1.0	8–12	Oral	Treatment of thyrotoxicosis
Chloral hydrate	10–15 mg/kg*	—	Oral	Sedative, gastric irritation
Chlorothiazide	10–40	12	Oral	Hypokalaemia caused
Chlorpromazine	2.0–2.5	6	Oral, im, iv	Drug withdrawal, seizures
Clonazepam	0.15 mg/kg*	—	iv	Intractable seizures
Cortisone	25–50	12–24	im or iv	Adrenal crisis treatment maintenance
Curare	0.3 mg/kg*	—	iv	Muscle relaxation for IPPV

* These drugs given only as a single dose and should not be ordered on a daily basis

Drug	*Dose* (mg/kg/day unless otherwise stated)	*Interval* (hours)	*Route*	*Comments*
Dexamethasone	0.25–1	6–12	im or iv	Cerebral oedema treatment
Diazepam	0.1–0.3 mg/kg*	6–8	im, iv, oral	Apnoea, jaundice side-effects
Diazoxide	5 mg/kg*	—	im	Emergency treatment of hypertension, causes hyperglycaemia
Digoxin†	30–50 μg/kg for digitalization 6–10 μg/kg for maintenance	 12	im or oral	Caution in preterm hypokalaemia, renal failure (see p. 237)
Dopamine	5–10 μg/kg/min		Infusion	For hypotension and reduced cardiac output
Edrophonium (Tensilon)	0.5–1 mg*	—	im or slow iv	Myasthenia test dose
Ferrous sulphate	10 (2 of elemental iron)	24	Oral	Start after 6 weeks
Flucytosine	50–150	6	Oral, iv over 30 min	For systemic candidiasis. Therapeutic serum levels 25–50 μg/ml. Diffuses into CSF (see p. 206)
Fludrocortisone	5 μg/kg/day	24	Oral	Salt-losing adrenal hyperplasia
Folic acid	0.25	24	Oral	
Frusemide	1 mg/kg*	—	im, iv, oral	Hypokalaemia, hypocalcaemia and bilirubin displacement caused

* These drugs given only as a single dose and should not be ordered on a daily basis

† Digitalization 30–50 μg/kg daily for 1 day; give one-third dose 8 hourly. Maintenance 6–10 μg/kg/day; give half of this 12 hourly. Watch for arrhythmias and measure serum levels if in doubt. Careful if hypokalaemic or hypercalcaemic. See also p. 237

Drug	*Dose* (mg/kg/day unless otherwise stated)	*Interval* (hours)	*Route*	*Comments*
Glucagon	0.03–0.30	6–12	im	For intractable hypoglycaemia
Heparin	1000 units/kg/day	6	iv	For anticoagulation
Hydralazine	1–6	8	iv, oral	For acute hypertension
Hydrocortisone	25–50	4–6	im, iv	For cerebral oedema
Indomethacin	0.1–0.2 mg/kg*	—	Oral, iv	Renal problems as side-effect
Insulin	0.1 unit/kg*	—	iv, im	For hyperglycaemia and hyperkalaemia
Isoprenaline	0.1–0.5 μg/kg/min	Continuous infusion for hypotension		Caution: use dopamine in preference (see also p. 244)
Lignocaine	1 mg/kg/load 20–50 μg/kg/min	— Maintenance	iv infusion	To treat serious ventricular arrhythmias
Magnesium sulphate	50	24	im or slow iv	50% solution. Dilute before giving iv (p. 175)
Mannitol (20%)	7 ml/kg over 30 min		iv infusion	For acute cerebral oedema (p. 222)
Methyldopa	5–50	6–8	iv oral	Antihypertensive. Start with lower dose
Morphine	0.1 mg/kg*	—	iv, im	Apnoea and raised pulmonary vascular resistance are side-effects

* These drugs given only as a single dose and should not be ordered on a daily basis

Drug	*Dose* (mg/kg/day unless otherwise stated)	*Interval* (hours)	*Route*	*Comments*
Naloxone	10–20 μg/kg*	—	iv, im	Best given iv, short acting
Neostigmine	0.15	8	im, iv, oral	For myasthenia maintenance
Nitroprusside	2.5–5.0 μg/kg/min		Infusion	Light-sensitive, causes hypotension
Paraldehyde	0.1 mg/kg*	12	im	Last resort, *glass syringe*, malodorous
Paregoric	0.3 ml/kg/day	4	Oral	For drug withdrawal (p. 20)
Pethidine	1 mg/kg*	—	iv, im	See morphine
Phenobarbitone	20 mg/kg loading dose; 5 mg maintenance	8–12	iv, im, oral	Depression especially with diazepam. Therapeutic serum level 10–20 μg/ml (p. 226)
Phenoxybenzamine	0.5–1.0	—	Slow iv over 1 hour	α-Blocker
Phenytoin	5–10	8–12	Oral, iv	ECG monitor if iv, not absorbed im. Therapeutic serum levels 10–20 μg/ml (p. 226)
Phytomenadione (Konakion, K_1)	0.3	24	im, oral	Increased doses can cause haemolysis
Potassium chloride	2 mmol/kg/day	8	Oral	1 mmol ≡ 75 mg
Potassium iodide (10%)	8	8	Oral	For neonatal thyrotoxicosis (p. 18)
Prednisone	1–2	6–12	Oral	Hypokalaemia can occur

* These drugs given only as a single dose and should not be ordered on a daily basis

Drug	*Dose* (mg/kg/day unless otherwise stated)	*Interval* (hours)	*Route*	*Comments*
Propranolol	0.5–3.0	6–8	iv, oral	Cardiac arrhythmia and bronchoconstriction are side effects
Prostaglandin (PGE_2)	0.1 μg/kg/min	—	infusion	Maintenance dose 1/4 (p. 242)
Prostigmine	3–10	4–6	Oral	Maintenance for myasthenia gravis
Protamine sulphate	0.1 ml/100 units heparin	—	Slow iv	Reverse heparin anticoagulation
Pyrimethamine	0.1–1.0 for 3 days 0.5 for 1 month	12	Oral	Given with sulphadiazine for toxoplasmosis (p. 194)
Sodium bicarbonate	2 mmol/kg*	—	iv, oral	About 1 mmol sodium per ml iv hyperalimentation in preterm if >8 mmol/kg/day
Sodium polystyrene sulphonate	1 g/kg/day	6	Oral, rectal	For hyperkalaemia (p. 178)
Spironolactone	3.5	6	Oral	For salt-losing adrenal hyperplasia
Theophylline	(See aminophylline)			4 mg theophylline = 5 mg aminophylline
Thyroxine	25 μg	24	Oral	Cautious increase in dose (p. 271)
Tolazoline	1–2 mg/kg stat. dose 1–2 mg/kg/h	—	Infusion	Bleeding and hypotension side-effects

* These drugs given only as a single dose and should not be ordered on a daily basis

Appendix V. Antibiotic doses

Antibiotic	*Infants less than 7 days*		*Infants over 7 days*	
	Dose (mg/kg/day)	*Interval* (hours)	*Dose* (mg/kg/day)	*Interval* (hours)
Penicillins				
Benzylpenicillin (Penicillin G)*	50–100 000 units‡	12	100 000 units‡	8
Ampicillin	50–100	12	100–200	6–8
Cloxacillin	30–100	12	100–150	6–8
Methicillin	50–100	12	100–150	6–8
Mezlocillin	150	12	225	8
Carbenicillin	200–250	12	300–400	6–8
Ticarcillin	150	12	225–300	6–8
Aminoglycosides				
Gentamicin	5	12	7.5	8
Tobramycin	4	12	6	8
Amikacin	15–20	12	20–30	8
Netilmicin	5–6	12	6	8
Others				
Chloramphenicol	25	24	25–50	8–12
Fucidin†	20–50	12	20–50	8
Rifampicin	10	12–24	10	12–24
Vancomycin	20–30	12	30–45	8
Clindamycin	50	12	50	8
Newer cephalosporins				
Cefotaxime	100	12	150	8
Cephradine	100	12	150	8
Ceftazidime	25–60	12	25–60	12
Cefuroxime	50–100	12	100–150	8
Latamoxef	100	12	100–150	8

Where two figures are given, e.g. 100–200 mg/kg/day or 6–8 hourly, use lower amount and reduced frequency for intants under 2000 g birth weight and higher ones for those over 2000 g. The preferred route is parenteral, either im or by slow iv infusion over 15–20 min for the penicillins and over 60 min for the aminoglycosides

* Double dose for meningitis

† Use 20 mg/kg/day iv, 50 mg/kg/day orally

Appendix VI. Normal echocardiographic measurements

	Mean ± sd
Left atrial to aorta ratio (LA/Ao)	1.1 ± 0.1
Left atrial dimension preterm (LAD)	0.7 ± 0.1 cm
Left ventricular end-diastolic dimension to aorta ratio (LVEDD/Ao)	1.8 ± 0.3
Left ventricular end-diastolic dimension preterm (LVEDD)	1.2 ± 0.3 cm
Percent shortening of internal dimension of LV (% SID)*	36 ± 3%
Mean velocity of circumferential fibre shortening (mean V_{cf})†	
Term	1.5 ± 0.3 cm/sec
Preterm	2.0 ± 0.3 cm/sec
Systolic time intervals	
LPEP/LVET	0.35 ± 0.04
RPEP/RVET‡	0.45 − 0.25

From Halliday *et al.* (1979a)

See Chapters 17 and 24

* $\% \text{ SID} = \frac{\text{LVEDD} - \text{LVESD}}{\text{LVEDD}} \times 100\%$

† $\text{Mean } V_{cf} = \frac{\% \text{ SID}}{\text{LVET}} \times 10 \text{ cm/sec}$

‡ RPET/RVET decreases with increasing postnatal age

Appendix VII. Patient daily information card

History may be written in pen but other sections should be pencilled in and updated daily.

NAME: DATE:

1. History wks , g , DOB , Del. Obst.
   Place , AS / , Resus Init. Diag.

2. Respiratory Diag. , % O , Press / , R , PH , CO_2
   Comps O_2

3. Fluids / nutr. Type Vol. (ml / kg / day) Cal / kg / day
   Oral
   IV, % Dextrose
   Vamin
   % Intralipid
   TOTAL

4 Elects. Na , K , Urea , Ca , Mg ,
   Treat , , ----- , , mmol / kg

5. Hct % Treat , bili , umol/l PT at , Ex ,

6. PDA murmur , pulses , CXR , Echo ,

7. CNS / apnoea, seizures , OFC , apnoea ,

8. Infection, sympts , WCC , Bands , Plates
   Cults Gastric ASP , Drugs

9. Coagulation PT PTT Plates

10. Social

Appendix VIII. Growth charts

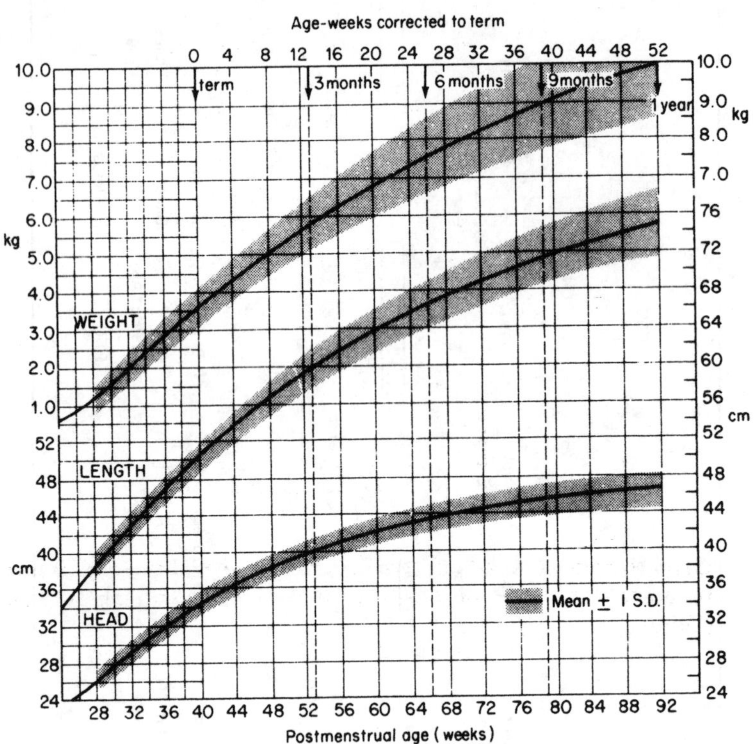

Growth chart of weight, length and head circumference related to gestational and postnatal age for both sexes. From Babson *et al.* (1970) with kind permission of the authors and the editor of *Pediatrics*.

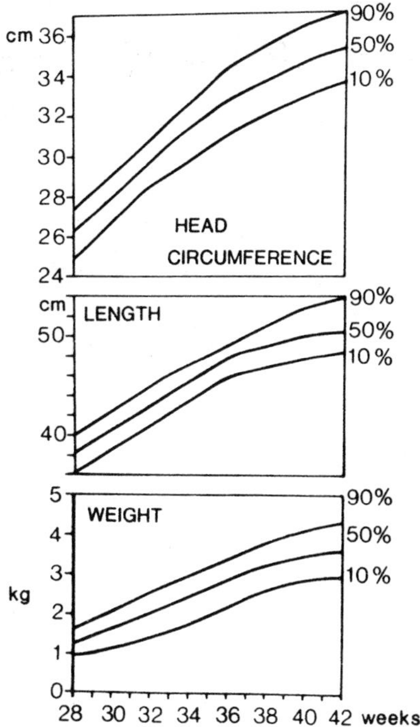

Growth chart of head circumference, weight and length related to gestational age for both sexes. After Usher and McLean (1969).

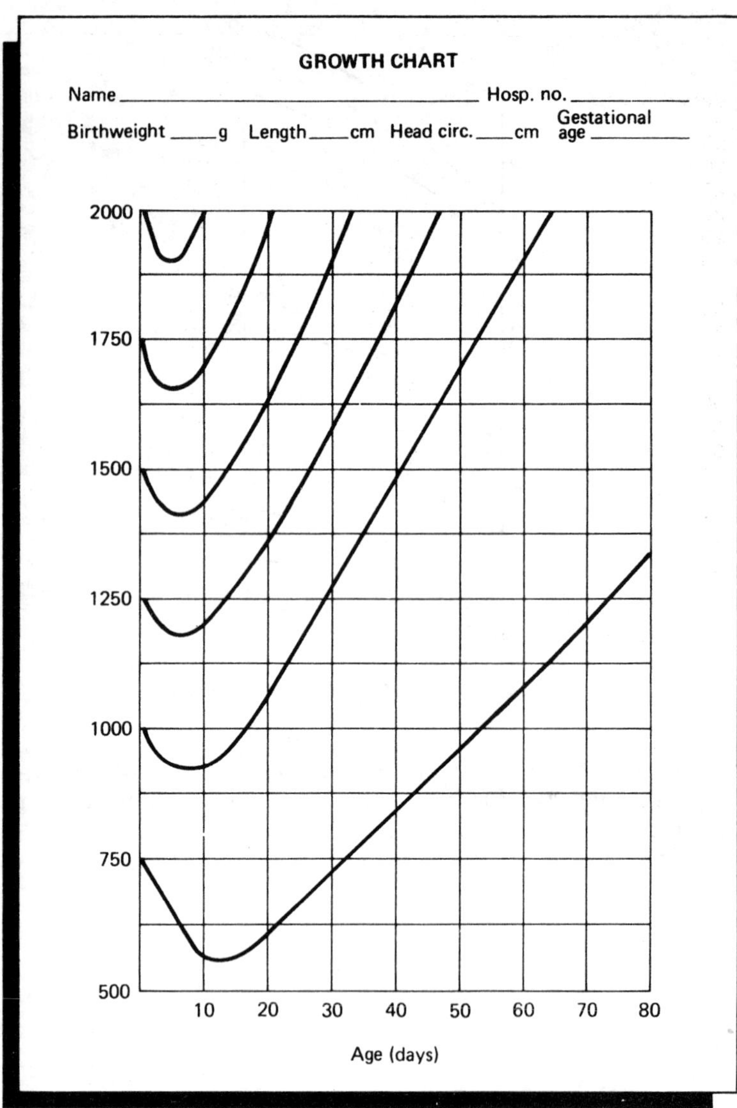

From Dancis *et al.* (1948) with kind permission of the publishers C. V. Mosby.

Birth weight and gestational age

Gestation (weeks)	*Weight* (g)		
	Mean	*5th*	*95th*
25	850	650	1050
26	935	705	1165
27	1015	745	1285
28	1115	815	1415
29	1230	900	1560
30	1375	1025	1725
31	1540	1140	1940
32	1725	1275	2175
33	1900	1400	2400
34	2115	1555	2675
35	2345	1715	2975
36	2590	1890	3290
37	2870	2120	3620
38	3135	2335	3935
39	3360	2500	4220
40	3480	2560	4400
41	3565	2615	4515
42	3515	2555	4475
43	3415	2445	4385
44	3385	2415	4355

After Usher and McLean (1969)

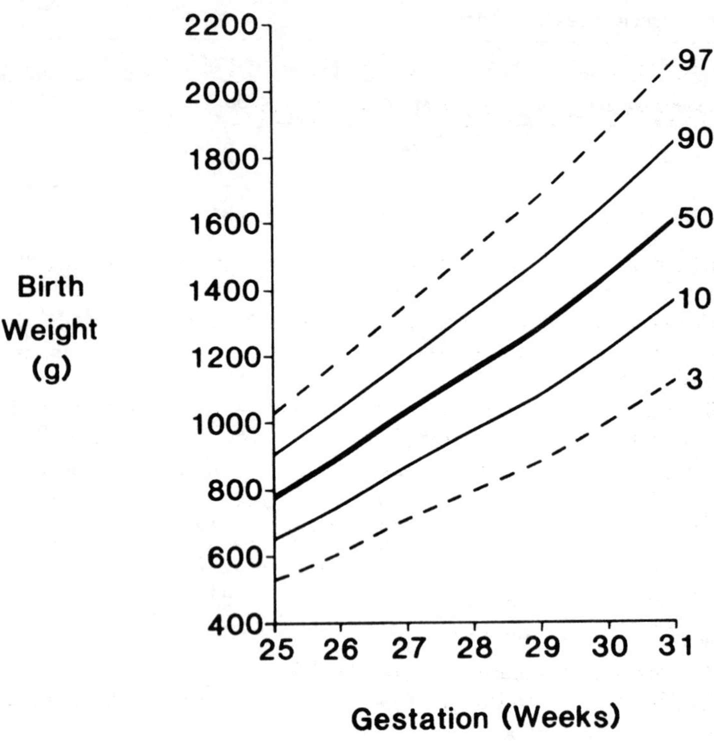

Birth weight centiles for babies of 25–31 weeks.

Appendix IX. Amniotic fluid or gastric aspirate 'shake test'

Surfactant in amniotic fluid or gastric aspirate forms stable surface films.

Shake with ethanol to remove proteins, bile salts or free fatty acids which also form stable foam. If heavy meconium or blood staining, discard.

0.5 ml fluid added to 0.5 ml isotonic saline in a clean test tube. Then add 1.0 ml 95% ethanol and cap with a clean stopper.

Shake vigorously by hand for 15 sec (timed) and set upright in rack for 15 min.

Then examine surface for bubbles:

1. Positive test: bubbles form complete ring
2. Negative test: no bubbles present
3. Doubtful: some bubbles, incomplete ring

Negative test means reasonable risk of RDS.

Doubtful test reduced risk of RDS and unlikely to need assisted ventilation.

Appendix X. Normal blood chemistry values of infants 1500–1750 g birth weight

	1 week	*3 weeks*	*5 weeks*
Sodium (mmol/l)	133–146	129–142	133–148
Potassium (mmol/l)	4.6–6.7	4.5–7.1	4.5–6.6
Chloride (mmol/l)	100–117	102–116	100–115
Urea (mmol/l) (mean)	1.0–8.5 (3.1)	0.7–10.4 (4.4)	0.6–8.8 (4.4)
Calcium (mmol/l)	1.5–2.9	2.0–2.8	2.1–2.6
Phosphorus (mmol/l)	1.9–3.7	2.1–3.0	1.9–2.7
Total protein (g/l)	44–63	43–67	41–69
Albumin (g/l)	33–45	32–53	32–43
Globulin (g/l)	9–22	6–29	5–15

From Thomas and Reichelderfer (1968) with kind permission of The American Association for Clinical Chemistry

Appendix XI. Notifiable Diseases as at 1 October 1988

Under the Public Health (Control of Disease) Act 1984:

Cholera
Plague
Relapsing fever
Smallpox
Typhus

Under the Public Health (Infectious Diseases) Regulations 1988:

Acute encephalitis
Acute poliomyelitis
Anthrax
Diphtheria
Dysentery (amoebic or bacillary)
Leprosy
Leptospirosis
Malaria
Measles
Meningitis
Meningococcal septicaemia (without meningitis)
Mumps
Ophthalmia neonatorum
Paratyphoid fever
Rabies
Rubella
Scarlet fever
Tetanus
Tuberculosis
Typhoid fever
Viral haemorrhagic fever
Viral hepatitis
Whooping cough
Yellow fever

Appendix XII. Normal coagulation values in the newborn

Factor/measurement	*Term infant*	*Preterm infant*	*Adult value*
Fibrinogen (mg %)	200–500	200–250	200–400
Factor II (%)	40	25	50–100
Factor V (%)	90	60–75	75–125
Factor VII (%)	50	35	75–125
Factor VIII (%)	100	80–100	50–150
Factor IX (%)	24–40	25–40	50–150
Factor X (%)	50–60	25–40	50–150
Factor XI (%)	30–40	25–40	75–125
Factor XII (%)	50–100	50–100	75–125
Factor XIII (titre)	1:16	1:8	1:8
Plasminogen	43	24	61–126
AT III	60	27	98
Partial thromboplastin time (s)	40–70	50–90	30–50
Prothrombin time (PT) (s)	12–18	14–20	10–20
Thrombin time (TT) (s)	12–16	13–20	10–12
α-Macroglobulin*	250	230	200–400
α-Antitrypsin*	100	90	275
Antithrombin*	12	12	20–35

* Plasma inhibitors of proteolytic enzymes

Appendix XIII. Conversion tables

TEMPERATURE

°F	°C
96	35.6
97	36.1
98	36.7
99	37.2
100	37.8
101	38.3
102	38.9
103	39.4
104	40.0
105	40.6
106	41.1

°C	°F
35.5	95.9
36.0	96.8
36.5	97.7
37.0	98.6
37.5	99.5
38.0	100.4
38.5	101.3
39.0	102.2
39.5	103.1
40.0	104.0
40.5	104.9

LENGTH

1 in = 2.54 cm
1 cm = 0.3937 in

WEIGHT

1 kg = 2.2 lb
1 lb = 0.45 kg

POUNDS AND OUNCES TO GRAMS CONVERSION TABLE

	Pounds											
Ounces	*1*	*2*	*3*	*4*	*5*	*6*	*7*	*8*	*9*	*10*	*11*	*12*
0	455	905	1360	1810	2265	2720	3170	3625	4075	4530	4985	5435
1	480	935	1385	1840	2290	2745	3200	3650	4105	4560	5010	
2	510	960	1415	1870	2320	2775	3225	3680	4135	4585	5040	
3	540	990	1445	1895	2350	2800	3255	3710	4160	4615	5065	
4	565	1020	1470	1925	2375	2830	3285	3735	4190	4645	5095	
5	595	1045	1500	1955	2405	2860	3310	3765	4220	4670	5125	
6	625	1075	1530	1980	2435	2885	3340	3795	4245	4700	5155	
7	650	1105	1555	2010	2460	2915	3365	3820	4275	4730	5180	
8	680	1130	1585	2025	2500	2945	3395	3850	4305	4755	5210	
9	710	1160	1610	2065	2530	2975	3425	3880	4335	4785	5290	
10	740	1190	1640	2095	2555	3000	3455	3905	4360	4815	5265	
11	765	1200	1670	2120	2585	3030	3480	3935	4390	4840	5295	
12	795	1245	1695	2150	2605	3060	3510	3965	4420	4870	5325	
13	825	1275	1725	2180	2635	3085	3540	3990	4445	4900	5350	
14	850	1305	1755	2210	2660	3115	3565	4020	4475	4925	5380	
15	880	1330	1785	2235	2690	3145	3595	4050	4500	4955	5410	

CONVERSION NOMOGRAMS

Conversion nomograms for various measurements appear on the following pages. Shading indicates the normal range where appropriate. To convert from 'old' to 'new' units, multiply by the conversion factor at the foot of each column.

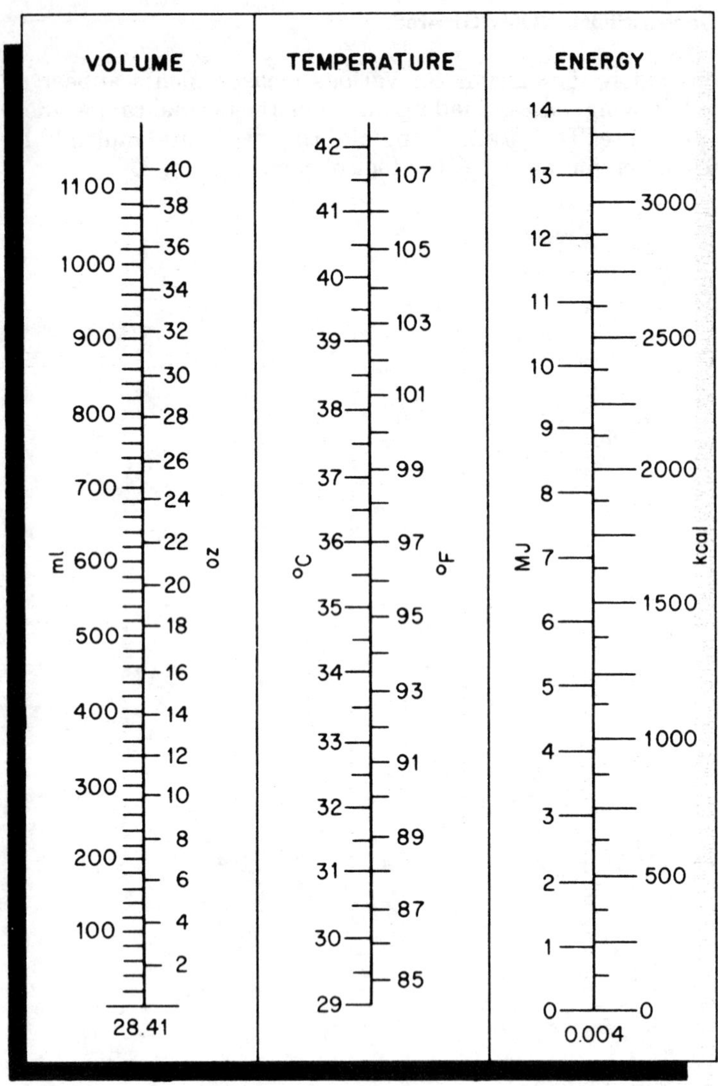
VOLUME
TEMPERATURE
ENERGY
ml
oz
28.41
°C
°F
MJ
kcal
0.004
1100
1000
900
800
700
600
500
400
300
200
100
40
38
36
34
32
30
28
26
24
22
20
18
16
14
12
10
8
6
4
2
42
41
40
39
38
37
36
35
34
33
32
31
30
29
107
105
103
101
99
97
95
93
91
89
87
85
14
13
12
11
10
9
8
7
6
5
4
3
2
1
0
3000
2500
2000
1500
1000
500
0

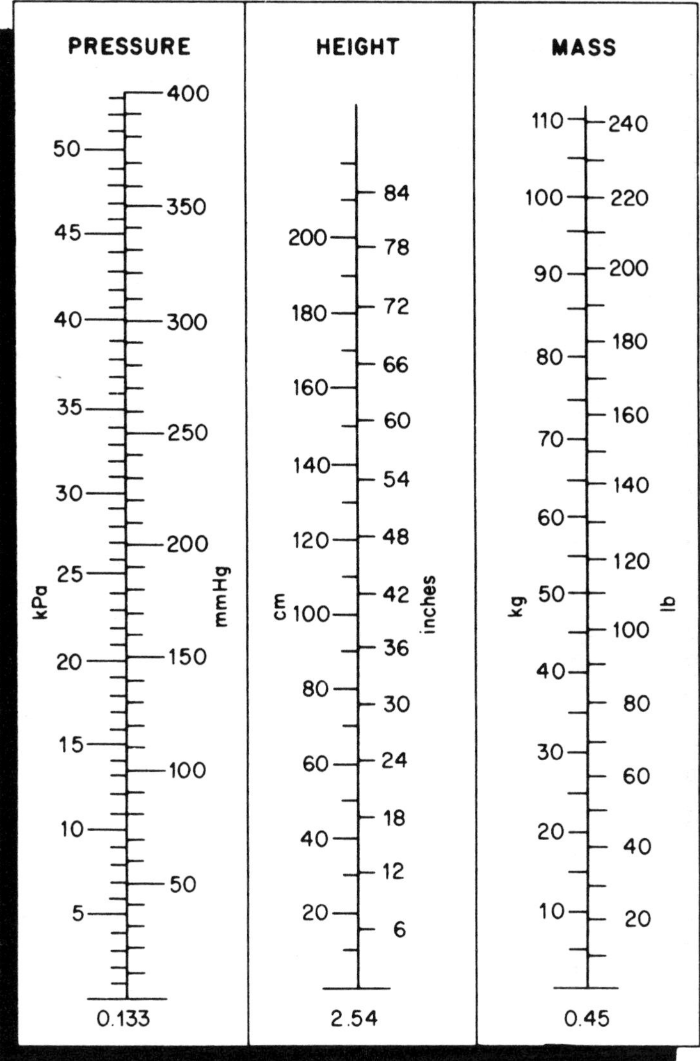
PRESSURE
HEIGHT
MASS
kPa
mmHg
cm
inches
kg
lb
50
45
40
35
30
25
20
15
10
5
400
350
300
250
200
150
100
50
200
180
160
140
120
100
80
60
40
20
84
78
72
66
60
54
48
42
36
30
24
18
12
6
110
100
90
80
70
60
50
40
30
20
10
240
220
200
180
160
140
120
100
80
60
40
20
0.133
2.54
0.45

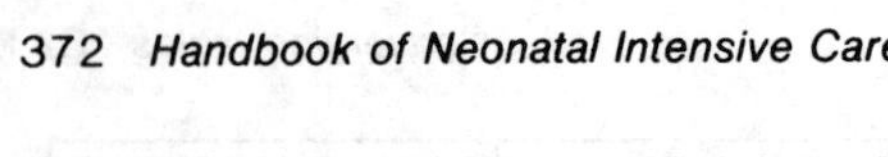

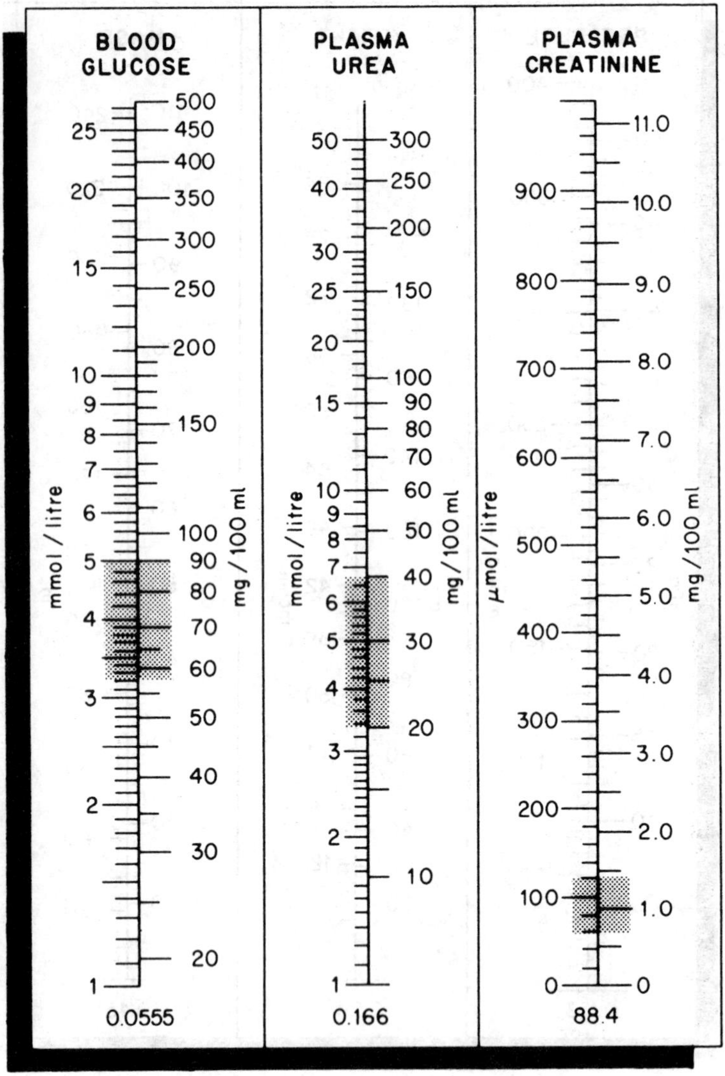

BLOOD GLUCOSE

mmol / litre: 25, 20, 15, 10, 9, 8, 7, 6, 5, 4, 3, 2, 1

mg / 100 ml: 500, 450, 400, 350, 300, 250, 200, 150, 100, 90, 80, 70, 60, 50, 40, 30, 20

0.0555

PLASMA UREA

mmol / litre: 50, 40, 30, 25, 20, 15, 10, 9, 8, 7, 6, 5, 4, 3, 2, 1

mg / 100 ml: 300, 250, 200, 150, 100, 90, 80, 70, 60, 50, 40, 30, 20, 10

0.166

PLASMA CREATININE

μmol / litre: 900, 800, 700, 600, 500, 400, 300, 200, 100, 0

mg / 100 ml: 11.0, 10.0, 9.0, 8.0, 7.0, 6.0, 5.0, 4.0, 3.0, 2.0, 1.0, 0

88.4

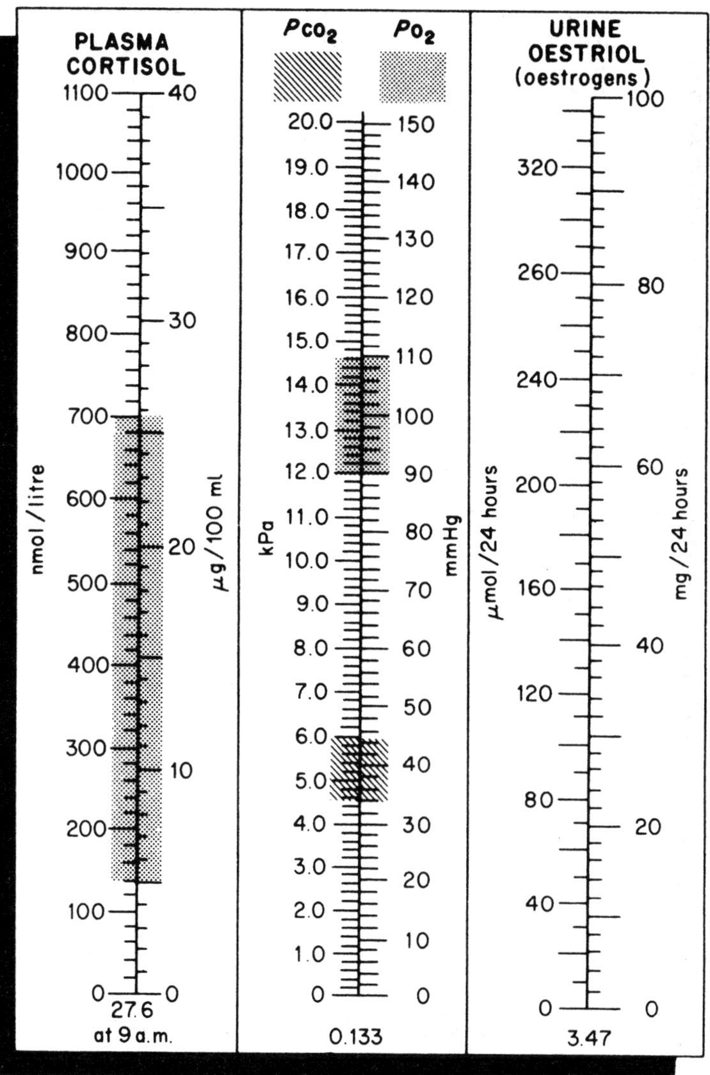
PLASMA CORTISOL
1100
1000
900
800
700
600
500
400
300
200
100
0
40
30
20
10
0
nmol/litre
µg/100 ml
27.6
at 9 a.m.
P_{CO_2}
P_{O_2}
20.0
19.0
18.0
17.0
16.0
15.0
14.0
13.0
12.0
11.0
10.0
9.0
8.0
7.0
6.0
5.0
4.0
3.0
2.0
1.0
0
150
140
130
120
110
100
90
80
70
60
50
40
30
20
10
0
kPa
mmHg
0.133
URINE OESTRIOL (oestrogens)
320
260
240
200
160
120
80
40
0
100
80
60
40
20
0
µmol/24 hours
mg/24 hours
3.47

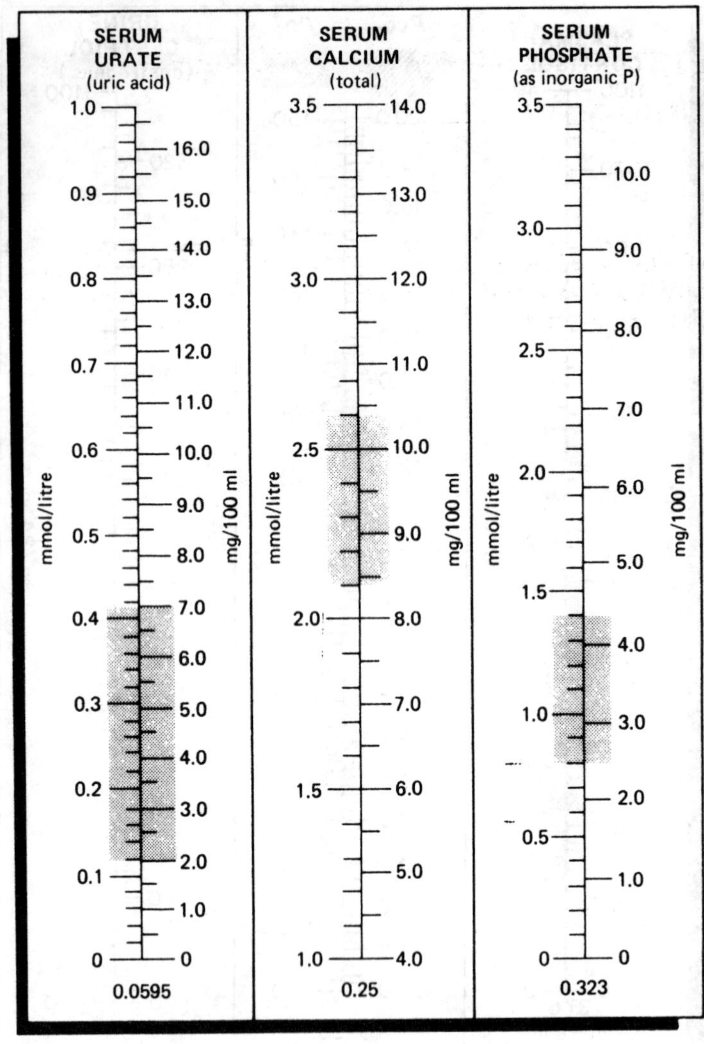
SERUM URATE (uric acid)
mmol/litre
mg/100 ml
1.0
0.9
0.8
0.7
0.6
0.5
0.4
0.3
0.2
0.1
0
16.0
15.0
14.0
13.0
12.0
11.0
10.0
9.0
8.0
7.0
6.0
5.0
4.0
3.0
2.0
1.0
0
0.0595
SERUM CALCIUM (total)
mmol/litre
mg/100 ml
3.5
3.0
2.5
2.0
1.5
1.0
14.0
13.0
12.0
11.0
10.0
9.0
8.0
7.0
6.0
5.0
4.0
0.25
SERUM PHOSPHATE (as inorganic P)
mmol/litre
mg/100 ml
3.5
3.0
2.5
2.0
1.5
1.0
0.5
0
10.0
9.0
8.0
7.0
6.0
5.0
4.0
3.0
2.0
1.0
0
0.323

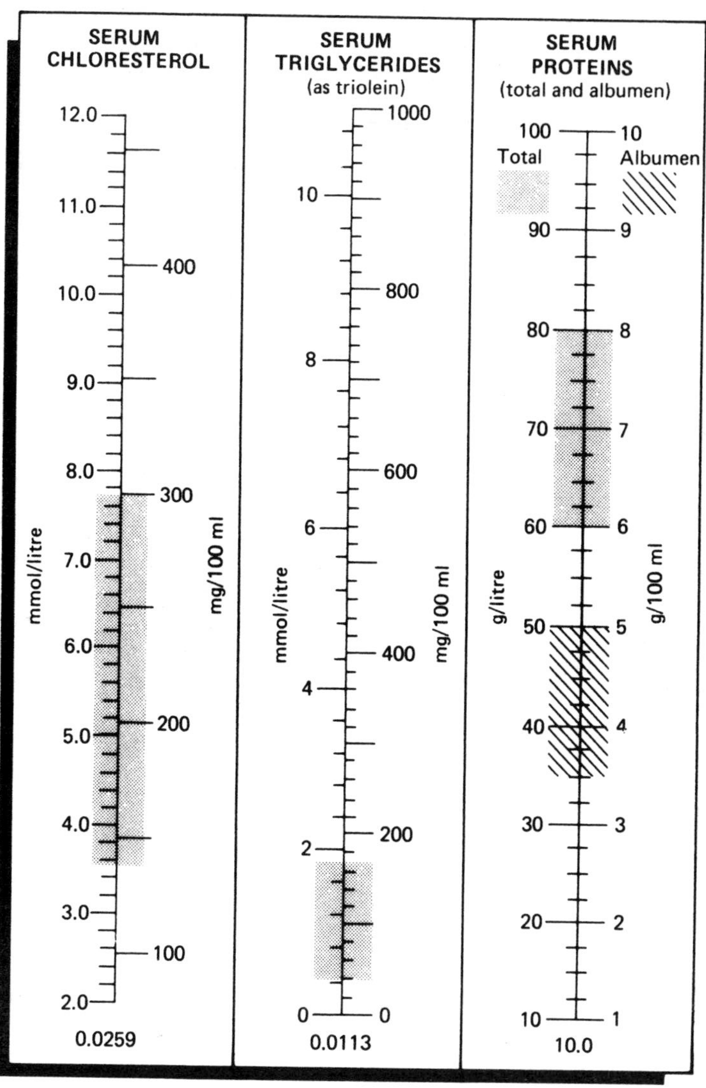
SERUM CHLORESTEROL
12.0
11.0
10.0
9.0
8.0
7.0
6.0
5.0
4.0
3.0
2.0
400
300
200
100
mmol/litre
mg/100 ml
0.0259
SERUM TRIGLYCERIDES
(as triolein)
1000
800
600
400
200
0
10
8
6
4
2
0
mmol/litre
mg/100 ml
0.0113
SERUM PROTEINS
(total and albumen)
Total
Albumen
100
90
80
70
60
50
40
30
20
10
10
9
8
7
6
5
4
3
2
1
g/litre
g/100 ml
10.0

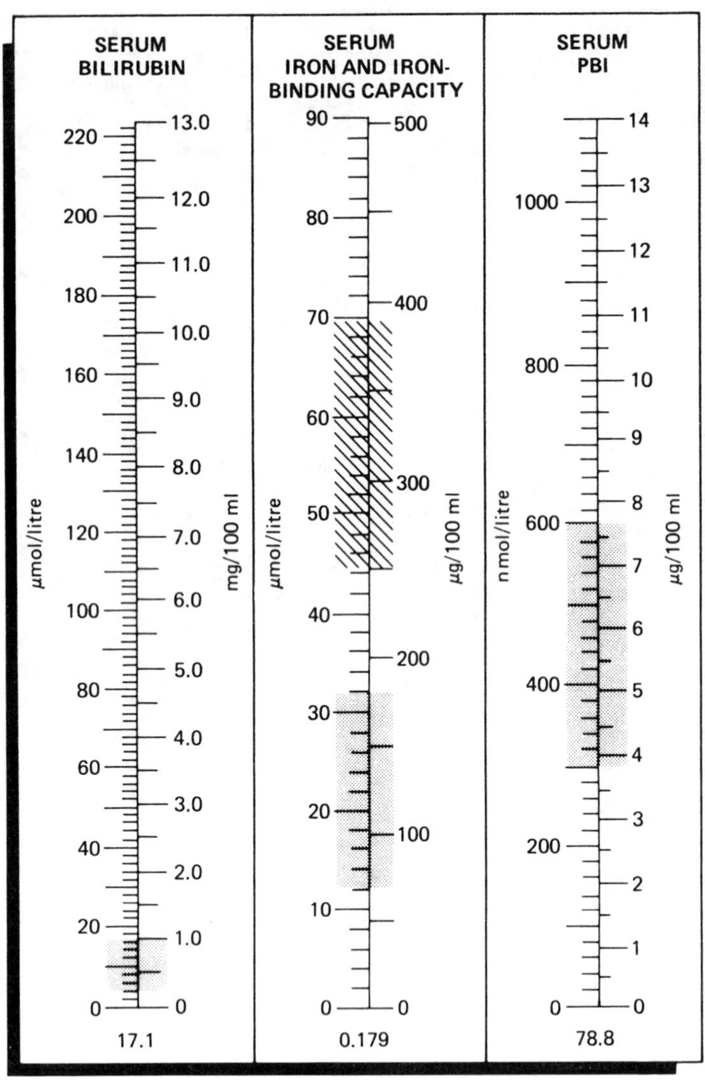
SERUM
BILIRUBIN
µmol/litre
mg/100 ml
220
200
180
160
140
120
100
80
60
40
20
0
13.0
12.0
11.0
10.0
9.0
8.0
7.0
6.0
5.0
4.0
3.0
2.0
1.0
0
17.1
SERUM
IRON AND IRON-
BINDING CAPACITY
µmol/litre
µg/100 ml
90
80
70
60
50
40
30
20
10
0
500
400
300
200
100
0
0.179
SERUM
PBI
n mol/litre
µg/100 ml
1000
800
600
400
200
0
14
13
12
11
10
9
8
7
6
5
4
3
2
1
0
78.8

Appendix XIV. Equipment and drugs needed for resuscitation

1. Resuscitation table:
   radiant warmer
   adequate light
   easy access to baby
2. Piped air/oxygen supply:
   up to 10 litre/min
   O_2 concentration variable 25–100%
   blow-off valve 40–60 cmH_2O
3. Vacuum supply for suction:
   negative pressure up to 200 cmH_2O
   suction catheters 5, 6, 8 FG
   Also have DeLee suction trap (mucus extractor) as standby
4. Stop-clock and stethoscope
5. Bag and mask system with mask sizes 0, 1 and 2
6. Oropharyngeal airways sizes 000, 00 and 0
7. Neonatal laryngoscope with straight blades sizes 0, 1 and 2
8. Endotracheal tubes and adapters:
   straight Portex sizes 2.5, 3.0, 3.5 mm
   shouldered (Cole's) sizes 2.5, 3.0, 3.5 mm
9. Umbilical vessel catheterization tray (see p. 96)
10. Drugs:
    4.2% bicarbonate for dilution (see p. 28)
    naloxone 20 μg/ml
    For occasional use:
    adrenaline 1:10 000
    calcium gluconate 10%
    atropine
    frusemide

Appendix XV. Weights and lengths of newborn infants, and organ weights related to gestational age and body weight at birth

Gestational age*	Number of cases	Body length (cm)	Body weight (g)	Heart (g)	Lungs, combined (g)	Spleen (g)	Liver (g)	Adrenal glands, combined (g)	Kidneys combined (g)	Thymus (g)	Brain (g)
24	108	31.3	638	4.9	17	1.7	32	2.9	6.4	2.7	92
		±3.7	±240	±1.6	±6	±1.1	±15	±1.4	±2.6	±1.4	±31
26	143	33.3	845	6.4	18	2.2	39	3.4	7.9	3.0	111
		±3.6	±246	±2.0	±6	±1.5	±15	±1.5	±2.9	±2.3	±39
28	139	36.0	1020	7.6	23	2.6	46	3.7	10.4	3.8	139
		±4.2	±340	±2.3	±7	±1.4	±16	±1.7	±3.6	±2.1	±48
30	148	37.8	1230	9.3	28	3.4	53	4.2	12.3	4.6	166
		±3.7	±340	±3.3	±11	±2.0	±19	±2.2	±3.9	±2.3	±55
32	150	40.5	1488	11.0	34	4.1	65	4.3	14.5	5.5	209
		±4.5	±335	±3.7	±11	±2.1	±22	±2.3	±4.8	±2.3	±44
34	104	42.8	1838	13.4	40	5.2	74	5.5	17.7	7.5	246
		±4.5	±530	±3.9	±13	±2.1	±27	±2.3	±5.3	±3.8	±58
36	87	45.0	2165	15.1	46	6.7	87	6.4	21.6	8.1	288
		±4.6	±600	±4.8	±16	±3.0	±33	±3.0	±6.7	±4.2	±62
38	102	47.2	2678	18.5	53	8.8	111	8.4	23.8	9.7	349
		±4.6	±758	±5.5	±15	±4.2	±40	±3.5	±7.0	±4.8	±56
40	220	49.8	3163	20.4	56	10.0	130	8.6	25.6	9.5	362
		±3.9	±595	±5.3	±15	±3.9	±45	±3.4	±6.5	±4.4	±55
42	112	50.3	3263	21.9	56	10.2	139	9.1	25.8	10.4	105
		±3.6	±573	±6.2	±18	±4.3	±45	±4.0	±7.5	±4.4	±54
44	42	52.8	3690	25.8	60	11.2	149	9.3	28.4	10.3	417
		±2.8	±800	±4.5	±17	±4.1	±35	±4.4	±7.5	±4.7	±55

* Gestational age is expressed in weeks from the last menstrual cycle

Body weight (g)	*Number of cases*	*Body length* (cm)	*Heart* (g)	*Lungs combined* (g)	*Spleen* (g)	*Liver* (g)	*Adrenal glands, combined* (g)	*Kidneys combined* (g)	*Thymus* (g)	*Brain* (g)	*Gestational age* *
											Weeks, Days
500	317	29.4	5.0	12	1.3	26	2.6	5.4	2.2	70	23, 5
		±2.5	±1.6	±5	±0.8	±10	±1.7	±2.1	±0.8	±18	±2, 3
750	311	32.9	6.3	19	2.0	39	3.2	7.8	2.8	107	26, 0
		±3.0	±1.8	±6	±1.2	±12	±1.5	±2.6	±1.3	±27	±2, 6
1000	295	35.6	7.7	24	2.6	47	3.5	10.4	3.7	143	27, 5
		±3.1	±2.0	±8	±1.5	±12	±1.6	±3.4	±2.0	±34	±3, 1
1250	217	38.4	9.6	30	3.4	56	4.0	12.9	4.9	174	29, 0
		±3.0	±3.3	±9	±1.8	±21	±1.7	±3.9	±2.1	±38	±3, 0
1500	167	41.0	11.5	34	4.3	65	4.5	14.9	6.1	219	31, 3
		±2.7	±3.3	±11	±2.0	±18	±1.8	±4.2	±2.7	±52	±2, 3
1750	148	42.6	12.8	40	5.0	74	5.3	17.4	6.8	247	32, 4
		±3.1	±3.2	±13	±2.5	±20	±2.0	±4.7	±3.0	±51	±2, 6
2000	140	44.9	14.9	44	6.0	82	5.3	18.8	7.9	281	34, 6
		±2.8	±4.2	±13	±2.7	±23	±2.0	±5.0	±3.4	±56	±3, 2
2250	124	46.3	16.0	48	7.0	88	6.0	20.2	8.2	308	36, 4
		±2.9	±4.3	±15	±3.3	±24	±2.3	±4.9	±3.4	±49	±3, 0
2500	120	47.3	17.7	48	8.5	105	7.1	22.6	8.3	339	38, 0
		±2.3	±4.2	±14	±3.5	±21	±2.8	±5.5	±4.4	±50	±3, 2
2750	138	48.7	19.1	51	9.1	117	7.5	24.0	9.6	362	39, 2
		±2.9	±3.8	±15	±3.6	±26	±2.7	±5.4	±3.8	±48	±2, 2
3000	144	50.0	20.7	53	10.1	127	8.3	24.7	10.2	380	40, 0
		±2.9	±5.3	±13	±3.3	±30	±2.9	±5.3	±4.3	±55	±2, 1
3250	133	50.7	21.5	59	11.0	145	9.2	27.3	11.6	395	40, 4
		±2.6	±4.3	±18	±4.0	±33	±3.4	±6.6	±4.4	±53	±1, 6

* Gestational age is expressed in weeks from the last menstrual cycle

Body weight (g)	*Number of cases*	*Body length* (cm)	*Heart* (g)	*Lungs combined* (g)	*Spleen* (g)	*Liver* (g)	*Adrenal glands, combined* (g)	*Kidneys combined* (g)	*Thymus* (g)	*Brain* (g)	*Gestational age* *
											Weeks, Days
3500	106	51.8	22.8	63	11.3	153	9.8	28.0	12.8	411	40, 4
		±3.0	±5.9	±17	±3.6	±33	±3.5	±6.5	±5.1	±55	±1, 5
3750	57	52.1	23.8	65	12.5	159	10.2	29.5	13.0	413	40, 6
		±2.3	±5.1	±15	±4.1	±40	±3.3	±6.8	±4.8	±55	±2, 3
4000	31	52.4	25.8	67	14.1	180	10.8	30.2	11.4	420	41, 4
		±2.7	±5.3	±20	±4.0	±39	±3.4	±6.2	±3.2	±62	±1, 3
4250	15	53.2	26.5	68	13.0	197	12.0	30.7	11.7	415	41, 2
		±2.5	±5.3	±16	±2.5	±42	±3.7	±5.8	±3.7	±38	±2, 1

* Gestational age is expressed in weeks from the last menstrual cycle

From Gruenwald and Minh (1960) with kind permission of the editor of *American Journal of Clinical Pathology*

Appendix XVI. Categories of Babies Receiving Neonatal Care

(a) *Intensive care*:

1. Babies receiving assisted ventilation (intermittent positive ventilation (IPPV), intermittent mandatory ventilation (IMV), constant positive airway pressure (CPAP)), and in the first 24 hours following its withdrawal
2. Babies receiving total parenteral nutrition
3. Cardiorespiratory disease which is unstable, including recurrent apnoea requiring constant attention
4. Babies who have had major surgery, particularly in the first 24 postoperative hours
5. Babies of less than 30 weeks gestation during the first 48 hours after birth
6. Babies who are having convulsions
7. Babies transported by the staff of the unit concerned. This would usually be between hospitals, or for special investigations or treatment
8. Babies undergoing major medical procedures, such as arterial catheterization, peritoneal dialysis or exchange transfusion.

(b) *Special care*:

1. Babies who require continuous monitoring of respiration or heart rate, or by transcutaneous transducers
2. Babies who are receiving additional oxygen
3. Babies who are receiving intravenous glucose and electrolyte solutions
4. Babies who are being tube fed
5. Babies who have had minor surgery in the previous 24 hours
6. Babies with a tracheostomy
7. Dying babies.
8. Babies who are being barrier nursed

9. Babies receiving phototherapy
10. Babies who receive special monitoring (for example frequent glucose or bilirubin estimations)
11. Other babies receiving constant supervision (for example babies whose mothers are drug addicts)
12. Babies receiving antibiotics
13. Babies with conditions requiring radiological examination or other methods of imaging

---

From British Paediatrics *Arch. Dis. Child* (1985), **60**: 599.

Appendix XVII. Drugs and Breast Feeding

Not safe for breast feeding (see also current BNF)

aloe
amantadine
anthraquinone
antineoplastic drugs
antithyroid drugs, e.g.
carbimazole, thiouracil
*atropine
bromides
*carbamazepine
cathartics, e.g. cascara
chloral hydrate
*chloramphenicol
*clindamycin
cortisone
cyclophosphamide
diazepam (high dose)
*dicoumarol
dihydrotachysterol
ergot/ergotamine
gold salts
heroin (diamorphine)
indomethacin
iodides
lithium
meprobamate
methadone
*metronidazole (high dose)
novobiocin
oestrogens
phenindione
phenothiazines (high dose)
*phenylbutazone
primidone
propranolol
pyrimethamine
radioactive agents
(radioiodine)
reserpine
*tetracyclines
thiouracil
tolbutamide
trimethoprim
vitamins A, D (high dose)

* Short courses of these drugs may not be harmful

The following drugs are excreted in breast milk in minimal or harmless amounts and are *probably safe for breast feeding*:

ACTH
alcohol (moderate intake)
ampicillin
antacids
anti-emetics
antihistamines
barbiturates (except high
dose)
benzodiazepines (low dose)
β-blockers

bisacodyl
bulk laxatives
caffeine
captopril
carbenicillin
cephaloridine
cephalosporins
chlordiazepoxide
chlormethiazole (low dose)
chloroquine
chlorothiazide
chlorpromazine
cimetidine
cloxacillin
codeine
corticosteroids
cromoglycate
dextropropoxyphene
diazepam (low dose)
diclofenac
digoxin
ephedrine
erythromycin
ethambutol
ethinyloestradiol
ethosuximide
fenbufen
flufenamic acid
folic acid
frusemide
gentamicin
guanethidine
heparin
hydralazine
ibuprofen
insulins
iron
isoniazid
kanamycin
kaolin compounds
ketoprofen
labetalol
lincomycin
mefenamic acid
methotrexate
methyldopa
metoclopramide
metronidazole (low dose)
mexiletine
milk of magnesia
morphine
naproxen
netilmicin
nitrofurantoin
oxyphenbutazone
paracetamol
para-aminosalicylic acid (PAS)
penicillins
pentazocine
pethidine
phenothiazines (low dose)
phenytoin
progestogens
quinidine
quinine
ranitidine
rifampicin
senna
salicylates (low dose)
sodium valproate
spironolactone
streptomycin
sulphonamides (unless jaundiced)
terbutaline
thiazides
thyroxine
tricyclic antidepressants
vitamins A, D (low dose)
vitamins B, C
warfarin

The milk from mothers taking these drugs *may be used to feed* the premature newborn.

Appendix XVIII. Role and Functions of Regional Perinatal Centres

1. Management of certain pregnancies with maternal or fetal complications (high-risk pregnancies). Such pregnancies may be booked at the perinatal centre or subsequently referred there, having been booked at another maternity unit (antenatal referral)
2. Provision of an intensive care service for the newborn, including the transfer of ill babies from other maternity units
3. Provision of a wide range of genetic services, including antenatal diagnosis, and genetic counselling
4. Provision of support services, including paediatric pathology, radiology, biochemistry, haematology, and bacteriology, which cater for a range of clinical problems peculiar to the perinatal period
5. Liaison with other paediatricians in the region in the developmental follow-up of preterm and other babies who have received intensive care so that long-term outcome is prospectively monitored on a regional basis
6. Collection and analysis of perinatal statistics such that, in collaboration with the regional health authority, a continuous programme of audit is maintained
7. Research in perinatal physiology, clinical perinatology, and related fields
8. Training and education in perinatal medicine for doctors, nurses, and midwives and those working in a wide range of essential support services

From: Medical Care of the Newborn in England and Wales, Royal College of Physicians of London, 1988

Appendix XIX. Guidelines for Training Towards a Career as Consultant Neonatal Paediatrician*

Most doctors pursuing a career as a consultant neonatal paediatrician will have satisfied the training programme for accreditation in paediatrics but will have included an additional 1 or 2 years training relevant to neonatal paediatrics as indicated below.

GENERAL PROFESSIONAL TRAINING

A vital ingredient in the training of a neonatal paediatrician is resident experience in a major maternity unit providing intensive care for the fetus and newborn infant. The following resident posts should be included during general professional training:

1. Six months in a paediatric house officer post
2. Six months in an obstetric house officer post
3. Six months as a neonatal paediatric house officer in a unit undertaking intensive care

HIGHER SPECIALIST TRAINING

This period will *normally* occupy 5 to 6 years. The following is *obligatory* experience:

---

* This is summarized from the guidelines of the Joint Committee on Higher Medical Training. Those guidelines refer to the specialty as 'perinatal paediatrics'.

1. In-patient and out-patient care of ill children including emergency work
2. Developmental and handicap assessment and surveillance, including some experience in the care and rehabilitation of handicapped children
3. At least 2 years directly responsible to a consultant for the running of a referral intensive care unit

The following is *recommended* experience:

1. Up to 2 years in research or in study of a specific aspect of perinatal medicine (e.g. perinatal physiology, pharmacology, developmental neurology)
2. A further period working in either obstetrics, perinatal pathology, paediatric surgery, perinatal epidemiology, adult intensive care or community paediatrics

Index

D

N

O

S

T